T0294583

Multiparametric Ultrasound for the Assessment of Diffuse Liver Disease

A Practical Approach

RICHARD G. BARR, MD, PhD
Professor of Radiology
Northeastern Ohio Medical University
Rootstown, OH, United States

GIOVANNA FERRAIOLI, MD
Researcher
Department of Clinical, Surgical, Diagnostic
and Pediatric Sciences
Medical School University of Pavia,
Pavia, Italy

ELSEVIER

Elsevier
1600 John F. Kennedy Blvd.
Ste 1800
Philadelphia, PA 19103-2899

Notice

Practitioners and researchers must always rely on their own experience and knowledge in evaluating and using any information, methods, compounds or experiments described herein. Because of rapid advances in the medical sciences, in particular, independent verification of diagnoses and drug dosages should be made. To the fullest extent of the law, no responsibility is assumed by Elsevier, authors, editors or contributors for any injury and/or damage to persons or property as a matter of products liability, negligence or otherwise, or from any use or operation of any methods, products, instructions, or ideas contained in the material herein.

ISBN: 9780323874793

Content Strategist: Melanie Tucker
Content Development Specialist: Malvika Shah
Publishing Services Manager: Shereen Jameel
Project Manager: Nadhiya Sekar
Design Direction: Amy Buxton

Printed in India

Last digit is the print number: 9 8 7 6 5 4 3 2 1

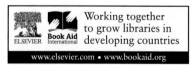

Working together to grow libraries in developing countries

www.elsevier.com • www.bookaid.org

Ultrasound in medicine is facing an unprecedented rapid evolution thanks to technological improvements and innovations. Hepatology is one of the specialties that is most benefiting from the novel ultrasound-based method that became and will become available in the near future. From being a rather simple anatomical imaging method (i.e., gray-scale ultrasound), ultrasonography evolved into a real-time tool to detail blood flow characteristics. Doppler-based techniques remain a backbone of ultrasound assessment in chronic liver disease, being the only real-time technique that is able to address hepatic hemodynamics; standard spectral, color, and power Doppler have been recently enriched by vector Doppler and ultrafast Doppler. More recently, contrast-enhanced ultrasound entered clinical practice providing, for the first time, a tool to address perfusion in focal liver lesions and to characterize their nature in most cases. Ultrasound elastography added a new dimension to the characterization of diffuse liver disease, providing, for the first time, a measurement of a physical property of the liver tissue unrelated to its morphology. Elastography, ranging from transient elastography to point shear wave and two-dimensional shear wave elastography, has become a mature technique and has been integrated in several pathways of care[1] and decision algorithms.[1,2] This has changed clinical practice and dramatically reduced the need for invasive techniques such as liver biopsy and endoscopic screening of gastroesophageal varices. Liver stiffness not only noninvasively defines the stage of liver fibrosis, but also provides important information on the risk of clinical decompensation and other relevant events, independent of clinical variables and of liver function tests.[2]

In an era of high prevalence of obesity and metabolic syndrome worldwide (which explains why nonalcoholic fatty liver disease–related end-stage liver disease and liver cancer have already become the first indication for liver transplantation) novel methods to quantify fat content, and potentially to characterize inflammation are being developed, and are the subject of specific studies. Ultrasound in hepatology has become undoubtedly multiparametric, and patients can benefit from a very large set of information gathered during a "one stop" examination. Miniaturization and web-based solutions will further prompt the use of ultrasound in clinical practice, and mastering the many techniques that now allow a comprehensive characterization of diffuse liver disease will be key for the next generation of radiologists and hepatologists.

Getting used to novel techniques and applications requires getting familiar with a large amount of published data, and learning how to appropriately apply these novel techniques. It is not surprising that radiologists and physicians who were used to performing standard ultrasound examinations might feel overwhelmed by this complexity. However, hepatologists who are not performing ultrasound themselves need to be updated on what can be asked of the ultrasound physician and what information needs to be provided as a minimal background to allow a correct diagnosis.

In this context, the book that you have in your hands is very valuable. Richard Barr and Giovanna Ferraioli joined forces as editors to guide physicians interested in ultrasound for diffuse liver diseases into the complexity of multiparametric ultrasound in a pragmatic and practical approach. You will find answers to several of your questions: how to use each of the existing techniques at its best to characterize your patient's liver disease, how to deal with the limitations of each of these techniques, and what to ask (and not ask) of your devices and software. The book presents an overview of conventional ultrasound findings in chronic liver disease and portal hypertension, and presents the basic concepts and protocols needed to measure liver stiffness, entering into the details of tips and tricks, artifacts, applications, and guidelines of liver ultrasound elastography. In other chapters the latest ultrasound techniques to assess liver steatosis and focal liver lesions are reviewed.

The editors and the experts who wrote this book provide a state-of-the-art review of the published data in a direct, concise, and organized way. In addition, they present high quality images and suggest practical hints based on their own experience—something that cannot be easily found—and that often helps solving difficult cases.

As an enthusiastic supporter of "ultrasound first" in patients with liver disease, I am convinced that this book will become useful to many colleagues and will represent a very valuable support both to those who aim to learn multiparametric ultrasound imaging, and to those who want to know more on how to integrate the results of multiparametric ultrasound in their clinical practice. I commend Dr. Barr and Dr. Ferraioli and the authors for their efforts and thank them for having invited me to write this foreword.

References

1. European Association for the Study of the Liver. EASL Clinical Practice Guidelines on non-invasive tests for evaluation of liver disease severity and prognosis - 2021 update. *J Hepatol.* 2021;75:659-689.
2. de Franchis R, Bosch J, Garcia-Tsao G, Reiberger T, Ripoll C; Baveno VII Faculty. Baveno VII - Renewing consensus in portal hypertension. *J Hepatol.* 2022;76:959-974.

Annalisa Berzigotti, MD, PhD

Chronic liver disease is a substantial worldwide problem. Ultrasound (US) plays a major role in the diagnostic armamentarium of patients with chronic liver disease. It is a noninvasive imaging technique with no exposure to ionizing radiation, therefore repeatable over short periods of time without any harm to the patient. Over the years, besides B-mode US, other US-based techniques have been introduced, leading to the possibility of a multiparametric approach for the evaluation of chronic liver disease. These include Doppler techniques, contrast-enhanced ultrasound, elastography, quantification of liver fat content, and shear wave dispersion. Each of these techniques evaluates a physical/biological/biomechanical property of the liver tissue or of the blood flow and leads to unique information about the state of the liver disease. However, it is of utmost importance to use them in an appropriate manner to obtain the most reliable information. Moreover, in order to properly interpret the results, it is important to be aware not only of the advantages but also of the limitations of each specific technique. As there are several techniques, how to appropriately use each of these and how to correlate them can be confusing.

These are the reasons why we undertook the task of writing this book. The experience of leading experts in the US technique, our own experience, and evidence from literature were combined in the effort of giving not only the most recent updates but also practical information on how to use each of these techniques and how to interpret them.

Each chapter stands on its own; hence, it can be read independently from the others and is a guidance for the use of the US-based techniques in the everyday practice. For each chapter, a summary is given at beginning whereas at the end, besides the conclusions, there is a "key-point" paragraph that outlines the most important take-away points of that chapter. Tips and tricks on the use of these new techniques are given, as well as how to deal with difficult-to-interpret cases.

We strongly feel that the content of the book will be helpful not only to colleagues who perform US studies but also to clinicians willing to understand the fundamental role played by multiparametric US in the management of patients with chronic liver disease.

CONTRIBUTORS

Richard G. Barr, MD, PhD
Professor of Radiology
Northeastern Ohio Medical University
Rootstown, OH,
USA

Jonathan R. Dillman, MD, Msc
Associate Professor; Associate Chief, Research
Department of Radiology
Cincinnati Children's Hospital Medical
    Center,
Cincinnati, OH,
USA

Giovanna Ferraioli, MD
Researcher
Department of Clinical, Surgical, Diagnostic
    and Pediatric Sciences
Medical School University of Pavia,
Pavia,
ITA

Guadalupe Garcia-Tsao, MD
Professor of Medicine
Internal Medicine/Digestive Diseases
Yale University,
New Haven, CT,
USA
Chief of Digestive Diseases
Internal Medicine
VA-CT Healthcare System,
West Haven,
CT,
USA

Christina D. Merrill, BSc, CRGS, CRVS, RDMS, RVT
Lead Sonographer, CEUS department
Foothills Medical Center, 1403 29
St NW, Calgary,
CAN

Spencer Moavenzadeh, PhD
Associate in Research
Department of Biomedical Engineering
Duke University,
Durham, NC,
USA

Guillermo A. Ortiz, MD
Gastroenterologist
Digestive Diseases Section, Department of
    Medicine
Yale University,
New Haven, CT,
USA

Mark Palmeri, MD, PhD
Professor of the Practice
Biomedical Engineering
Duke University,
Durham, NC,
USA

Davide Roccarina, PhD
Associate Professor, Sheila Sherlock Liver
    Unit and UCL Institute for Liver and
    Digestive Health, Royal Free Hospital,
London,
UK
Internal Medicine and Hepatology
    Consultant
Internal Medicine and Hepatology
Azienda Ospedaliero-Universitaria Careggi,
Florence,
ITA

Anna S. Samuel
Research Student
Foothills Medical Center,
Calgary,
CAN

Katsutoshi Sugimoto, MD, PhD
Associate Professor
Gastroenterology and Hepatology
Tokyo Medical University,
Tokyo,
JPN

Stephanie R. Wilson, MD, FAIUM, FSRU
Clinical Professor
Radiology
University of Calgary,
Calgary, Alberta,
CAN

CONTENTS

CHAPTER 1

Introduction

Guillermo A. Ortiz ■ Guadalupe Garcia-Tsao

The Burden of Chronic Liver Disease

Chronic liver disease (CLD) is a significant cause of morbidity and mortality and an important contributor to the burden of disease and health care utilization worldwide. It is estimated that CLD accounts for approximately 2 million deaths per year in the world: 1 million related to complications of cirrhosis and 1 million related to viral hepatitis and hepatocellular carcinoma (HCC); this is approximately 3.5% of all deaths worldwide.[1] In a global estimation from 2019, CLD appeared in the top 10 causes of disability-adjusted life-years in men and ranked 16 in the general population.[2] The current mortality attributed to liver disease as well as the prevalence of CLD and cirrhosis may be systematically underestimated in the United States.[3]

The Global Burden of Disease study shows that age standardized incidence rate of CLD and cirrhosis has increased by 13% from 2000 to 2017.[4] This increase is driven mostly by incidence of cirrhosis in Europe, high-income populations in Asia Pacific, East Asia, Southeast Asia, and South Asia. In the United States, a recent study suggests that, between 2007 and 2017, there has been a 30% increase in the incidence of cirrhosis and liver cancer.[5] The driving force behind the reported increase in CLD is likely related to the raising rates of metabolic syndrome and alcohol misuse.

The epidemiology and distribution of the different causes of CLD varies geographically by ethnicity and by age group and is rapidly changing. From the 1.5 billion persons estimated to be affected with CLD worldwide in 2017, nonalcoholic fatty liver disease (NAFLD) accounted for 60%, hepatitis B 29%, hepatitis C 9%, and alcoholic liver disease 2%.[6] Other far less common causes of CLD include autoimmune and cholestatic-related diseases such as autoimmune hepatitis, primary biliary cholangitis, primary sclerosing cholangitis, and metabolic/genetic diseases such as hemochromatosis.

NAFLD has a wide spectrum of disease including simple steatosis, nonalcoholic steatohepatitis (NASH), and cirrhosis. It is difficult to estimate the prevalence of the stages of NAFLD in the general population; based on radiological diagnosis (which cannot differentiate between simple steatosis, fibrosis, or cirrhosis), there is a worldwide estimated prevalence of 25% in NAFLD with the highest prevalence in the Middle East (32%), South America (31%), and Asia (34%).[7] On a recent systematic review and metaanalysis of the prevalence of NAFLD in the United States, it is estimated that approximately one in three U.S. residents has steatosis, with higher rates seen in Hispanics; the prevalence of NASH among patients with NAFLD in the United States has been estimated to be around 32.4% based on histology and transaminases; and based on 11 studies assessing advanced fibrosis in patients with NAFLD, the prevalence was estimated to be close to 19%.[8]

ALD also has a wide spectrum of disease, including alcoholic hepatitis, simple steatosis, steatohepatitis, and cirrhosis. The progression through these stages depends on continued alcohol use, comorbid liver disease, and other risk factors like female sex and genetic susceptibility.[9] It is estimated that alcohol misuse accounts for 27% of deaths from liver disease and 30% of liver cancers in the world.[10,11] With an increase in alcohol consumption around the world, it is estimated that the burden of ALD will continue to increase.[12]

Staging of Liver Fibrosis

CLD is characterized by progressive and diffuse deposition of fibrous tissue as a response of sustained liver injury or inflammation. This diffuse liver damage leads to architectural changes and replacement of the normal lobular structure of the liver parenchyma leading to the development of cirrhosis.

Histologically, fibrosis is a continuum, which has been graded in different stages; the most widely used staging system is the METAVIR fibrosis score, which is essentially the same as the NASH fibrosis score,[13] and classifies the degree of fibrosis into five progressive stages: F0, no fibrosis; F1, portal fibrosis (or periportal fibrosis); F2, portal and periportal fibrosis with some septa formation; F3, bridging fibrosis; and F4, cirrhosis, characterized by the formation of nodules surrounded by fibrous tissue (Fig. 1.1).[14,15]

Stages of fibrosis, particularly stages 3 and 4 (cirrhotic stage), are important prognostically and are therefore important in identifying patients with CLD who would benefit from referral to a liver specialist, who would need to be prioritized for treatments of the underlying etiology of CLD, and in whom screening strategies would be initiated to prevent complications of CLD, specifically the development of complications of portal hypertension (ascites, variceal hemorrhage, encephalopathy) and the development of HCC.

Biopsy is the gold standard for staging of fibrosis. However, biopsies are an imperfect test. The accuracy of biopsy can be compromised by inadequate sampling, sampling variation, and interobserver variability at the time of interpretation. Sampling variation is the result of heterogenicity in inflammation and fibrosis across different etiologies of liver disease, and it has been shown to be a relevant issue in NAFLD, PBC, HCV, and HBV.[16-19] Interobserver variability is not surprisingly an issue given that interpretation of liver histology is often complex; the degree of concordance varies according to the feature analyzed with degree of fibrosis and, although an adequate kappa (k) statistic of around 0.8 has been described for mostly viral etiologies of CLD,[13,20,21] a more recent study showed important interobserver variability in the staging of fibrosis in patients with NASH.[22] Furthermore, biopsies are an invasive procedure and, as such, they have been associated with complications such as pain, bleeding, bile duct injury, perforation of adjacent organs, infections, etc.[23]

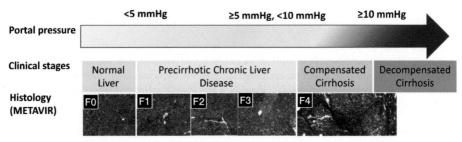

Fig. 1.1 Natural history of chronic liver disease (CLD). With persistent liver injury, independent of the etiology, there is progressive deposition of fibrous tissue with distortion of the normal liver parenchyma. The METAVIR fibrosis score categorizes fibrosis into five possible stages: F0 = no fibrosis, F1 = portal fibrosis without septa, F2 = portal fibrosis with rare septa, F3 = numerous septa without cirrhosis, and F4 = cirrhosis. Cirrhosis is the end stage of CLD; there are two clinical stages for cirrhosis: compensated and decompensated. A patient with cirrhosis is said to have decompensated cirrhosis after developing variceal bleeding, ascites, or hepatic encephalopathy. Decompensation is triggered by an increase in portal pressure, typically when the patients develop clinically significant portal hypertension (CSPH) (i.e., portal pressure ≥10 mmHg). Differentiating between F3 and F4 is challenging, particularly when utilizing noninvasive means for staging of fibrosis; the concept of compensated, advanced CLD has been coined to refer to patients with advanced liver fibrosis who are at risk of CSPH and its complications. CLD is a dynamic process: to a certain degree, treatment of the underlying etiology of CLD may reverse histological features and decrease portal pressure.

Stages of Cirrhosis

Cirrhosis, which is the end stage of CLD of any etiology, is a histologic diagnosis based on the severity and burden of fibrosis, as described previously. Most complications of CLD, including liver-related complications (ascites, variceal hemorrhage, encephalopathy, or jaundice), HCC, and death, occur once the patient has reached a cirrhotic stage. Although patients with advanced fibrosis (F3) have also been described as having higher complication and mortality rates than those with earlier stages of fibrosis (F1, F2), the relevant fibrosis stage is the cirrhotic stage in which complications and liver-related mortality are highest.[24,25]

Clinically, cirrhosis has been classified into two main stages: compensated and decompensated.[26,27] Decompensation in cirrhosis is defined by the development of overt ascites (not one identified only by ultrasound), variceal hemorrhage, and overt (not subclinical) hepatic encephalopathy and jaundice.[26] Of these, those related to portal hypertension (ascites and variceal hemorrhage) are most common, whereas those related to liver insufficiency (encephalopathy and jaundice) occur more infrequently as, in the pathogenesis of cirrhosis, portal hypertension occurs first and liver insufficiency appears later on in the course of the disease. Once a patient develops one of these complications, the survival rate decreases significantly.[26-28] In fact, the main determinant of death in patients with cirrhosis is the development of decompensation.[29] The median survival in patients with compensated cirrhosis is typically greater than 12 years, as long as these subjects remain compensated, whereas the median survival rate in decompensated patients is under 2 years.[28]

Compensated cirrhosis represents the long, asymptomatic stage of cirrhosis. Because these patients do not have overt complications of portal hypertension/liver insufficiency, the diagnosis is challenging. Several simple laboratory tests including platelet count, international normalized ratio (INR), albumin levels, and aspartate aminotransferase (AST) to alanine aminotransferase (ALT) ratio, as well some other clinical findings such as splenomegaly, nodular liver, and presence of collaterals have varying predictive value in making a diagnosis of compensated cirrhosis.[30] These parameters have been combined in different clinical scores like the Lok index, the FIB-4, or the NAFLD fibrosis scores to estimate the probabilities of cirrhosis.[31-33] Although these variables/indices are valuable at ruling in cirrhosis, they are not optimal at ruling it out, resulting in the continued need to obtain a liver biopsy.

The diagnosis of cirrhosis in a decompensated patient is not as challenging; patients present with overt decompensating events, and, at this stage, they are more likely to have physical examination findings that support the presence of cirrhosis (e.g., palmar erythema, telangiectases, palpable left lobe of the liver, splenomegaly).

Another stage of cirrhosis that could be proposed is that of "regression" of cirrhosis. The process of fibrosis is dynamic, and cirrhosis is no longer considered an irreversible and progressive disease.[34] There is evidence that, with treatment of the underlying liver disease (e.g., alcohol abstinence, antiviral therapy, immunosuppression in autoimmune diseases), fibrosis can regress, and in some cases of early cirrhosis it may regress to a precirrhotic stage.[35-37] Patients with prior decompensated events can recompensate if the cause of disease is removed.

Clinically Significant Portal Hypertension

Within the compensated stage, two substages have been recently identified based on the severity of portal hypertension.

The pathogenic substrate of decompensation in cirrhosis is related to portal hypertension. The structural change in the cirrhotic liver (fibrosis) together with active intrahepatic vasoconstriction lead to an increase in resistance to portal flow. This leads to mild portal hypertension, which, in turn, leads to splanchnic vasodilation with resultant increase portal venous inflow that further increases portal pressure.

Portal pressure can be measured indirectly by the hepatic venous pressure gradient (HVPG), which is a measure of hepatic sinusoidal pressure obtained by wedging (or balloon occluding) a catheter introduced via the jugular vein (or femoral vein) into one of the major hepatic veins (usually the right hepatic vein). In order to correct the wedged (occluded) pressure with a systemic pressure, a "free" pressure (with the catheter unwedged or with the balloon deflated) is subtracted from the wedged (occluded) pressure. Therefore the result is a gradient obtained by subtracting free from the wedged pressure.[38] A normal HVPG is 3–5 mmHg. In most patients with cirrhosis, the HVPG is greater than 5 mmHg. When the HVPG reaches a threshold of ≥10 mmHg, patients with CLD have fourfold risk of decompensation compared to patients with cirrhosis and HVPG <10 mmHg.[39] This HVPG ≥10 mmHg has also been associated to a greater probability of developing varices, HCC, postsurgical complications, and death. Therefore it is referred to as clinically significant portal hypertension (CSPH).[40-44]

Patients with compensated cirrhosis are now subclassified into those with mild portal hypertension (HVPG >5 mmHg but <10 mmHg) and those with CSPH (HVPG >10 mmHg), with the latter being those more likely to decompensate and those in whom drugs that decrease portal venous inflow more effective.

In fact, the PREDESCI trial showed that, in patients with compensated cirrhosis and CSPH, decompensation can be prevented by using beta-blockers to decrease the portal pressure.[45] Therefore the stratification of patients with advanced CLD, as those with CSPH and those without CSPH, has key implications for management of cirrhosis.

In the setting of compensated cirrhosis, elimination of the etiological agent delays decompensation of cirrhosis and progression of CLD, as mentioned, but it also has been proven to have a positive effect on HVPG, particularly in early stages of cirrhosis when patients have a lower degree of portal hypertension.[46] However, it has been shown in subjects with cirrhosis related to HCV that, although there is an improvement in portal pressure, CSPH persists in the majority of patients, and therefore these patients appear to be at continued risk of decompensation and HCC.[47,48]

As of now, the diagnosis of CSPH is established via hepatic vein catheterization. This is an invasive procedure that carries a risk, albeit small, of complications; furthermore, HVPG is a nuanced technique and appropriate, reliable measurements are not obtained in centers that do not perform the measurements routinely.[49]

In conclusion, both the diagnosis of cirrhosis and that of CSPH require invasive procedures. The use of noninvasive means for staging, screening, and monitoring CLD, mainly the use of ultrasound-based technologies to determine liver stiffness, is currently favored and has become a cornerstone in the armamentarium of hepatologists around the world. Noninvasive means provide the advantages of safe longitudinal monitoring and the possibility of applying it to larger populations.

The objective of this book, therefore, will be to review the applications of parametric ultrasound in the context of the diagnosis, staging, and management of CLDs.

References

1. Asrani SK, Devarbhavi H, Eaton J, Kamath PS. Burden of liver diseases in the world. *J Hepatol.* 2019;70:151-171.
2. Diseases GBD, Injuries C. Global burden of 369 diseases and injuries in 204 countries and territories, 1990–2019: a systematic analysis for the Global Burden of Disease Study 2019. *Lancet.* 2020;396:1204-1222.
3. Asrani SK, Larson JJ, Yawn B, Therneau TM, Kim WR. Underestimation of liver-related mortality in the United States. *Gastroenterology.* 2013;145:375-382.
4. Wong MCS, Huang JLW, George J, et al. The changing epidemiology of liver diseases in the Asia-Pacific region. *Nat Rev Gastroenterol Hepatol.* 2019;16:57-73.

5. Paik JM, Golabi P, Younossi Y, Saleh N, Nhyira A, Younossi ZM. The growing burden of disability related to chronic liver disease in the United States: data from the Global Burden of Disease Study 2007–2017. *Hepatol Commun.* 2021;5:749-759.

6. Disease GBD, Injury I, Prevalence C. Global, regional, and national incidence, prevalence, and years lived with disability for 354 diseases and injuries for 195 countries and territories, 1990–2017: a systematic analysis for the Global Burden of Disease Study 2017. *Lancet.* 2018;392:1789-1858.

7. Younossi ZM, Koenig AB, Abdelatif D, Fazel Y, Henry L, Wymer M. Global epidemiology of nonalcoholic fatty liver disease-meta-analytic assessment of prevalence, incidence, and outcomes. *Hepatology.* 2016;64:73-84.

8. Rich NE, Oji S, Mufti AR, et al. Racial and ethnic disparities in nonalcoholic fatty liver disease prevalence, severity, and outcomes in the United States: a systematic review and meta-analysis. *Clin Gastroenterol Hepatol.* 2018;16:198-210.

9. Crabb DW, Im GY, Szabo G, Mellinger JL, Lucey MR. Diagnosis and treatment of alcohol-associated liver diseases: 2019 practice guidance from the American Association for the Study of Liver Diseases. *Hepatology.* 2020;71:306-333.

10. Rehm J, Samokhvalov AV, Shield KD. Global burden of alcoholic liver diseases. *J Hepatol.* 2013;59:160-168.

11. GBD 2016 Causes of Death Collaborators. Global, regional, and national age-sex specific mortality for 264 causes of death, 1980–2016: a systematic analysis for the Global Burden of Disease Study 2016. *Lancet.* 2017;390:1151-1210.

12. *Global Hepatitis Report 2017.* Geneva: World Health Organization; 2017. Available at: https://apps.who.int/iris/bitstream/handle/10665/255016/9789241565455-eng.pdf;jsessionid=614316A7CDDB72987F9D845B0CE31136?sequence=1.

13. Kleiner DE, Brunt EM, Van Natta M, et al. Design and validation of a histological scoring system for nonalcoholic fatty liver disease. *Hepatology.* 2005;41:1313-1321.

14. Goodman ZD. Grading and staging systems for inflammation and fibrosis in chronic liver diseases. *J Hepatol.* 2007;47:598-607.

15. Intraobserver and interobserver variations in liver biopsy interpretation in patients with chronic hepatitis C. The French METAVIR Cooperative Study Group. *Hepatology.* 1994;20(1 Pt 1):15-20.

16. Ratziu V, Charlotte F, Heurtier A, et al. Sampling variability of liver biopsy in nonalcoholic fatty liver disease. *Gastroenterology.* 2005;128:1898-1906.

17. Garrido MC, Hubscher SG. Accuracy of staging in primary biliary cirrhosis. *J Clin Pathol.* 1996;49:556-559.

18. Regev A, Berho M, Jeffers LJ, et al. Sampling error and intraobserver variation in liver biopsy in patients with chronic HCV infection. *Am J Gastroenterol.* 2002;97:2614-2618.

19. Ekiz F, Yuksel I, Arikok AT, et al. Will a second biopsy sample affect treatment decisions in patients with chronic hepatitis B? *Hepatol Int.* 2016;10:602-605.

20. Bedossa P, Poynard T, Naveau S, Martin ED, Agostini H, Chaput JC. Observer variation in assessment of liver biopsies of alcoholic patients. *Alcohol Clin Exp Res.* 1988;12:173-178.

21. Goldin RD, Goldin JG, Burt AD, et al. Intra-observer and inter-observer variation in the histopathological assessment of chronic viral hepatitis. *J Hepatol.* 1996;25:649-654.

22. Davison BA, Harrison SA, Cotter G, et al. Suboptimal reliability of liver biopsy evaluation has implications for randomized clinical trials. *J Hepatol.* 2020;73:1322-1332.

23. Neuberger J, Cain O. The need for alternatives to liver biopsies: non-invasive analytics and diagnostics. *Hepat Med.* 2021;13:59-69.

24. Dulai PS, Singh S, Patel J, et al. Increased risk of mortality by fibrosis stage in nonalcoholic fatty liver disease: systematic review and meta-analysis. *Hepatology.* 2017;65:1557-1565.

25. Taylor RS, Taylor RJ, Bayliss S, et al. Association between fibrosis stage and outcomes of patients with nonalcoholic fatty liver disease: a systematic review and meta-analysis. *Gastroenterology.* 2020;158:1611-1625.

26. D'Amico G, Garcia-Tsao G, Pagliaro L. Natural history and prognostic indicators of survival in cirrhosis: a systematic review of 118 studies. *J Hepatol.* 2006;44:217-231.

27. D'Amico G, Pasta L, Morabito A, et al. Competing risks and prognostic stages of cirrhosis: a 25-year inception cohort study of 494 patients. *Aliment Pharmacol Ther.* 2014;39:1180-1193.

28. Gines P, Quintero E, Arroyo V, et al. Compensated cirrhosis: natural history and prognostic factors. *Hepatology.* 1987;7:122-128.

29. Ripoll C, Bari K, Garcia-Tsao G. Serum albumin can identify patients with compensated cirrhosis with a good prognosis. *J Clin Gastroenterol.* 2015;49:613-619.
30. Udell JA, Wang CS, Tinmouth J, et al. Does this patient with liver disease have cirrhosis? *JAMA.* 2012;307:832-842.
31. Wai CT, Greenson JK, Fontana RJ, et al. A simple noninvasive index can predict both significant fibrosis and cirrhosis in patients with chronic hepatitis C. *Hepatology.* 2003;38:518-526.
32. Vallet-Pichard A, Mallet V, Nalpas B, et al. FIB-4: an inexpensive and accurate marker of fibrosis in HCV infection. Comparison with liver biopsy and fibrotest. *Hepatology.* 2007;46:32-36.
33. Angulo P, Hui JM, Marchesini G, et al. The NAFLD fibrosis score: a noninvasive system that identifies liver fibrosis in patients with NAFLD. *Hepatology.* 2007;45:846-854.
34. Ramachandran P, Iredale JP, Fallowfield JA. Resolution of liver fibrosis: basic mechanisms and clinical relevance. *Semin Liver Dis.* 2015;35:119-131.
35. Marcellin P, Gane E, Buti M, et al. Regression of cirrhosis during treatment with tenofovir disoproxil fumarate for chronic hepatitis B: a 5-year open-label follow-up study. *Lancet.* 2013;381:468-475.
36. Takahashi H, Shigefuku R, Maeyama S, Suzuki M. Cirrhosis improvement to alcoholic liver fibrosis after passive abstinence. *BMJ Case Rep.* 2014;2014:bcr2013201618.
37. Czaja AJ, Carpenter HA. Decreased fibrosis during corticosteroid therapy of autoimmune hepatitis. *J Hepatol.* 2004;40:646-652.
38. Groszmann RJ, Wongcharatrawee S. The hepatic venous pressure gradient: anything worth doing should be done right. *Hepatology.* 2004;39:280-282.
39. Ripoll C, Groszmann R, Garcia-Tsao G, et al. Hepatic venous pressure gradient predicts clinical decompensation in patients with compensated cirrhosis. *Gastroenterology.* 2007;133:481-488.
40. Zipprich A, Garcia-Tsao G, Rogowski S, Fleig WE, Seufferlein T, Dollinger MM. Prognostic indicators of survival in patients with compensated and decompensated cirrhosis. *Liver Int.* 2012;32:1407-1414.
41. Groszmann RJ, Garcia-Tsao G, Bosch J, et al. Beta-blockers to prevent gastroesophageal varices in patients with cirrhosis. *N Engl J Med.* 2005;353:2254-2261.
42. Ripoll C, Groszmann RJ, Garcia-Tsao G, et al. Hepatic venous pressure gradient predicts development of hepatocellular carcinoma independently of severity of cirrhosis. *J Hepatol.* 2009;50:923-928.
43. Garcia-Tsao G, Abraldes JG, Berzigotti A, Bosch J. Portal hypertensive bleeding in cirrhosis: risk stratification, diagnosis, and management: 2016 practice guidance by the American Association for the Study of Liver Diseases. *Hepatology.* 2017;65:310-335.
44. Bruix J, Castells A, Bosch J, et al. Surgical resection of hepatocellular carcinoma in cirrhotic patients: prognostic value of preoperative portal pressure. *Gastroenterology.* 1996;111:1018-1022.
45. Villanueva C, Albillos A, Genesca J, et al. Beta blockers to prevent decompensation of cirrhosis in patients with clinically significant portal hypertension (PREDESCI): a randomised, double-blind, placebo-controlled, multicentre trial. *Lancet.* 2019;393:1597-1608.
46. Mandorfer M, Kozbial K, Schwabl P, et al. Sustained virologic response to interferon-free therapies ameliorates HCV-induced portal hypertension. *J Hepatol.* 2016;65:692-699.
47. Lens S, Alvarado-Tapias E, Marino Z, et al. Effects of all-oral anti-viral therapy on HVPG and systemic hemodynamics in patients with hepatitis C virus-associated cirrhosis. *Gastroenterology.* 2017;153:1273-1283.
48. Lens S, Baiges A, Alvarado-Tapias E, et al. Clinical outcome and hemodynamic changes following HCV eradication with oral antiviral therapy in patients with clinically significant portal hypertension. *J Hepatol.* 2020;73:1415-1424.
49. Suk KT. Hepatic venous pressure gradient: clinical use in chronic liver disease. *Clin Mol Hepatol.* 2014;20:6-14.

CHAPTER 2

Conventional Ultrasound Findings in Chronic Liver Disease

Richard G. Barr

Introduction

Chronic liver disease (CLD) is a substantial worldwide problem. Any disease that incites liver inflammation can lead to liver fibrosis, which can then progress to cirrhosis.

The stage of liver fibrosis is important to determine prognosis, surveillance, progression, or regression of disease. The process of fibrosis is dynamic, and regression of fibrosis is possible up to the stage of early cirrhosis with treatment of the underlying conditions.[1] Therefore it is important to detect the presence of the disease before the development of decompensated cirrhosis. Worldwide there is a significant increase in fatty liver disease, which can lead to cirrhosis, and noninvasive methods to detect steatosis and monitor progress or regression of the disease are needed.

With increasing fibrosis, the liver becomes stiffer and eventually portal hypertension develops. Previously, the only method of quantifying the degree of fibrosis was a random liver biopsy, which is an imperfect reference standard.[1] Although conventional ultrasound (US) is limited in the detection of fibrosis stages less than cirrhosis, it is a widely used screening examination. Conventional US is used as a screening tool for assessment of steatosis because it is noninvasive, lacks radiation, and is widely available. Other methods such as shear wave elastography are more accurate in the assessment of the stage of fibrosis, and new US techniques are becoming available for fat quantification, which are discussed in other chapters of this book.

For liver stiffness and fat quantification, high quality B-mode images are required for accurate measurements. This chapter reviews the conventional US techniques and how to optimize both B-mode and Doppler images, eliminate artifacts, and use these features in CLD.

The use of B-mode imaging for liver stiffness measurements is discussed in Chapter 4, portal hypertension in Chapter 8, and fat quantification in Chapter 11. Details about Doppler studies for the evaluation of portal hypertension are given in Chapter 8. Detection and characterization of focal liver lesions in CLD are presented in Chapter 13. A review of the normal anatomy of the liver can be found elsewhere.[2,3]

B-Mode Imaging

OPTIMIZING B-MODE IMAGES

When evaluating patients with suspected CLD, a complete US evaluation of the liver should be performed. The entire liver should be evaluated in two planes to reconstruct its three-dimensionality. In adults the examination should be performed with a curved transducer optimized for abdominal imaging, usually with a range of 2 MHz to 6 MHz. The frequency of the transducer should be adjusted as needed for the patient's body habitus. Most modern transducers are wideband and have the ability to adjust the center frequency to optimize the imaging. Most systems have a RES

TABLE 2.1 ■ **Typical Scanning Protocol for Patients with Chronic Liver Disease**

Mode		Anatomic Location	Key Findings
B-mode	Curved	Entire liver	Echo pattern
Use of spatial	linear	Bile ducts/gallbladder	Capsule nodularity
compounding	probe	Spleen	Liver size (right lobe and caudate lobe)
and harmonic			Focal liver lesions
imaging			Spleen size
	Linear probe		Liver capsule—smooth or nodular
Color Doppler		Portal vein	Portal vein diameter and flow pattern
with spectral		Hepatic vein	Hepatic vein flow pattern
analysis		Hepatic Artery	(RI 0.55–0.7)
		Splenic vein	Varices present or not
		Inferior vena cava	
		Aorta	
Elastography		Liver stiffness	Liver stiffness
		? Spleen stiffness	? Spleen stiffness in patients with advanced chronic liver disease

RI, Resistive index.

(resolution) setting using higher frequencies in easy-to-scan patients, a GEN (general) setting using mid-range frequencies, and a PEN (penetration) setting using lower frequencies in difficult-to-scan patients. Spatial compounding and harmonic imaging also improve the quality of the image by decreasing artifacts and clutter. Using these settings appropriately will improve the image quality. Generally, the left lobe of the liver is best imaged in a supine position using a subcostal approach whereas the right lobe is best imaged using a left lateral decubitus position using both a subcostal approach and through an intercostal window. Having the patient take a deep inspiration may be required to visualize the dome of the liver. A small sector probe also can be helpful in anatomically difficult locations and in pediatric patients. Vascular landmarks should be included in the images to allow identification of the segment according to the Couinaud classification.[4] Color Doppler, power Doppler, or microvascular flow techniques are used to evaluate vessel patency and flow dynamics. Optimization of the Doppler images should be performed, including selecting the appropriate scanning frequency and filters. The biliary system including the gallbladder and intrahepatic and extrahepatic bile ducts also should be evaluated for masses, strictures, or areas of dilation. An examination for CLD should include evaluation of the liver echotexture, evaluation of the liver capsule to assess for nodularity using a high-frequency linear probe, and assessment of the size of the right lobe of the liver and caudate lobe and portal vein diameter. Doppler evaluation with spectral analysis of the portal vein and hepatic veins is required to assess for portal hypertension or hepatic venous outflow obstruction (see Chapter 8). Detection and characterization of focal liver lesions should be included as there is a risk for hepatocellular carcinoma in patients with severe fibrosis/liver cirrhosis, which is discussed in Chapter 13. The spleen size should be estimated and the possible presence of varices should be evaluated, particularly in patients with advanced chronic liver disease (ACLD) as these are signs of clinically significant portal hypertension. Table 2.1 lists the conventional US protocol for CLD.

FATTY LIVER DISEASE

Diffuse fatty infiltration results in increased echogenicity of the liver, thus the sound transmission is progressively and more markedly reduced from the proximal to the distal portions of the liver. This leads to poor or nonvisualization of the diaphragm, intrahepatic vessels, and posterior portion of the right hepatic lobe. It is important to remember that different US systems may have a more grainy or less grainy appearance of the liver, and learning the appearance of the liver echotexture on the system being used is important.

The main features to take into consideration for a qualitative estimate of liver fat content are liver–kidney contrast, diaphragm definition, and vessel blurring.

Liver–Kidney Contrast

The echogenicities of liver and kidney are almost equivalent in normal subjects. However, the liver appears hyperechoic as the fat deposition in the liver causes increased echogenicity. The contrast between the liver and parenchyma of the right kidney is therefore increased in liver steatosis (Fig. 2.1).[5] Due to the increased attenuation of the ultrasonic waves in a steatotic liver, the diaphragm, intrahepatic vessels, and the posterior part of the right lobe are poorly or nonvisualized.[6] As an increased liver echogenicity leads to a decreased acoustic impedance between the liver parenchyma and other echogenic structures like portal vein walls, liver capsule, and gallbladder walls, those structures are depicted with difficulty (Fig. 2.2).[7] In rare cases, patients with liver steatosis may show a paradoxical lack of posterior attenuation on US images due to scattering in attenuation of the US beam seen in fatty livers (Fig. 2.3).[8]

Using a combination of some of the aforementioned parameters, the degree of steatosis may be qualitatively assessed as discussed later.[6,7,9]

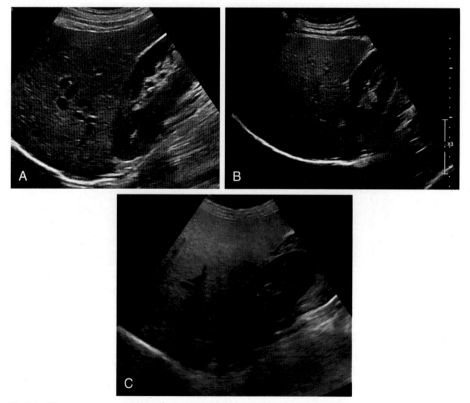

Fig. 2.1 Three cases comparing the echogenicity of the kidney to the liver. Increasing fat deposition going from (A) normal, (B) moderate fatty infiltration of the liver, and (C) marked fatty infiltration of the liver. Note the difference in echogenicity between the liver and kidney in these cases.

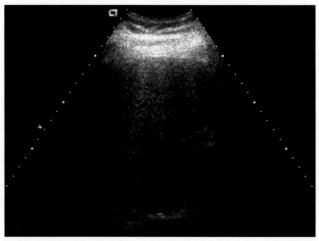

Fig. 2.2 In this case of marked fatty infiltration of the liver, the decreased acoustic impedance between the liver parenchyma and other echogenic structures like portal vein walls, liver capsule, and gallbladder walls result in these structures being difficult to identify.

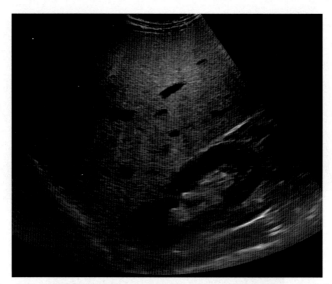

Fig. 2.3 In this patient with a markedly fatty liver (attenuation coefficient of 1.0 dB/cm/MHz), there is still good visualization of the deep structures. This is one of the rare cases in which the attenuation does not dramatically affect the imaging.

Diaphragm Definition

Diaphragm visualization is an important indicator for diagnosing liver steatosis. It can be visualized normally in mild liver steatosis. The echogenicity of the diaphragm is discontinuous in moderate liver steatosis, and it is not visualized in patients with severe liver steatosis.[5]

Vessel Blurring

Intrahepatic vessels are sharply demarcated in normal liver. Vessel blurring is an indicator of moderate liver steatosis, and it is based on an impaired visualization of the borders of the intrahepatic vessels and narrowing of their lumen. There are two major reasons for vessel blurring in fatty liver: attenuation of acoustic wave and intrahepatic vascular remodeling.[10] These two reasons can exist alone or at the same time. Intrahepatic vascular remodeling contributes to high resistance and constricted sinusoidal vessels, even to the extent to which intrahepatic vascular shunts develop.[11] Among the various criteria used to diagnose liver steatosis, vascular attenuation, which includes both portal vein and hepatic vein blurring, has lower sensitivity and specificity compared with hepatorenal echo contrast and bright liver.[12]

The assessment of hepatic steatosis on US is subjective, leading to intra- and interreader variability. The features of large hepatic vein blurring, liver–kidney contrast, and overall impression have the highest intrareader, intertransducer, and interreader agreement. Large hepatic vein blurring has the highest accuracy for classifying dichotomized hepatic steatosis grade.[5] Large hepatic vein blurring (intraclass correlation coefficient [ICC]: 0.76), liver–kidney contrast (ICC: 0.78), and overall impression (ICC: 0.75) have the highest mean intrareader agreement, whereas liver echo texture (ICC: 0.43) have the lowest mean intrareader agreement, also depending on the frequency of the transducer. Among individual imaging features, large hepatic vein blurring has the highest diagnostic accuracy (71%) for classifying dichotomized hepatic steatosis (80% sensitivity, 63% specificity) using histological grade as the reference standard. Large hepatic vein blurring provided nominally similar accuracy as overall impression for classifying dichotomized hepatic steatosis with higher specificity but lower sensitivity point estimates.[5]

Grading Liver Steatosis

An accurate estimate of the fat in the liver is a crucial component in the diagnostic work-up of patients with nonalcoholic fatty liver disease (NAFLD) because liver steatosis is associated with metabolic syndrome and the degree of fatty degeneration is directly proportional to the cardiovascular risk.[13]

Based on the features discussed previously, US allows for a subjective estimate of the degree of fatty infiltration in the liver. Grading of liver steatosis can be made using a qualitative grading system of absent, mild, moderate, or severe. Absent (Grade 0) is when the echotexture of the liver is normal. Grade 1 (mild) is represented by a mild diffuse increase in liver echogenicity with normal visualization of the diaphragm and intrahepatic vessel borders (mainly portal vein). Grade 2 (moderate) is represented by a moderate diffuse increase in liver echogenicity with slightly impaired visualization of the portal vein and diaphragm. Grade 3 (marked) is represented by a marked increase in liver echogenicity with poor or no visualization of the intrahepatic vessel borders, diaphragm, and posterior portion of the right lobe of the liver (Fig. 2.4).[6,7,14] In mild hepatic steatosis, the liver size is normal and the edge is relatively sharp. In severe hepatic steatosis, the liver is enlarged and the edge is blunt. The liver size of moderate steatosis is in between.[15] Numerous other studies have dealt with the US-based semiquantitative classification of fatty liver.[16-21]

The Hamaguchi score and the Ultrasound Fatty Liver Indicator scores combine several US findings assigning a number to each of them, therefore a semiquantitative estimate of liver fat content is obtained. They are presented in detail in Chapter 11. Conventional US is particularly accurate when there is no other underlying liver disease. The sensitivity and specificity of sonography for the detection of moderate to severe steatosis using histology as a reference standard are 80%–89% and 87%–97%, respectively.[22-26] If all degrees of steatosis are considered, the sensitivity and specificity decrease to 65% and 81%, respectively.[22] A metaanalysis based on 49 studies has shown a high accuracy of US for the diagnosis of moderate to severe steatosis.[27] However, US accuracy is highly operator dependent, and its sensitivity is reduced when steatosis infiltration is lower than 30% or in morbidly obese patients.[28] Furthermore, the quantification of hepatic steatosis is subjective and could be influenced by the heterogeneity seen in some patients with NAFLD. Due to substantial inter- and intraobserver variability and the reduced sensitivity in assessing mild steatosis, the four-point visual scale evaluation has clear limitations.[6,7,23]

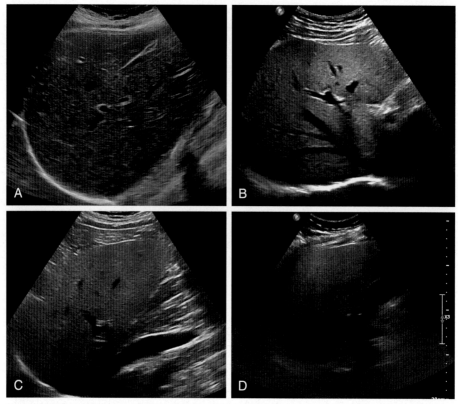

Fig. 2.4   With increasing steatosis (fatty deposition) the echogenicity of the liver increases and visualization of the vascular structures and diaphragm changes. (A) Normal. (B) Grade 1. (C) Grade 2. (D) Grade 3. Note the difference in visualization of the vessels and diaphragm at the various grades of liver steatosis.

As a diagnostic tool for the detection of fatty liver, US showed a sensitivity and specificity of 85% and 94%, respectively, as a large metaanalysis of 49 studies with 4720 patients found in which histology served as the gold standard.[25] Computed tomography has inferior diagnostic value (low sensitivity for mild cases and intermachine variability) and exposes the patient to radiation, limiting it for screening. Magnetic resonance spectroscopy (MRS) allows for quantification of hepatic fat. Magnetic resonance imaging–derived proton density fat fraction (MRI-PDFF) is a quantitative noninvasive biomarker that objectively estimates the liver fat content and has been accepted as an alternative to the histological assessment of liver steatosis in patients with NAFLD.[29,30]

Hepatorenal Index

A semiquantitative method of grading liver steatosis is the sonographic hepatorenal index (HRI)[6,31] (Fig. 2.5). This is based on comparison of the echogenicity of the liver to the normal kidney. The effectiveness of steatosis detection can be increased by quantification of liver brightness as compared to the kidney brightness. On a US image showing segment VI of the liver and the right kidney (usually the upper pole), two regions of interest should be selected: one in the liver parenchyma, far from vessels and bile ducts, and the other in the renal cortex (between the pyramids) at the same field depth. The mean brightness of each region of interest is determined using numerical values assigned to gray-scale pixels. The HRI is the mean liver brightness

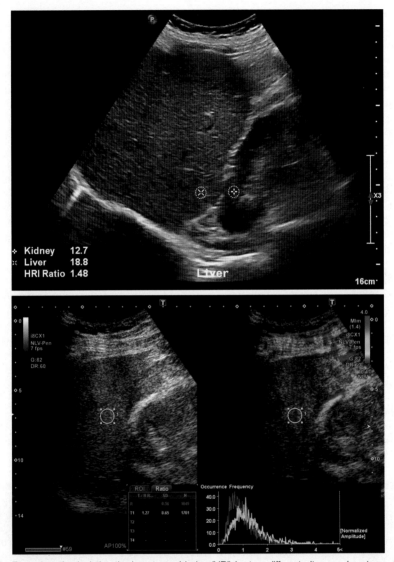

Fig. 2.5 Examples of calculating the hepatorenal index (HRI) by two different ultrasound systems. In both cases a region of interest was placed in the renal cortex and one in the liver parenchyma at the same depth. The system then calculated the ratio of signal intensity between the two tissues using the raw data. When using post processed images for the calculation, gain and other factors can affect the signal intensity of the tissues making the calculation less accurate.

divided by the mean renal cortex brightness. A histogram analysis of the echogenicity can be performed directly on some US systems or may be exported to freeware available online as JPEGs. The results seem to be better if the histogram is performed on DICOM images downloaded from the PACS.[14]

Significant correlation between histological steatosis and the HRI has been found in several studies.[32] The accuracy of the HRI for the diagnosis of mild steatosis (≥5%) was excellent

(AUROC 0.99) with 100% sensitivity and 91% specificity using a cutoff of 1.49.[33] Further studies have confirmed that the HRI had excellent accuracy for the detection of steatosis (negative predictive value = 94%−100% with cutoffs ranging from 1.24 to 1.34).[34] In addition, for the prediction of steatosis grades less than moderate or severe, HRI is superior to qualitative grading.

Several studies have found this technique to have significant correlation to histologic steatosis. A recent study using 3 Tesla magnetic resonance imaging as the gold standard found that cutoff values of 1.21, 1.28, and 2.15 had 100% sensitivity for diagnosis of greater than 5%, 25%, and 50%, respectively, with a specificity of greater than 70%.[31] It is important to note that each vendor has its own method of assessing the HRI, and cutoff values may vary between vendors.

In some studies, histogram analyses of the echogenicity ratio of liver and renal cortex were performed.[33,35] The software-based histogram analyses significantly increased the diagnostic accuracy of sonography for a degree of fat ≥5% (AUROC >0.90).[33] In another study, a sensitivity of 100% and a specificity of 54% were achieved for the detection of a degree of fat ≥5% with an HRI of ≥1.28.[31] A more recent study by the same working group was able to achieve a sensitivity of 92% and a specificity of 85% for the detection of low-grade fatty degeneration (≥5%) using new software for an HRI calculation and a cutoff value of ≥1.34.[36] Like the other previously mentioned scores, the HRI has not yet been sufficiently validated for clinical routine.

Focal Fatty Infiltration Patterns

Hepatic steatosis may present with different patterns of deposition and sparing. In the literature six patterns of liver steatosis are described: diffuse, geographic, focal, subcapsular, multifocal, and perivascular.[15] Diffuse fatty liver deposition is the most prevalent form of fatty liver disease. Geographic fatty liver disease is often encountered and can be attributed to specific causes (vascular or inflammatory) (Fig. 2.6). Focal fat deposition and focal fatty sparing are less frequent and occur predominately in specific areas (i.e., perivascular and subcapsular regions abutting the hepatic hilum or falciform ligament) and can mimic a tumor (Fig. 2.7).[6]

Focal Fatty Sparing

Focal fatty sparing appears as focal hypoechoic areas within the liver (Fig. 2.8). It has been suggested that less portal venous blood flow and/or regional dilution of portal venous blood

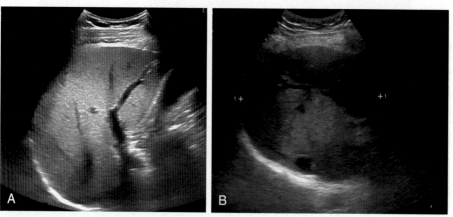

Fig. 2.6 Two cases of geographic fat distribution are presented here. The areas of geographic fat deposition are echogenic compared to the normal liver echogenicity. Note that blood vessels are not displaced. (A) is from a 63-year-old patient referred for ultrasound for elevated liver function tests. (B) is from a 26-year-old patient referred for routine screening for Fontan surgery.

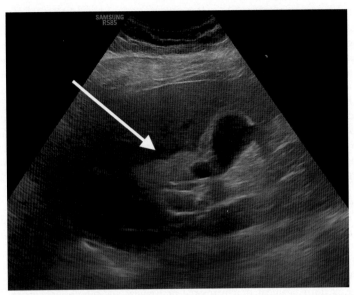

Fig. 2.7 A case of focal fatty infiltration adjacent to the gallbladder *(arrow)*. The area of focal fatty infiltration is well defined and increased in echogenicity compared to the normal liver parenchyma. This is a common place for both focal fatty deposition and focal fatty sparing.

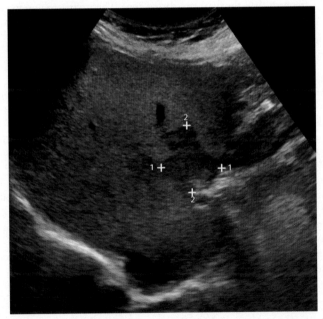

Fig. 2.8 Focal fatty sparing can be identified as a well circumscribed area of decreased echogenicity compared to the rest of the liver. The rest of the liver has increased fat content, making it more echogenic. Focal fatty sparing can appear as a mass lesion but can be identified as the normal liver vasculature is not displaced. If there is concern of a mass lesion, a contrast-enhanced ultrasound can confirm this is normal liver tissue as it will have the same enhancement in all vascular phases.

secondary to anatomical variations of supplying vessels are present, therefore providing regional hepatocytes with less fatty substrates than the remaining parenchyma. In liver areas with reduced focal fat accumulation, fibrous tissue remodeling may occur, which seems to be caused by a different vascular supply compared with the rest of the liver.[5,37-45] However, the exact cause is unknown. The prevalence of these pseudo-lesions has been reported to be as low as 5.3%–19.8%[45-48] and may reach near 100% in patients with significant steatosis.[38] On US these areas are hypoechoic to the rest of the liver and occur mainly in liver segments IV and V, adjacent to the gallbladder fossa and falciform ligament or ventral to the portal vein.[42,49] Focal fatty sparing does not have mass effect. Identifying the lesions in the typical locations and lack of mass effect can help in making the diagnosis. If focal fat-sparing areas occur in atypical locations, they may be difficult to distinguish from solid liver tumors.[50] In these cases, a contrast-enhanced US can help confirm the diagnosis.

Focal Fatty Infiltration

Regions of focal fatty infiltration are hyperechoic compared to the rest of the liver. Histologically, there is a larger number of fat-filled vacuoles in these zones.[39,51,52] They differ from space-consuming lesions by their typical location and lack of mass effect.[53] The cause is not clearly understood, but arterial tissue hypoxia with compensatory stronger portal venous supply has been proposed. Areas of focal fatty infiltration are often located around the gallbladder bed, the medial aspect of the falciform ligament, or in periportal, perivenular, and subcapsular regions.[54] They can be multifocal nodular, round, or oval and may mimic liver metastases in B-mode US. The lack of mass effect and typical location are helpful to make the diagnosis. If there is still concern of a mass lesion, contrast-enhanced US can make the diagnosis as focal fatty infiltration or focal fatty sparing will have an enhancement pattern of a normal liver. The focal fatty infiltration zone is significantly less frequent than the focal fat-sparing zone. These appear in up to 40% of patients taking corticosteroids (Fig. 2.7).[52]

Limitations of B-Mode Ultrasound in the Evaluation of Hepatic Steatosis

There are several limitations of B-mode US in the evaluation of hepatic steatosis.

1. The performance of B-mode US imaging for the detection of mild steatosis (fat content between 5% and 20%) is quite variable (sensitivity of 55%–90%),[55] and most of the studies reported low sensitivities (60.9%–65%).[14] US was found to have acceptable diagnostic accuracy for detecting moderate or severe hepatic steatosis (>20%–30% steatosis) in adults, with pooled sensitivities ranging from 86% to 99% and pooled specificities ranging from 85% to 92%.[56]
2. Hepatic fibrosis may also increase liver echogenicity, thus the presence of underlying CLD may reduce the accuracy of conventional US in the diagnosis of hepatic steatosis.[14,23]
3. In obese patients with a body mass index >46 kg/m², US is an unreliable tool for screening for steatosis with sensitivities of 40%–65%.[55] US artifacts due to thick layers of subcutaneous fat account for these low performances.[7,14,55]
4. Conventional US is highly dependent on the operator expertise with significant intra- and interobserver variability.

FIBROSIS

Fibrosis is a common pathway for numerous causes of hepatic inflammation leading to cirrhosis. The cause of the hepatic inflammation can be from infectious diseases, metabolic disease, toxins, autoimmune diseases, or other causes. Fibrosis is an abnormal increase in collagen fibers and other components of the extracellular matrix in response to chronic injury. Cirrhosis is a diffuse process characterized by fibrosis and the conversion of normal liver architecture into structurally abnormal nodules.[57]

The speckle pattern of the liver changes with both steatosis and fibrosis. Acoustic structure quantification (ASQ), a vendor specific application, can be used to assess the speckle pattern. ASQ does not perform as well as shear wave elastography techniques in staging fibrosis but can be used for quantification of steatosis.[58]

Conventional US features that have been used to stage liver fibrosis include liver parenchymal echotexture, liver surface, liver edge, liver size, portal vein diameter, spleen size, and portal vein flowmetry with Doppler technique. The liver parenchymal echotexture becomes coarse with the development of fibrosis. However, this finding is subjective, operator dependent, a function of the equipment, and complicated when fatty infiltration of the liver is present. Therefore this sign is neither sensitive nor specific.[59]

As fibrosis progresses to cirrhosis, the liver becomes nodular.[60] It has been reported that liver surface nodularity is the most specific sign for the diagnosis of cirrhosis. In a study that included 300 consecutive asymptomatic patients with elevated transaminase values undergoing liver biopsy, the accuracy of liver surface nodularity, caudate lobe hypertrophy, and pattern of hepatic venous blood flow were investigated. The study found that liver surface nodularity had the highest diagnostic accuracy, with specificity of 95%. Of note, of the 107 patients with severe fibrosis or definite cirrhosis, 28 (26%) were negative for liver surface nodularity and caudate lobe hypertrophy and had normal hepatic venous flow. Therefore the sensitivity of this sign is not high.

The B-mode and Doppler findings of liver cirrhosis and portal hypertension are discussed in detail in Chapter 8.

Doppler Features

OPTIMIZING DOPPLER IMAGING

Selecting the proper tissue-specific preset is important to set the Doppler parameters for the appropriate application. The choice of the setting should be based on the flow characteristics of the vessels being evaluated. Since both the portal system and hepatic veins have slow flow, it is important to set the flow optimization parameters to maximize for slow flow and use low wall filters. Increasing persistence for these vessels can provide a smoother image with less noise. Most systems allow for selecting the mean Doppler frequency of the transducer and for selecting a lower Doppler frequency if the vessel is deep to improve visualization. Most systems also allow the selection of a flow-optimization setting with a speed setting (higher frame rate at the expense of image quality) or a general setting (compromise between speed and quality) and a resolution setting (slow frame rate with higher resolution). Note this is different than the frequency selection. Since the vessels being interrogated are mostly slow-flow venous vessels, selecting the general setting or resolution flow optimization setting is appropriate. Power Doppler is more sensitive than color Doppler and can improve vascular evaluation at the expense of the loss of direction information. Some US systems have a directional power Doppler that provides direction information. Microvascular flow is now available on many US systems and can provide visualization of smaller vessels with a substantial decrease in blooming. For pulsed-wave Doppler, setting the gate to approximately half of the vessel diameter and placing it in the center of the vessel are important to limit artifacts. Many US systems can add chroma coloring to the waveforms for improved visualization. All systems allow for measuring the flow velocity, the resistive index (RI), and other parameters.

DOPPLER EVALUATION IN CHRONIC LIVER DISEASE

Hepatic Veins

The normal flow profile of the three hepatic veins is triphasic (Fig. 2.9). The hepatic vein flow can change with concomitant cardiological and respiratory disease. It is also influenced by histological changes in liver tissue and changes with the severity of liver fibrosis.[40,61-65] Some

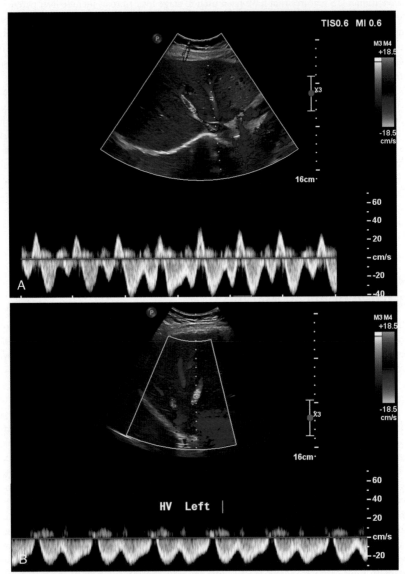

Fig. 2.9   The normal hepatic venous waveforms are triphasic. This occurs because there is no valve between the right atrium and the hepatic veins. Therefore the pressure changes due to contraction and relaxation of the right atrium are transmitted to the hepatic veins. The majority of the flow is directed toward the heart. Two examples (A and B) are presented here.

studies have shown that a monophasic flow profile of the hepatic veins is often associated with fatty liver and much less with liver cirrhosis[40,65,66] and can be observed in completely normal patients as well.[66] The typical flow profile in liver cirrhosis is biphasic due to the arterialization of the liver vascularity.[40] In patients with chronic hepatitis C infection with and without liver cirrhosis, it was found that a monophasic flow profile in the right hepatic vein was less associated with the degree of fibrosis and inflammation than with the degree of (histological) fatty degeneration of the liver.[38] In this study, the fat content of hepatocytes was the only independent variable that influenced the hepatic vein flow pattern: 90% of the patients with a liver fat content of more than 50% showed a monophasic flow profile, but only 5% of the patients with a fat content of less than 25% did. Another study observed a significant inverse correlation between the sonographic degree of hepatic steatosis (none, mild, moderate, severe) and the phasicity of the liver vein flow profile.[67] The etiology of liver disease does not appear to directly influence the hepatic venous flow profile.[40,62] The mechanism of origin of this sign is still unclear. It may be due to a compliance loss of the hepatic veins caused by fibrosis and fat infiltration: the rigidity of the surrounding liver tissue leads to a flattening of the flow profile.[67,68] Other authors assume a compression of the hepatic veins by the (inflammatory) hypertrophy of liver cells or by fat accumulation.[40,61,62,69]

Hepatic Artery

The hepatic artery normally has a low resistive (RI between 0.55 and 0.70) arterial flow pattern with hepatopetal flow (Fig. 2.10). The measurement of the hepatic artery resistive index (HARI) has been studied in the context of fatty liver and fibrosis progression.[70,71] It was shown that HARI was inversely correlated with the severity of steatosis and positively correlated with the degree of fibrosis measured by the NAFLD Fibrosis Score (NFS) in NAFLD.[71] In patients with an NFS >0.67, the HARI was significantly above the range of the control group (mean HARI value = 0.98 ± 0.02 in NAFLD patients vs. 0.88 ± 0.03 in controls, $P < .05$). This indicates that fibrous and fat-accumulated tissue of varying quantity can lead to rigidity of the arterial vessel walls and

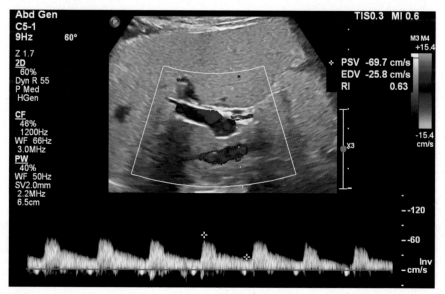

Fig. 2.10 In this example of a normal hepatic artery pulsed Doppler, there is a low resistive arterial flow pattern (RI = 0.63) with flow directed toward the liver. *RI,* Resistive index.

thus to an increase in flow resistance. However, only a few studies are available, and further prospective studies are necessary to investigate the added value of HARI in the context of fatty liver evaluation.

Portal Vein

The normal portal venous peak systolic velocities range between 15 cm/s and 40 cm/s. Flow velocity <15 cm/s, together with an enlargement of the main portal vein diameter, are suggestive of increased portal pressure. Monophasic deformation is an unspecific sign of steatosis but not correlated to the amount of intrahepatic fat deposition (Fig. 2.11). A pronounced undulation in the portal vein was associated with portal inflammation but not with other parameters of the histologic activity index or the intrahepatic fat deposition.[40] The velocity and direction of flow are important in the evaluation of portal hypertension and are discussed in detail in Chapter 8.

Acute Hepatitis and Budd-Chiari Syndrome

In addition to CLD, there are several acute diffuse liver diseases that may have similar findings. These include acute viral hepatitis and acute Budd-Chiari syndrome. In acute hepatitis of any cause, hepatomegaly, hypoechoic parenchyma, and increased periportal echoes may be seen. Color Doppler and spectral Doppler findings usually remain within normal limits. It should be noted that for viral causes, only chronic infections progress to fibrosis. While 5%–15% of hepatitis B acute infections in adults become chronic, 75%–85% of acute hepatitis C infections become chronic.[72]

Acute Budd-Chiari syndrome is characterized by hepatomegaly and heterogeneity of the liver due to congestion (Fig. 2.12). The hepatic vein(s) occlusion will be identified on Doppler imaging with color and spectral analysis. There may be development of small intrahepatic venous collaterals with flow reversal. In chronic Budd-Chiari syndrome there is usually peripheral liver atrophy with central hypertrophy and regenerating nodules. The caudate lobe can be markedly enlarged because the venous drainage is independent from the rest of the liver. See also Chapter 8 for more details.

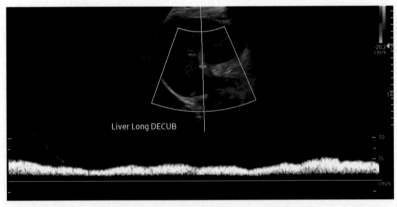

Liver Long DECUB

Fig. 2.11 The Doppler evaluation of portal venous blood flow provides information on the degree of portal hypertension and is an important part of any ultrasound performed for chronic liver disease. The flow normally has mild respiratory variation with velocities of between 15 cm/s and 40 cm/s as noted in this figure. The arterial waveform superimposed on the venous waveforms is from the hepatic artery. Including the hepatic artery in the Doppler gate can help confirm the direction of flow of the portal vein as the hepatic artery flow is always hepatopetal.

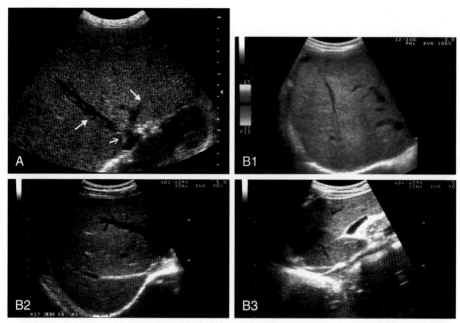

Fig. 2.12 (A) In this case of Budd-Chiari syndrome, the right and mid hepatic veins are occluded with echogenic material within them. (B) Chronic Budd-Chiari syndrome in 45-year-old woman with breast cancer and diagnosed with cirrhosis of unknown origin. In B1, reversal of hepatic venous flow is noted. In B2, the white linear line is occlusion of the right hepatic vein. An enlarged caudate lobe with enlarged caudate vein is present in B3.

KEY POINTS

1. Conventional US is a widely available, radiation-free, and noninvasive technique.
2. Conventional US can be used as a screening technique for the detection of fatty infiltration of the liver, however, it is limited in the detection of mild levels of steatosis, and new techniques described in Chapter 11 are significant improvements in the assessment of liver fat content.
3. Mild to moderate levels of fibrosis are difficult to detect with conventional US, and elastographic techniques discussed in Chapter 7 are more accurate in assessing the stage of fibrosis. Moreover, even in advanced fibrosis, the liver may appear quite normal on B-mode imaging.
4. The changes of ACLD that can be detected with conventional US are discussed in this chapter. The complication of decompensated cirrhosis, ascites, recanalization of the umbilical vein, portal vein thrombosis, etc. are easily visualized on conventional US. Changes in the diameter and blood flow pattern of the portal vein can help determine if significant portal hypertension is present (see Chapter 8).
5. B-mode US is also the preferred screening method for focal liver lesions in patients with CLD. Characterization of focal liver lesions can be made with high accuracy using contrast-enhanced US (see Chapter 13).
6. The combination of several US techniques (i.e., multiparametric US) discussed in this book is a very powerful method of assessing CLD.

References

1. Barr RG, Ferraioli G, Palmeri ML, et al. Elastography assessment of liver fibrosis: Society of Radiologists in Ultrasound Consensus Conference Statement. *Ultrasound Q.* 2016;32:94-107.
2. Majno P, Mentha G, Toso C, Morel P, Peitgen HO, Fasel JH. Anatomy of the liver: an outline with three levels of complexity—a further step towards tailored territorial liver resections. *J Hepatol.* 2014;60:654-662.
3. Elsayes KM, Shaaban AM, Rothan SM, et al. A comprehensive approach to hepatic vascular disease. *Radiographics.* 2017;37:813-836.
4. Fasel JH, Schenk A. Concepts for liver segment classification: neither old ones nor new ones, but a comprehensive one. *J Clin Imaging Sci.* 2013;3:48.
5. Hong CW, Marsh A, Wolfson T, et al. Reader agreement and accuracy of ultrasound features for hepatic steatosis. *Abdom Radiol (NY).* 2019;44:54-64.
6. Gerstenmaier JF, Gibson RN. Ultrasound in chronic liver disease. *Insights Imaging.* 2014;5:441-455.
7. Lupşor-Platon M, Stefănescu H, Mureşan D, et al. Noninvasive assessment of liver steatosis using ultrasound methods. *Med Ultrason.* 2014;16:236-245.
8. Davies RJ, Saverymuttu Sh, Fallowfield M, Joseph AE. Paradoxical lack of ultrasound attenuation with gross fatty change in the liver. *Clin Radiol.* 1991;43:393-396.
9. Castera L, Friedrich-Rust M, Loomba R. Noninvasive assessment of liver disease in patients with non-alcoholic fatty liver disease. *Gastroenterology.* 2019;156:1264-1281.e4.
10. Jesper D, Klett D, Schellhaas B, et al. Ultrasound-based attenuation imaging for the non-invasive quantification of liver fat - a pilot study on feasibility and inter-observer variability. *IEEE J Transl Eng Health Med.* 2020;8:1800409.
11. Lee JS, Semela D, Iredale J, Shah VH. Sinusoidal remodeling and angiogenesis: a new function for the liver-specific pericyte? *Hepatology.* 2007;45:817-825.
12. Dasarathy S, Dasarathy J, Khiyami A, Joseph R, Lopez R, McCullough AJ. Validity of real time ultrasound in the diagnosis of hepatic steatosis: a prospective study. *J Hepatol.* 2009;51:1061-1067.
13. Guth S, Leise U, Bamberger CM, Windler E. Ultrasonographic hepatic steatosis as a surrogate for atherosclerosis. *Ultrasound Int Open.* 2016;2:E27-E31.
14. Ferraioli G, Soares Monteiro LB. Ultrasound-based techniques for the diagnosis of liver steatosis. *World J Gastroenterol.* 2019;25:6053-6062.
15. Decarie PO, Lepanto L, Billiard JS, et al. Fatty liver deposition and sparing: a pictorial review. *Insights Imaging.* 2011;2:533-538.
16. Saverymuttu SH, Joseph AE, Maxwell JD. Ultrasound scanning in the detection of hepatic fibrosis and steatosis. *Br Med J (Clin Res Ed).* 1986;292:13-15.
17. Saadeh S, Younossi ZM, Remer EM, et al. The utility of radiological imaging in nonalcoholic fatty liver disease. *Gastroenterology.* 2002;123:745-750.
18. Tominaga K, Kurata JH, Chen YK, et al. Prevalence of fatty liver in Japanese children and relationship to obesity. An epidemiological ultrasonographic survey. *Dig Dis Sci.* 1995;40:2002-2009.
19. Henschke CI, Goldman H, Teele RL. The hyperechogenic liver in children: cause and sonographic appearance. *AJR Am J Roentgenol.* 1982;138:841-846.
20. Chan DF, Li AM, Chu WC, et al. Hepatic steatosis in obese Chinese children. *Int J Obes Relat Metab Disord.* 2004;28:1257-1263.
21. Arslan N, Buyukgebiz B, Ozturk Y, Cakmakci H. Fatty liver in obese children: prevalence and correlation with anthropometric measurements and hyperlipidemia. *Turk J Pediatr.* 2005;47:23-27.
22. Palmentieri B, de Sio I, La Mura V, et al. The role of bright liver echo pattern on ultrasound B-mode examination in the diagnosis of liver steatosis. *Dig Liver Dis.* 2006;38:485-489.
23. Lee SS, Park SH. Radiologic evaluation of nonalcoholic fatty liver disease. *World J Gastroenterol.* 2014;20:7392-7402.
24. Lee SS, Park SH, Kim HJ, et al. Non-invasive assessment of hepatic steatosis: prospective comparison of the accuracy of imaging examinations. *J Hepatol.* 2010;52:579-585.
25. Hernaez R, Lazo M, Bonekamp S, et al. Diagnostic accuracy and reliability of ultrasonography for the detection of fatty liver: a meta-analysis. *Hepatology.* 2011;54:1082-1090.
26. Bril F, Ortiz-Lopez C, Lomonaco R, et al. Clinical value of liver ultrasound for the diagnosis of nonalcoholic fatty liver disease in overweight and obese patients. *Liver Int.* 2015;35:2139-2146.
27. Hernaez R, Lazo M, Bonekamp S, et al. Diagnostic accuracy and reliability of ultrasonography for the detection of fatty liver: a meta-analysis. *Hepatology.* 2011;54:1082-1090.

28. Mottin CC, Moretto M, Padoin AV, et al. The role of ultrasound in the diagnosis of hepatic steatosis in morbidly obese patients. *Obes Surg.* 2004;14:635-637.
29. Middleton MS, Heba ER, Hooker CA, et al. Agreement between magnetic resonance imaging proton density fat fraction measurements and pathologist-assigned steatosis grades of liver biopsies from adults with nonalcoholic steatohepatitis. *Gastroenterology.* 2017;153:753-761.
30. Permutt Z, Le TA, Peterson MR, et al. Correlation between liver histology and novel magnetic resonance imaging in adult patients with non-alcoholic fatty liver disease—MRI accurately quantifies hepatic steatosis in NAFLD. *Aliment Pharmacol Ther.* 2012;36:22-29.
31. Marshall RH, Eissa M, Bluth EI, Gulotta PM, Davis NK. Hepatorenal index as an accurate, simple, and effective tool in screening for steatosis. *AJR Am J Roentgenol.* 2012;199:997-1002.
32. Borges VF, Diniz AL, Cotrim HP, Rocha HL, Andrade NB. Sonographic hepatorenal ratio: a noninvasive method to diagnose nonalcoholic steatosis. *J Clin Ultrasound.* 2013;41:18-25.
33. Webb M, Yeshua H, Zelber-Sagi S, et al. Diagnostic value of a computerized hepatorenal index for sonographic quantification of liver steatosis. *AJR Am J Roentgenol.* 2009;192:909-914.
34. Chauhan A, Sultan LR, Furth EE, Jones LP, Khungar V, Sehgal CM. Diagnostic accuracy of hepatorenal index in the detection and grading of hepatic steatosis. *J Clin Ultrasound.* 2016;44:580-586.
35. Tuma J, Novakova B, Schwarzenbach HR, et al. [Image analysis in the differential diagnosis of renal parenchyma lesions]. *Ultraschall Med.* 2011;32:286-292.
36. Shiralkar K, Johnson S, Bluth EI, Marshall RH, Dornelles A, Gulotta PM. Improved method for calculating hepatic steatosis using the hepatorenal index. *J Ultrasound Med.* 2015;34:1051-1059.
37. Arai K, Matsui O, Takashima T, Ida M, Nishida Y. Focal spared areas in fatty liver caused by regional decreased portal flow. *AJR Am J Roentgenol.* 1988;151:300-302.
38. Hirche TO, Ignee A, Hirche H, Schneider A, Dietrich CF. Evaluation of hepatic steatosis by ultrasound in patients with chronic hepatitis C virus infection. *Liver Int.* 2007;27:748-757.
39. Dietrich CF, Wehrmann T, Zeuzem S, Braden B, Caspary WF, Lembcke B. [Analysis of hepatic echo patterns in chronic hepatitis C]. *Ultraschall Med.* 1999;20:9-14.
40. Dietrich CF, Lee JH, Gottschalk R, et al. Hepatic and portal vein flow pattern in correlation with intrahepatic fat deposition and liver histology in patients with chronic hepatitis C. *AJR Am J Roentgenol.* 1998;171:437-443.
41. Marchal G, Tshibwabwa-Tumba E, Verbeken E, et al. "Skip areas" in hepatic steatosis: a sonographic-angiographic study. *Gastrointest Radiol.* 1986;11:151-157.
42. Zezos P, Tatsi P, Nakos A, et al. Focal fatty liver sparing lesion presenting as a "pseudotumour": case report. *Acta Gastroenterol Belg.* 2006;69:323-326.
43. Valls C, Iannaccone R, Alba E, et al. Fat in the liver: diagnosis and characterization. *Eur Radiol.* 2006;16:2292-2308.
44. Hashimoto M, Heianna J, Tate E, Nishii T, Iwama T, Ishiyama K. Small veins entering the liver. *Eur Radiol.* 2002;12:2000-2005.
45. Kratzer W, Akinli AS, Bommer M, et al. Prevalence and risk factors of focal sparing in hepatic steatosis. *Ultraschall Med.* 2010;31:37-42.
46. Strunk H, Mildenberger P, Jonas J. [The incidence of focal liver lesions in patients with colorectal carcinoma]. *Rofo.* 1992;156:325-327.
47. Kester NL, Elmore SG. Focal hypoechoic regions in the liver at the porta hepatis: prevalence in ambulatory patients. *J Ultrasound Med.* 1995;14:649-652.
48. Koseoglu K, Ozsunar Y, Taskin F, Karaman C. Pseudolesions of left liver lobe during helical CT examinations: prevalence and comparison between unenhanced and biphasic CT findings. *Eur J Radiol.* 2005;54:388-392.
49. Karcaaltincaba M, Akhan O. Imaging of hepatic steatosis and fatty sparing. *Eur J Radiol.* 2007;61:33-43.
50. Kyogoku S, Shiraishi A, Ozaki Y, Kurosaki Y. Focal sparing of segment 2 in fatty liver: US appearance. *Radiat Med.* 2004;22:342-345.
51. Caturelli E, Costarelli L, Giordano M, et al. Hypoechoic lesions in fatty liver. Quantitative study by histomorphometry. *Gastroenterology.* 1991;100:1678-1682.
52. Dietrich CF, Schall H, Kirchner J, et al. Sonographic detection of focal changes in the liver hilus in patients receiving corticosteroid therapy. *Z Gastroenterol.* 1997;35:1051-1057.
53. Siegelman ES, Rosen MA. Imaging of hepatic steatosis. *Semin Liver Dis.* 2001;21:71-80.
54. Bhatnagar G, Sidhu HS, Vardhanabhuti V, Venkatanarasimha N, Cantin P, Dubbins P. The varied sonographic appearances of focal fatty liver disease: review and diagnostic algorithm. *Clin Radiol.* 2012;67:372-379.

55. Khov N, Sharma A, Riley TR. Bedside ultrasound in the diagnosis of nonalcoholic fatty liver disease. *World J Gastroenterol.* 2014;20:6821-6825.
56. Bohte AE, van Werven JR, Bipat S, Stoker J. The diagnostic accuracy of US, CT, MRI and 1H-MRS for the evaluation of hepatic steatosis compared with liver biopsy: a meta-analysis. *Eur Radiol.* 2011;21:87-97.
57. Anthony PP, Ishak KG, Nayak NC, Poulsen HE, Scheuer PJ, Sobin LH. The morphology of cirrhosis: definition, nomenclature, and classification. *Bull World Health Organ.* 1977;55:521-540.
58. Ricci P, Marigliano C, Cantisani V, et al. Ultrasound evaluation of liver fibrosis: preliminary experience with acoustic structure quantification (ASQ) software. *Radiol Med.* 2013;118:995-1010.
59. Di Lelio A, Cestari C, Lomazzi A, Beretta L. Cirrhosis: diagnosis with sonographic study of the liver surface. *Radiology.* 1989;172:389-392.
60. Colli A, Fraquelli M, Andreoletti M, Marino B, Zuccoli E, Conte D. Severe liver fibrosis or cirrhosis: accuracy of US for detection—analysis of 300 cases. *Radiology.* 2003;227:89-94.
61. Arda K, Ofelli M, Calikoglu U, Olcer T, Cumhur T. Hepatic vein Doppler waveform changes in early stage (Child-Pugh A) chronic parenchymal liver disease. *J Clin Ultrasound.* 1997;25:15-19.
62. Bolondi L, Li Bassi S, Gaiani S, et al. Liver cirrhosis: changes of Doppler waveform of hepatic veins. *Radiology.* 1991;178:513-516.
63. Coulden RA, Britton PD, Farman P, Noble-Jamieson G, Wight DG. Preliminary report: hepatic vein Doppler in the early diagnosis of acute liver transplant rejection. *Lancet.* 1990;336:273-275.
64. Jequier S, Jequier JC, Hanquinet S, Le Coultre C, Belli DC. Orthotopic liver transplants in children: change in hepatic venous Doppler wave pattern as an indicator of acute rejection. *Radiology.* 2003;226:105-112.
65. von Herbay A, Frieling T, Haussinger D. Association between duplex Doppler sonographic flow pattern in right hepatic vein and various liver diseases. *J Clin Ultrasound.* 2001;29:25-30.
66. Scheinfeld MH, Bilali A, Koenigsberg M. Understanding the spectral Doppler waveform of the hepatic veins in health and disease. *Radiographics.* 2009;29:2081-2098.
67. Karabulut N, Kazil S, Yagci B, Sabir N. Doppler waveform of the hepatic veins in an obese population. *Eur Radiol.* 2004;14:2268-2272.
68. Colli A, Cocciolo M, Riva C, et al. Abnormalities of Doppler waveform of the hepatic veins in patients with chronic liver disease: correlation with histologic findings. *AJR Am J Roentgenol.* 1994;162:833-837.
69. Oguzkurt L, Yildirim T, Torun D, Tercan F, Kizilkilic O, Niron EA. Hepatic vein Doppler waveform in patients with diffuse fatty infiltration of the liver. *Eur J Radiol.* 2005;54:253-257.
70. Tana C, Schiavone C, Ticinesi A, et al. Hepatic artery resistive index as surrogate marker for fibrosis progression in NAFLD patients: a clinical perspective. *Int J Immunopathol Pharmacol.* 2018;32:2058738418781373.
71. Tana C, Tana M, Rossi S, Silingardi M, Schiavone C. Hepatic artery resistive index (HARI) and non-alcoholic fatty liver disease (NAFLD) fibrosis score in NAFLD patients: cut-off suggestive of non-alcoholic steatohepatitis (NASH) evolution. *J Ultrasound.* 2016;19:183-189.
72. Castaneda D, Gonzalez AJ, Alomari M, Tandon K, Zervos XB. From hepatitis A to E: a critical review of viral hepatitis. *World J Gastroenterol.* 2021;27:1691-1715.

CHAPTER 3

Liver Stiffness Measurement Techniques: Basics

Spencer Moavenzadeh ▪ Mark L. Palmeri ▪ Giovanna Ferraioli ▪
Richard G. Barr

Introduction to Stiffness

Liver diseases, such as nonalcoholic fatty liver disease (NAFLD)/nonalcoholic steatohepatitis (NASH), alcoholic liver disease, viral hepatitis as well others, may be characterized by the accumulation of extracellular matrix material (collagen, fibronectin, proteoglycans, and glycosaminoglycans), fats and triglycerides, or tissue scarring, all of which increase tissue stiffness.[1] Biologically, tissue stiffness is important for resisting forces at the cellular, intracellular, and super-cellular levels and for guiding the migration of cells via durotaxis.[2] Though chronic liver diseases can present with increased tissue stiffness, they often also present asymptomatically with normal laboratory tests and imaging results. Since the advent of objective measures of liver stiffness through elasticity imaging, liver stiffness has proven an accurate surrogate biomarker for many liver diseases.

In contrast to traditional B-mode ultrasound imaging, which detects reflections due to differences in the acoustic properties in the underlying tissue, elasticity imaging relies upon differences in mechanical properties of soft tissue.[3] Therefore, understanding elasticity imaging techniques requires understanding mechanical and acoustic properties of soft tissue, mechanisms to perturb tissue, and mechanisms to measure tissue displacement.

SOFT TISSUE MECHANICS

Material stiffness, or elasticity, is a measure of the degree of resistance to elastic deformation in response to an applied force. Stiffness is measured in terms of pressure in Pascals and is calculated as the ratio between the applied stress (applied force per unit area) and resulting strain (change in length per unit length) of a material.[4] Stress and strain are second-order tensor quantities and together completely describe the state of deformation of a material.[5] Elasticity imaging thereby relies upon disturbing soft tissue with an external force and measuring the tissue's displacement to calculate stiffness as a biomarker for disease.[4] Deriving tissue stiffness in terms of measurable quantities utilized by common imaging techniques follows.

Stress can be represented as

$$\sigma_{ij} = \int f_i \, dx_j = \int \rho \alpha_i \, dx_j \tag{1}$$

where $\vec{a}$ is particle acceleration, $\vec{f}$ represents applied force per unit volume, ρ is material density, and σ_{ij} is the stress tensor.[5] In elasticity imaging methods, the force is commonly applied using static external compression, acoustic radiation force, or an external vibration mechanism.[3] The material density is commonly assumed to be that of water and is not estimated from the imaging data.

The strain tensor, ε_{ij}, can be represented as

$$\varepsilon_{ij} = \frac{1}{2}\left(\frac{du_i}{dx_j} + \frac{du_j}{dx_i} + \frac{du_j}{dx_i}\frac{du_i}{dx_j} \right) \tag{2}$$

where $\vec{u}$ represents displacement. Displacement is commonly measured in ultrasonic imaging modalities by correlating time shifts using ultrasonic radio frequency data,[6] phase shifts of in-phase and quadrature (IQ) data[7,8] at a pulse repetition frequency of several kilohertz.[9]

However, for complex, nonhomogenous, nonlinear materials or for complex applied stress fields (e.g., those generated from focused acoustic radiation force), it can be difficult to derive stress–strain relations that model elasticity under any loading.[10] Soft tissues are viscoelastic (strain dependent on rate of stress application), nonhomogenous, and anisotropic (stress–strain response is orientation dependent).[11] To simplify modeling of soft tissue complexity, many assumptions are made to model linear, elastic behavior under loading used in imaging.

Assuming small strains, soft tissues can be described as linear, elastic solids.[11]

Three moduli are used to characterize the material's elastic properties: Young's modulus, E, which describes resistance to deformation uniaxially; shear modulus or rigidity, G or μ, which characterizes resistance to shear; bulk modulus, K, which measures a material's resistance to compression. Deformation orthogonal to the axis of loading is described by Poisson's ratio, v. Three linear elastic constitutive equations relate these four constants,

$$G = \mu = \frac{E}{\left(2\left(1+v\right)\right)} \tag{3}$$

$$v = \frac{E}{2G} - 1 \tag{4}$$

$$K = \frac{E}{3\left(1-2v\right)} \tag{5}$$

Assuming units of tissue are homogenous and isotropic further allows a single equation to be used to relate stress and strain because isotropic materials behave the same in every direction[4]; therefore all coefficients of stress and strain tensors as represented in equations (1) and (2) can be represented in terms of material coefficients and their relations in equations (3), (4), and (5). The constitutive equation arises from the derivation of Hooke's law in three dimensions and is represented as

$$\sigma_{ij} = \frac{E}{1+v}\varepsilon_{ij} + \frac{Ev}{(1+v)(1-2v)}\Sigma_i \Sigma_j \varepsilon_{ij} \tag{6}$$

$$\sigma_{ij} = 2\mu\varepsilon_{ij} + \lambda \Sigma_i \Sigma_j \varepsilon_{ij} \tag{7}$$

The two material coefficients, λ where $\lambda = K + 2\mu/3$, and μ is also the shear modulus, are known as the Lamé constants.[12]

Elastic materials can support two main modes of wave propagation.[13] In longitudinal or compressional waves, the wave particles oscillate in the direction of wave propagation, whereas in transverse or shear waves, the particles oscillate in the direction normal to the direction of wave propagation. The other principal wave modes, surface and plate waves, are not relevant unless the structures being imaged are considered "thin" (relative to the shear wavelength) or shear waves are incident on a structural boundary (e.g., the edge of an organ).[11] By taking the spatial derivative of equation (7) and decomposing it with respect to the Helmholtz theorem, two wave equations can separately describe the longitudinal and transverse wave propagation, represented respectively as

$$c_L = \sqrt{\frac{\lambda + 2\mu}{\rho}} \tag{8}$$

$$c_T = \sqrt{\frac{\mu}{\rho}} \tag{9}$$

where c_L and c_T are the longitudinal and shear wave speeds, respectively.[13] These equations can be related to material parameters instead of Lamé constants of soft tissue by

$$c_L = \sqrt{\frac{K}{\rho}} \tag{10}$$

$$c_T = \sqrt{\frac{G}{\rho}} \tag{11}$$

For incompressible materials, $\nu = 0.5$ and (3) reduces to $3G = E$. In soft tissues that have ultrasonic (compressional) wave speeds ranging between 1490–1540 m/s (instead of an infinite compressional wave speed for a truly incompressible material), the factor of 3 relating E and G is >99.9% accurate.

Accurately measuring shear waves is only possible in the far-field as in the near-field coupling between longitudinal and shear waves can occur.[14] In the case of viscoelastic materials like soft tissue, shear wave speed depends on elastic properties.[15] The shear modulus can be represented as

$$G = \frac{E}{3} = \rho c_T{}^2 \tag{12}$$

where ρ is roughly constant in soft tissues at 1000 kg/m^3. Combined with $3G = E$ under the assumption of incompressible materials, both Young's modulus and shear modulus can be represented in terms of shear velocity.[4]

To model the elastic properties of soft tissue in which stiffness is dependent upon strain magnitude and is time-dependent, the elastic model can be coupled with a viscous component to calculate a complex shear modulus.[16] Elasticity is often quantified by the magnitude of G whereas the real and imaginary components can be decomposed to the viscoelastic storage and loss components of deformation, respectively. Viscosity leads to a frequency-dependent shear modulus and can be a source of difference between different elasticity imaging methods.[17]

ACOUSTIC MECHANICS IN SOFT TISSUE

Acoustic radiation force imaging techniques transmit an acoustic wave into a region of interest, and the force is generated from the loss of momentum of the propagating wave in the attenuating soft tissue causing a phase shift between the pressure and particle velocities.[13] For the attenuating wave, the force can be derived from the Navier-Stokes equation and expressed for any location within the tissue as

$$\vec{f} = \frac{2\alpha \vec{I}}{c_L} \tag{13}$$

where α represents the absorption or attenuation coefficient and $\vec{I}$ is the time-averaged intensity.[17-20] The equation expresses that acoustic radiation force is a function of both attenuation and intensity. Attenuation in soft tissue is both frequency- and depth-dependent, where higher attenuation typically means more uniformly distributed force due to greater momentum transfer but lower peak force intensity.[21] Using equations (10), (11), and (12), the elastic material properties of soft tissue can be calculated from the measured displacement. The direction of the intensity vector, which dictates the direction of the applied force, is in the direction of the propagating acoustic wave, which is commonly assumed to be orthogonal to the face of the ultrasound transducer.[22]

Techniques

To measure tissue stiffness, the tissue's transient response (wave speed) to deformation needs to be observed after the applied force and excitation. Like palpating the body to determine tenderness, measurement requires inducing mechanical stress into the liver. The different approaches to induce mechanical stress can be categorized based on the source of excitation used to deform the tissue. There are two main means of disturbing tissue: external vibration and internally applied acoustic radiation force.

External sources include using a transducer to compress the skin such as in transient elastography (TE) and strain imaging, mechanical vibration to vibrate tissue at specific frequencies such as in sonoelastography and magnetic resonance elastography, and physiological sources such as cardiac motion, breathing, or arterial motion.[23-26] Furthermore, external sources can be categorized into static approaches and dynamic approaches in which dynamic approaches can be over a short period of time in TE or continuous in harmonic elastography.[2]

Although external sources provide powerful and controlled-frequency vibration, the mechanical waves couple with the skin surface and distort as they propagate through superficial tissues such as fat and muscle.[27] Internally applied acoustic radiation forces circumvent the challenges with external vibration; acoustic excitation delivers localized displacements within a region of interest in single or multiple focal zones of an ultrasonic excitation.

Elasticity imaging is also categorized by the technique used to record the response to deformation. The response can be recorded through ultrasound, magnetic resonance imaging (MRI), or tactile sensors.[2] The tissue response can be observed in various dimensions, including as a computed value (zero-dimensional), along a line (one-dimensional), on a plane (two-dimensional), or as a volume (three-dimensional). The results are often overlayed with an anatomical image of the liver to form a stiffness map or elastogram.

MAGNETIC RESONANCE ELASTOGRAPHY

Magnetic resonance elastography (MRE) is a phase-contrast–based MRI technique that can generate a three-dimensional elasticity map covering the entire liver.[16] There are three main components to MRE machines: (1) the generation of mechanical waves on the surface of the abdomen via a static, acoustic vibrator, (2) the phase-contrast pulse sequence with motion-encoding gradients (MEGs) to acquire data, and (3) the magnetic resonance inversion algorithm used to calculate liver stiffness from recovery times.

In typical MRE configurations, a pneumatic mechanical wave driver is located outside the MRE room and is connected to a passive acoustic driver. The passive driver is a static, acoustic, external vibrator that generates continuous, 60-Hz acoustic vibrations delivered through the abdomen and into the liver.[28] Either gradient-echo or spin-echo pulse sequences are used with transverse read-outs.[16] Tissue displacement is encoded by oscillating gradients, MEGs, either in synchrony with the mechanical driver or with shorter periods to reduce T2-signal relaxation time.[29] The MRI machine then processes the magnitude and phase data to generate elastograms of the liver with either quantitative values for liver stiffness in regions of interest or qualitative gradients of liver stiffness.[28] Shear wave images can be captured within minutes for three-dimensional field acquisition, allowing both breath-holding and free-breathing protocols with reproducibility.[30] Motion correction postprocessing helps reduce breathing artifacts in image registration.

There are some limitations with MRE. The harmonic excitations used in MRE result in coupling of longitudinal and shear waves, providing complications when calculating elasticity.[13] Secondly, MRE relies upon full penetration of the liver with harmonic vibrations[16]; insufficient penetration can lead to noise artifacts in image reconstruction.

TRANSIENT ELASTOGRAPHY

TE utilizes transient mechanical external vibration to induce tissue deformation and tracks the progression of the shear wave into the liver via ultrasound to produce a one-dimensional quantitative image of tissue stiffness.[15] The shear wave is tracked as it travels deeper within the tissue along the axis of the one-dimensional ultrasound beam.[31] The ultrasound images per time are then displayed in a two-dimensional diagram from which shear wave speed is calculated. The dynamic nature of the mechanical vibration allows decoupling of longitudinal and shear waves as shear wave speeds are much slower than longitudinal waves in soft tissue; the transient nature of the mechanical vibration and high frame rate of ultrasound allows temporal separation of longitudinal and shear waves.[31,32]

A typical TE configuration uses a single-element, disk-shaped transducer on a mechanical vibrator to induce shear waves at low frequency.[15] The most common utilization of TE is vibration-controlled transient elastography (VCTE), which implements controls on the transient vibration to ensure reproducibility. The force applied to the ultrasound probe, and consequently the mechanical actuator, remains constant during VCTE to prevent distortion of the vibration and ensure the vibration is transferred through the tissue with enough power. This is controlled via electro-dynamic feedback between tip sensors and the mechanical actuator. Excessive force would likely distort the excitation and decrease center frequency, resulting in a lower recorded stiffness measurement. The transient excitation center frequency and shape is also controlled to ensure quantitative stiffness thresholds remain constant and can be used for differentiating physiologically determinant values.

ACOUSTIC RADIATION FORCE IMAGING

There are two major types of elastography—strain elastography (SE) and shear wave elastography (SWE). SE can be performed either with a manual displacement technique or using acoustic radiation force (ARF). The manual displacement technique is performed by applying and releasing pressure with the transducer or by using the patient's normal breathing and heartbeat. Acoustic radiation force imaging (ARFI), a strain technique, refers to ultrasound imaging of tissue displacement in response to ARF excitation to create qualitative, two-dimensional images of relative displacement.[33] The displacement of the tissue following an acoustic impulse is measured along the axis of the pushed beam, and by pushing and tracking in multiple locations, a map of shear waves and tissue stiffness is generated.

ARFI techniques rely upon pulse-echo ultrasound measuring shifted signals before and after the excitation is triggered. Each axis in an ARFI typically requires three separate pulse types: a single B-mode tracking pulse pre–ARF stimulation, an impulsive ARFI push at a single or multiple focal depths along the axis (Fig. 3.1), and a series of postimpulse B-mode tracking pulses

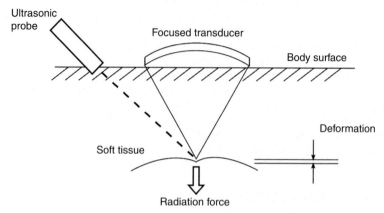

Fig. 3.1 General concept of acoustic radiation force-based elasticity imaging methods. A focused ultrasound transducer is used to generate sufficient acoustic radiation force to cause localized tissue displacements. The resulting deformation is monitored using the same or a separate remote device.[3]

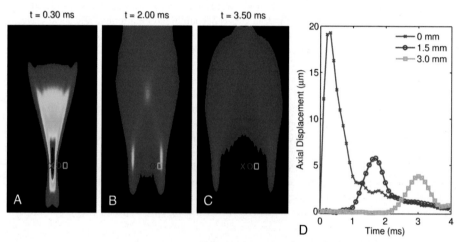

Fig. 3.2 Axial displacements depicted at three different time steps following excitation in (A) through (C) showing the propagation of shear waves away from the region-of-excitation and the displacement-through-time
profiles for each lateral location.[3] *t*, Time.

at high repetition frequency to track displacement and recovery of the tissue (Fig. 3.2).[27] Finally,
postprocessing phase-shift or cross-correlation analysis is performed to extract tissue stiffness.
ARFI sequences are then repeated at consecutive lateral positions across the transducer aperture
to generate a two-dimensional elastogram. The two-dimensional elastogram can be displayed in
terms of absolute displacements at given durations of recovery, maximum displacement, or time
elapsed until certain displacements.[3,34]

To generate sufficient displacement from the acoustic radiation force on the magnitude of
1–10 μm, ARFI often uses a focused transducer and longer acoustic pushes.[4] As a result of the
localized distribution of force within the region of interest, ARFI results in smaller strains than
compressive elastography and is not bounded by coupling of longitudinal and shear waves from
external stress sources.

The ARFI technique (i.e., the measure of the longitudinal displacement) is not used for estimation of liver stiffness. However, the manual displacement SE method has been used for liver stiffness measurements, sometimes combining with other sonographic features. Since the manual displacement SE has limited use, it is not discussed further in this book.

ACOUSTIC RADIATION FORCE–BASED TECHNIQUES

ARF-based techniques are similar to ARFI in that an impulsive ARF is transmitted into a region of interest to cause tissue displacement. However, the tracking pulse-echo beams are directed outside the region of interest at lateral positions from the beam axis to measure shear wave parameters directly, rather than using multiple pushes at different lateral locations and measuring on-axis deformation during ARFI.[2,35] Calculation of shear wave speed can be made in either the time or frequency domain. In the time domain, the time shift resulting in the maximum correlation between two signals represents the time delay during displacement,[36] and either linear regression between each lateral position or more complex implementations of compounded excitations, tracking, and directional filtering is used to calculate shear wave speed.[27] Frequency-domain measurements rely upon variations in center frequency of the received echo for each displacement estimate to calculate shear wave speed.[7] ARF-based techniques, as compared to ARFI, which does not involve direct shear wave measurement and can only estimate tissue stiffnesses through axial elasticity measurements, measure shear wave speed directly to calculate tissue stiffness.[37]

There are two common types of ARF-based techniques: point shear wave elastography (pSWE) and two-dimensional shear wave elastography (2D-SWE). In pSWE a singleton shear wave speed is reported for the region of interest as all propagation data in the region of interest are averaged for a representative metric.[34] In 2D-SWE, displacement is induced by ARFI using multiple focal zones at different lateral positions that are stressed sequentially. In some implementations, such as supersonic imaging (now Hologic imaging), the multiple focal zones are excited in very rapid succession to create a single shear wave front.[37] Other implementations, such as comb-push shear wave imaging, multiple lateral excitations are fired concurrently, and directional filtering is used to isolate the individual propagating shear wave components.[38] Two-dimensional regions of interest are then monitored to estimate the resultant tissue displacements and localized shear wave speeds to give a more localized map of tissue stiffness.[2]

KEY POINTS

1. The shear waves are attenuated as they traverse the liver. This can be seen in the displacement curves (Fig. 3.3). The shear waves are of too low amplitude within 5–10 mm for accurate measurement; therefore it is important to limit motion of both the patient and the transducer as small changes can lead to inaccurate measurements.
2. The ARF pulse focus in most systems is focused at 4.0–4.5 cm from the transducer (Fig. 3.4). This is the depth of the strongest shear waves. Taking measurements at this depth is preferred for best estimate of liver stiffness.
3. The ARF pulse can be reflected from the liver capsule if the transducer is not perpendicular to the liver capsule; this weakens the ARF pulse and therefore the shear wave amplitude, thus decreasing the signal to noise, which can lead to less accurate estimates of liver stiffness.
4. The ARF pulse in pSWE and 2D-SWE has a mean frequency and bandwidth. In all the chapters of this book we refer to these techniques as acoustic radiation force impulse (ARFI) or ARFI-based. As the pulses traverse the liver, the higher frequencies are attenuated faster than the lower frequencies so the mean ARF pulse changes with depth, particularly in steatotic and fibrotic livers. Therefore liver stiffness measurements may change with the depth of the measurement. Both VCTE and MRE can be used to obtain measurements at a fixed frequency and therefore do not have this depth dependence. These points are further discussed as they pertain to the protocol of acquiring liver stiffness measurements.

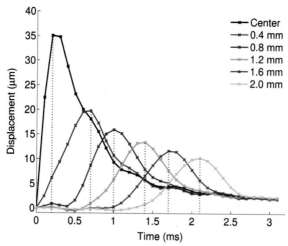

Fig. 3.3 Sample of the displacement curves from a liver stiffness measurement. Note that the tracking B-mode lines distances are in millimeters. By 2.0 mm, the shear wave has attenuated to less than half of the amplitude of the tracking pulse closest to the ARFI pulse. (From Palmeri ML, Wang MH, Dahl JJ, Frinkley KD, Nightingale KR. Quantifying hepatic shear modulus in vivo using acoustic radiation force. Ultrasound Med Biol. 2008;34(4):546-558.).

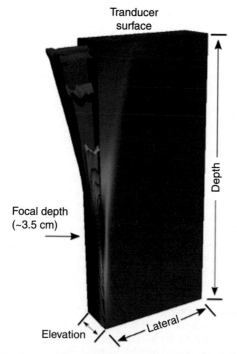

Fig. 3.4 Diagram of a slice profile of an acoustic radiation force imaging pulse. Note that the pulse has a focus usually at 3–5 cm deep. (From Barr RG, Ferraioli G, Palmeri ML, et al. Elastography assessment of liver fibrosis: Society of Radiologists in Ultrasound consensus conference statement. Radiology. 2015;276(3):845-861).

References

1. Schiff ER, Maddrey WC, Reddy KR. *Schiff's Diseases of the Liver.* Oxford: Wiley; 2018.
2. Chattopadhyay S, Raines RT. Review collagen-based biomaterials for wound healing. *Biopolymers.* 2014;101:821-833.
3. Doherty JR, Trahey GE, Nightingale KR, Palmeri ML. Acoustic radiation force elasticity imaging in diagnostic ultrasound. *IEEE Trans Ultrason Ferroelectr Freq Control.* 2013;60:685-701.
4. Mueller S. Liver stiffness and its measurement. In: Mueller S, ed. *Liver Elastography.* 1st ed. Switzerland: Springer Nature; 2020:495-508.
5. Lai WM, Rubin D, Krempel E. *Introduction to Continuum Mechanics.* Burlington, MA: Butterworth-Heinmann; 1999.
6. Pinton GF, Dahl JJ, Trahey GE. Rapid tracking of small displacements with ultrasound. *IEEE Trans Ultrason Ferroelectr Freq Control.* 2006;53:1103-1117.
7. Kasai C, Namekawa K, Koyano A, Omoto R. Real-time two-dimensional blood flow imaging using an autocorrelation technique. *IEEE Trans Ultrason Ferroelectr Freq Control.* 1985;32:458-464.
8. Loupas T, Peterson R, Gill R. Experimental evaluation of velocity and power estimation for ultrasound blood flow imaging by means of a two-dimensional autocorrelation approach. *IEEE Trans Ultrason Ferroelectr Freq Control.* 1995;42:689-699.
9. Palmeri ML, McAleavey SA, Trahey GE, Nightingale KR. Ultrasonic tracking of acoustic radiation force-induced displacements in homogeneous media. *IEEE Trans Ultrason Ferroelectr Freq Control.* 2006;53:1300-1313.
10. Fung YC. *Biomechanics: Mechanical Properties of Living Tissue.* 2nd ed. New York: Springer-Verlag; 1993.
11. Wells PN, Liang HD. Medical ultrasound: imaging of soft tissue strain and elasticity. *J R Soc Interface.* 2011;8:1521-1549.
12. Symon KR. In: *Mechanics.* Reading: Addison-Wesley; 1971.
13. Kino GS. *Acoustic Waves: Devices, Imaging, and Analog Signal Processing.* Englewood Cliffs: Prentice-Hall; 1987.
14. Sandrin L, Cassereau D, Fink M. The role of the coupling term in transient elastography. *J Acoust Soc Am.* 2004;115:73-83.
15. Sandrin L. Liver stiffness measurement using vibration-controlled transient elastography. In: Mueller S, ed. *Liver Elastography.* 1st ed. Switzerland: Springer Nature; 2020:495-508.
16. Hirsch S, Braun J, Sack I. *Magnetic Resonance Elastography: Physical Background and Medical Applications.* New Jersey, USA: Wiley-VCH; 2017.
17. Palmeri ML, Milkowski A, Barr R, et al. Radiological Society of North America/Quantitative Imaging Biomarker Alliance Shear wave speed bias quantification in elastic and viscoelastic phantoms. *J Ultrasound Med.* 2021;40:569-581.
18. Palmeri ML, Sharma AC, Bouchard RR, Nightingale RW, Nightingale KR. A finite-element method model of soft tissue response to impulsive acoustic radiation force. *IEEE Trans Ultrason Ferroelectr Freq Control.* 2005;52:1699-1712.
19. Nyborg W. Acoustic streaming. In: Mason W, ed. *Physical Acoustics.* Vol. IIB. New York: Academic; 1965:265-311.
20. Torr GR. The acoustic radiation force. *Am J Phys.* 1984;52:402-408.
21. Palmeri ML, Nightingale KR. Acoustic radiation force-based elasticity imaging methods. *Interface Focus.* 2011;1:553-564.
22. Palmeri ML, Qiang B, Chen S, Urban MW. Guidelines for finite-element modeling of acoustic radiation force-induced shear wave propagation in tissue-mimicking media. *IEEE Trans Ultrason Ferroelectr Freq Control.* 2017;64:78-92.
23. Lerner RM, Huang SR, Parker KJ. Sonoelasticity images derived from ultrasound signals in mechanically vibrated tissues. *Ultrasound Med Biol.* 1990;16:231-239.
24. Parker KJ. The evolution of vibration sonoelastography. *Curr Med Imaging Rev.* 2011;7:283-291.
25. Dickinson RJ, Hill CR. Measurement of soft tissue motion using correlation between A-scans. *Ultrasound Med Biol.* 1982;8:263-271.
26. de Korte CL, van der Steen AF. Intravascular ultrasound elastography: an overview. *Ultrasonics.* 2002;40:859-865.
27. Palmeri ML. Characterizing liver stiffness with acoustic radiation force. In: Mueller S, ed. *Liver Elastography.* 1st ed. Switzerland: Springer Nature; 2020:495-508.

28. Guglielmo FF, Venkatesh SK, Mitchell DG. Liver MR elastography technique and image interpretation: pearls and pitfalls. *Radiographics.* 2019;39:1983-2002.
29. Dittmann F, Hirsch S, Tzschätzsch H, Guo J, Braun J, Sack I. In vivo wideband multifrequency MR elastography of the human brain and liver. *Magn Reson Med.* 2016;76:1116-1126.
30. Hudert CA, Tzschätzsch H, Rudolph B, et al. Tomoelastography for the evaluation of pediatric nonalcoholic fatty liver disease. *Invest Radiol.* 2019;54:198-203.
31. Sandrin L, Tanter M, Gennisson JL, Catheline S, Fink M. Shear elasticity probe for soft tissues with 1-D transient elastography. *IEEE Trans Ultrason Ferroelectr Freq Control.* 2002;49:436-446.
32. Sandrin L, Fourquet B, Hasquenoph JM, et al. Transient elastography: a new noninvasive method for assessment of hepatic fibrosis. *Ultrasound Med Biol.* 2003;29:1705-1713.
33. Nightingale K, Palmeri N, Nightingale R, Trahey G. On the feasibility of remote palpation using acoustic radiation force. *J Acoust Soc Am.* 2001;110:625-634.
34. Palmeri ML, McAleavey SA, Fong KL, Trahey GE, Nightingale KR. Dynamic mechanical response of elastic spherical inclusions to impulsive acoustic radiation force excitation. *IEEE Trans Ultrason Ferroelectr Freq Control.* 2006;53:2065-2079.
35. Nightingale K, McAleavey S, Trahey G. Shear-wave generation using acoustic radiation force: in vivo and ex vivo results. *Ultrasound Med Biol.* 2003;29:1715-1723.
36. Bonnefous O, Pesqué P. Time domain formulation of pulse-Doppler ultrasound and blood velocity estimation by cross correlation. *Ultrason Imaging.* 1986;8:73-85.
37. Bercoff J, Tanter M, Fink M. Supersonic shear imaging: a new technique for soft tissue elasticity mapping. *IEEE Trans Ultrason Ferroelectr Freq Control.* 2004;51:396-409. [Erratum in: IEEE Trans Ultrason Ferroelectr Freq Control. 2020;67:1492-1494.]
38. Song P, Zhao H, Manduca A, Urban MW, Greenleaf JF, Chen S. Comb-push ultrasound shear elastography (CUSE): a novel method for two-dimensional shear elasticity imaging of soft tissues. *IEEE Trans Med Imaging.* 2012;31:1821-1832.

CHAPTER 4

Protocols for Liver Stiffness Acquisition

Giovanna Ferraioli ■ Richard G Barr

General Protocol

For all of the ultrasound (US) shear wave elastography (SWE) techniques (vibration controlled transient elastography [VCTE], point shear wave elastography [pSWE] and two-dimensional shear wave elastography [2D-SWE]), adherence to a strict protocol when assessing liver stiffness is required.[1-9] The recommended items and the quality criteria that must be used follow.

We use the convention that the region of interest (ROI) is the larger area (field of view [FOV]) where the color-coded values are displayed in 2D-SWE and the measurement box is the area selected where the measurement is taken.

ACOUSTIC RADIATION FORCE IMAGING–BASED TECHNIQUES

Patients Should Fast at Least 4 Hours Before the Examination

It should be kept in mind that SWE techniques assess tissue stiffness, which is directly correlated with liver fibrosis but can also increase due to several other factors including but not limited to congestion and inflammation. Within 5–30 minutes after a meal, blood flow to the digestive organs increases. This is a normal physiological phenomenon that lasts for up to 3 hours. The resultant increase of blood flow to the liver through the portal vein and hepatic artery leads to an increase of liver stiffness.

Several studies have demonstrated an increase of liver stiffness after ingestion of food.[10-12] A study in patients with chronic liver disease reported that liver stiffness significantly increased immediately after food intake for up to 60 minutes and normalized after 180 minutes. An increase of at least 1 kPa after food intake was found in more than half of patients who had baseline stiffness ≤10 kPa.[10]

Ingestion of food can only increase the liver stiffness; therefore, if patients are not in a fasting state and their stiffness value is normal, they have no or mild fibrosis.

Measurement Should Be Taken at an Intercostal Space with the Patient in the Supine or Slight Lateral Decubitus (30 Degree) Position with the Right Arm in Extension.

This is not an arbitrary recommendation or an expert opinion. In fact, the highest consistency and intra- and interobserver reproducibility of liver stiffness measurements and the highest accuracy are observed for measurement taken in the intercostal space.[13-17] This is likely due to factors related to both the operator and the patient. In utilizing the intercostal space, the effect of pushing with the transducer, which may lead to an increase of stiffness value due to compression of the organ, is somehow weakened by the ribs and the intercostal muscles.[18] Moreover, it is easier to maintain the transducer perpendicular to the liver capsule. On the contrary, measurement taken with a subcostal approach may be hampered by gas in the abdomen requiring a patient to take a deep breath to displace the gas, and external compression with the transducer is also applied; both may lead to an overestimation of liver stiffness. All these factors are subject to some degree of variability from patient to patient and affect the variability of measurement in an unpredictable manner. In addition, the reported rate of failure for measurements performed with a subcostal approach in patients with supposedly normal livers reached 62% in one study.[13] Measurements performed in the left lobe of the liver are hampered by motion due to the heartbeat, and higher stiffness values than those in the right liver lobe using an intercostal approach are obtained. Moreover, the measurement success rate is significantly higher in the right liver lobe (91%–98% vs. 77%–84%, respectively).[13,19] The agreement in stiffness values between the liver lobes has been reported to be moderate to poor.[13,19,20]

To increase the width of the intercostal space for a correct positioning of the transducer between the ribs, the patient should extend the right arm above the head in the supine position. The expert opinion is that a slight left lateral decubitus, not more than 30 degrees, might be of help in obese or difficult-to-scan subjects.[1] To keep the angle less than 30 degrees, a pillow just beneath the upper right side of the patient is of help. A higher degree of decubitus positioning is not recommended because it has been shown that it affects the portal vein blood flow and therefore causes stiffness (Figs. 4.1 and 4.2).[21]

In liver transplant patients with a left-lobe graft, the epigastric approach can be used. However, the higher variability and higher stiffness values for measurements taken in the left liver lobe should be considered; therefore the stiffness can be overestimated using the cutoffs that were obtained in the right liver lobe through an intercostal approach. In these cases, the change over time of the baseline stiffness value may help overcome this issue, allowing the monitoring of the efficacy of the treatment or the progression of the disease.[4]

It is important to have the transducer perpendicular to the liver capsule in both the superior/inferior and right/left planes. The liver capsule should be a bright fine white line. When the

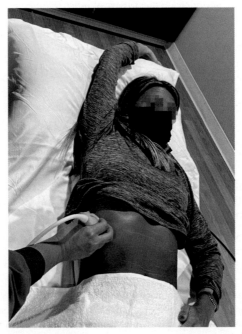

Fig. 4.1 Image showing the positioning of the right arm to increase the intercostal space to allow for improved acoustic imaging. Note the arm is extended above the head.

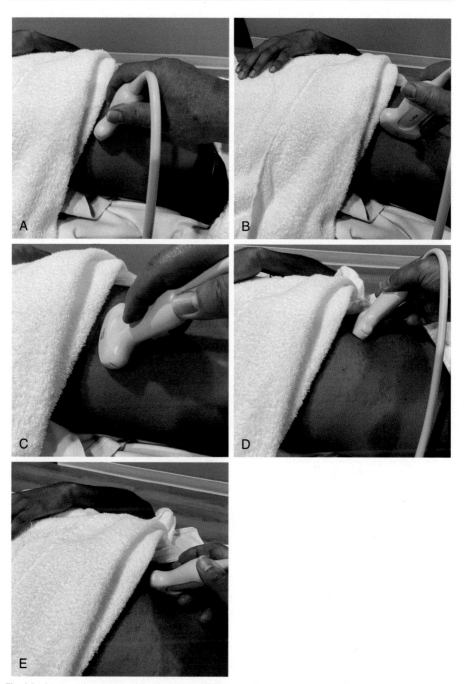

Fig. 4.2 Images showing the (A) correct and (B through E) incorrect positioning of the transducer when performing liver elastography. The transducer should not be placed across the ribs (B), angled to the liver capsule (C), substernal scanning (D), or angling to obtain liver stiffness values from the left lobe of the liver (E).

transducer is angled to the liver capsule, the ARFI pulse is refracted and therefore weakened. This causes weaker shear waves with the resultant decrease in signal-to-noise leading to more error in the measurement (Figs. 4.3 and 4.4).

Measurements Should Be Taken at Neutral Breathing During a Breath Hold

Generally, patients undergoing an US examination of the upper abdomen know that they will be asked to take deep breaths for better visualization of the liver. Hence, they may be expecting that when the operator is exploring the liver for the best acoustic window for liver stiffness measurement they should take a deep breath and hold it.

It is suggested to instruct the patients before taking a stiffness measurement, advising quiet breathing while looking for the optimal scanning window and then asking them to stop breathing when the image on the monitor is free of vessels or ligaments.

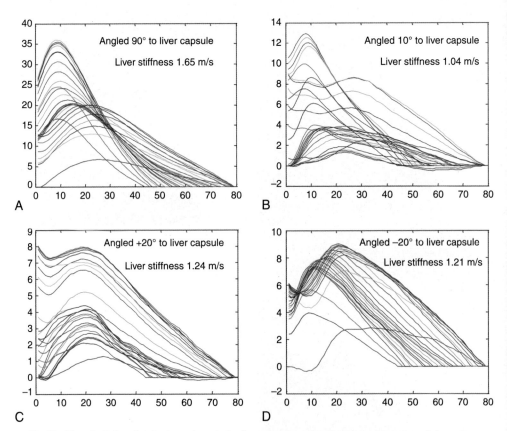

Fig. 4.3 The effect of angling the transducer to the liver capsule on the displacement curves and shear wave speed on a patient is demonstrated in this figure. The degree of angling to the liver capsule is presented in the upper right-hand corner of each image. Note the amplitude of the maximum displacement curve decreases from (A) 36 units to (B) 13 units on angling the transducer 10 degrees to the liver capsule and down to less than (C, D) 10 units on angling the transducer 20 degrees either to the right or left of the liver capsule. The shear wave speed is listed centrally in each image. Note that the family of curves also becomes abnormal. Note that there is a significant change in the shear wave speed obtained when the transducer is angled.

It is the expert opinion that breath hold (a few seconds) during quiet breathing leads to the most optimal results. Taking a deep breath or using a Valsalva maneuver or deep expiration changes hepatic venous pressures, which can affect the stiffness measurement (Fig. 4.5).

Of note, a study found that deep inspiration significantly increased stiffness values by 13%.[14]

When using a pSWE technique in patients unable to hold their breath, the stiffness values can be measured at the end of the expiratory phase when there is an automatic pause with almost

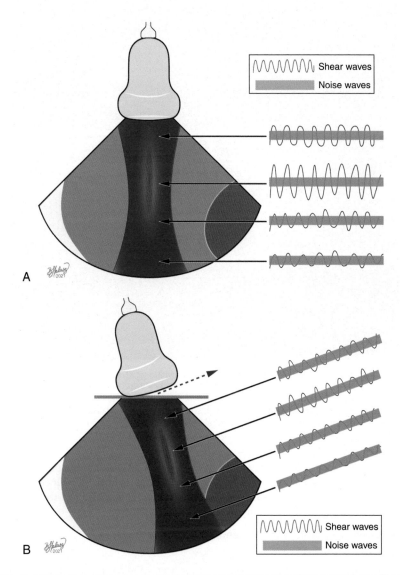

Fig. 4.4   Illustration of the effect when the transducer is perpendicular (A) and not perpendicular (B) to the liver capsule. Note that the shear waves have higher amplitude when the transducer is perpendicular to the liver capsule. When the transducer is angled to the liver capsule, the shear waves are generated perpendicular to the acoustic radiation force imaging (ARFI) pulse, and their amplitude is decreased because of refraction of energy *(dotted red arrow)* weakening the ARFI pulse. Both factors lead to inaccurate measurements of liver stiffness.

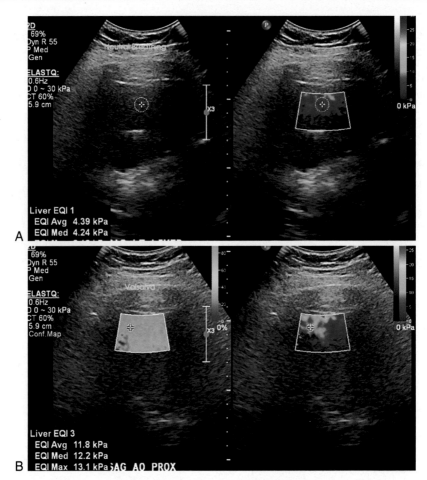

Fig. 4.5 The effect of performing liver stiffness in a neutral breathing position and with a Valsalva maneuver done within a minute. Note the marked increase in the liver stiffness value when the measurement is done with a Valsalva maneuver. In neutral breathing (A) this patient has a liver stiffness value of 4.39 kPa. During a Valsalva maneuver (B) the stiffness measurement increases to 11.8 kPa, demonstrating the effect that can be seen when measurements are not taken in a neutral breathing position.

no motion for two seconds. This is not possible with 2D-SWE because the elastogram may take a slightly longer time to stabilize. In this case, as suggested for children (see Measurements in Pediatric Patients with the ARFI Techniques), a cine loop can be recorded and the image with the most stable pattern can be utilized for the stiffness measurement.

ROI Placement to Avoid Liver Vessels and/or Bile Ducts and Rib Shadows

The ROI must be placed in a homogeneous area of the liver, avoiding vessels and/or bile ducts as well as artifacts. Using 2D-SWE, the inclusion of small vessels at the edges of the ROI is acceptable; however, the measurement box must always be placed at least 5 mm away from them.

There could be a false increase of liver stiffness adjacent to vessels (Figs. 4.6 and 4.7). In 2D-SWE, these artifacts can be identified and avoided. Depending on the US's vendor, artifacts may

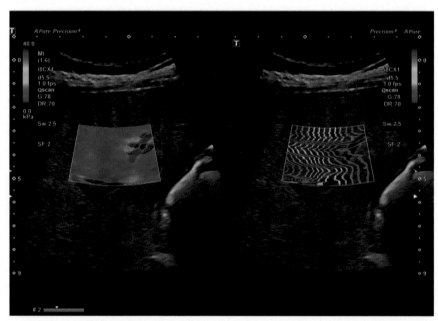

Fig. 4.6 The hepatic veins included in the sample box cause a local false increase of stiffness *(green, yellow, and red colors on the elasticity map)*. The lines in the propagation map (right side of the image) are distorted.

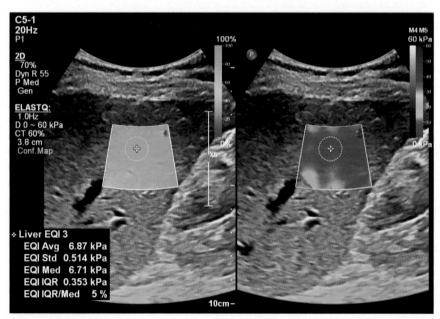

Fig. 4.7 A vessel is included in the region of interest at the distal portion of the image. The elasticity map *(mostly blue)* shows an increase of stiffness *(light green)* around the vessel *(gray/black)*. The confidence map *(green)* shows mild yellow but the artifacts are larger as visualized in the elasticity map. The measurement box is placed in an area free of artifacts. The quality map does not identify all artifacts, therefore it is recommended to look at both the confidence map and the elasticity map.

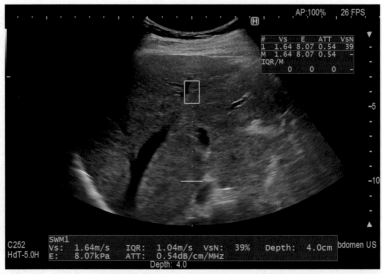

Fig. 4.8 Wrong acquisition: a vessel appears inside the region of interest. In this case the manufacturer's quality factor, *VsN*, indicates a poor-quality acquisition (VsN: 39%). This measurement must be rejected.

not be color-coded or appear as areas of increased stiffness. These areas must be avoided when placing the measurement box. These artifacts are not visualized in pSWE, and therefore measurements must be obtained at least 5 mm from these structures (Fig. 4.8).

Measurement Location

Measurement should be taken at least 15–20 mm below the liver capsule in pSWE. The 2D-SWE ROI can be positioned closer to the liver capsule if reverberation artifacts are avoided.

Using 2D-SWE it is quite common to find reverberation artifacts when the proximal edge of the ROI is too close to the liver capsule (Figs. 4.9 and 4.10). These artifacts are presented in detail in Chapter 6. Because they are well visualized in 2D-SWE, the operator can avoid them and not include them in the measurement box. With pSWE the reverberation artifact is not visualized, therefore the operator must avoid positioning the sample box up to 15–20 mm below the liver capsule (Fig. 4.11).

Of note, a study performed early in the evaluation of the first commercially available pSWE technique found a statistically significant difference between the mean shear wave velocity values obtained at 5.5 cm from the liver capsule and that obtained immediately under the liver surface (1.56 vs. 1.90 m/s).[22]

Location of Maximum ARFI Push Pulse

In most systems, the maximum ARFI push pulse is at 4–4.5 cm from the transducer, which is the optimal location for obtaining measurements.

Most vendors have placed the focus of the ARFI pulse between 4 and 5 cm from the transducer. This is the region of highest energy deposition, and therefore shear waves with the highest amplitude are generated. This recommendation is also based on the results obtained with studies on phantoms,[23,24] which have shown that the results with the lowest variability are obtained at a depth of 4–5 cm with a convex probe. The acoustic push pulse is progressively attenuated as it traverses

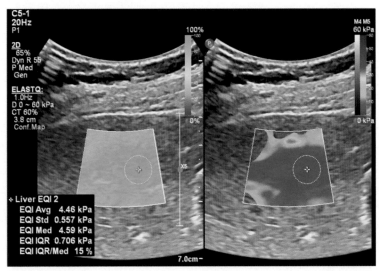

Fig. 4.9 The upper part of the sample box is positioned close to the liver capsule. Reverberation artifacts *(gray areas)* can be seen in the elasticity map *(mainly blue)*. They appear as a false increase of liver stiffness. The confidence map *(mainly green)* gives a warning *(yellow color)*. The measurement box should not include the reverberation artifacts.

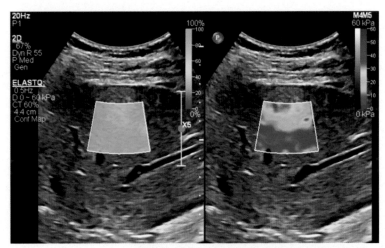

Fig. 4.10 The confidence map *(mainly green)* does not identify all artifacts *(yellow areas)*, and both the confidence map and the elasticity map should be evaluated for artifacts. In fact, since the reverberation artifacts are very stable, sometimes the confidence map fails in identifying them.

the tissue. The amplitude of the shear waves is proportional to the strength of the push pulse. Therefore measurements taken at deeper depths will have lower amplitude shear waves leading to less signal-to-noise ratio in the estimate of the shear wave speed (SWS; Fig. 4.12).

Studies on phantoms have also reported that the influence of the depth on estimating liver stiffness is not negligible. In viscoelastic phantoms, the deepest focal depth (7.0 cm) generated the greatest intersystem variability for each phantom, reaching a maximum of 17.7% as evaluated

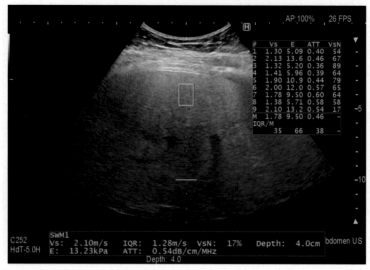

Fig. 4.11 Point shear wave elastography does not have an elasticity map, therefore the reverberation artifacts cannot be visualized. In this case the very high variability between consecutive measurements is explained by the inclusion of artifacts in the sample box.

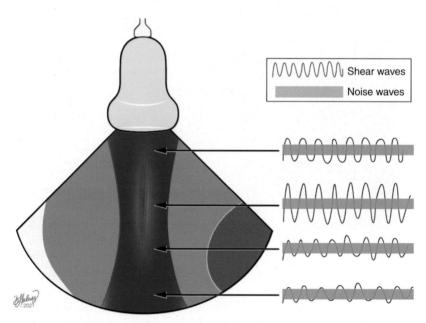

Fig. 4.12 Figure showing the change in amplitude of shear waves with depth and noise. Note that the acoustic radiation force imaging pulse has an area of maximum push *(red)*. This is where the strongest shear waves are generated. In general, this is usually at 4.0–4.5 cm from the transducer. Note at greater depths the signal-to-noise ratio is very small, leading to inaccurate measurements.

by the interquartile range.[24] On the other hand, although most vendors allow measurements up to 8 cm from the transducer, it should be underscored that the ARFI push pulse is attenuated by 6–7 cm, limiting adequate shear wave generation.

It should also be pointed out that the SWS is proportional to the mean ARFI frequency. For the US systems using ARFI technique there is a bandwidth of the ARFI pulse. Especially in steatotic or stiff livers, the mean ARFI frequency will change with depth as the higher frequency components will be attenuated sooner, leading to a change in the liver stiffness value measurement. Therefore, when performing follow-up examinations in addition to using the same US system and transducer, the same depth of measurement should be maintained. For VCTE and magnetic resonance elastography (MRE), this does not occur as the measurements are taken at a fixed frequency (no bandwidth).

As of July 2021, Siemens Healthineers is the only vendor that has designed and commercialized a transducer (Deep Abdominal Transducer, DAX) able to penetrate deeper into the abdomen, up to 40 cm. It has been designed to work in all advanced modes including SWE. It allows for SWE measurements up to 14 cm. In addition, the lower frequency of the transducer allows for SWE measurements in some patients with high body mass index in whom other systems may not be able to obtain accurate SWE measurements (Fig. 4.13).[25] However, it must be emphasized that studies aimed at assessing the intraobserver and interobserver variability and the accuracy of stiffness measurement obtained with this new transducer are not yet available.

Attenuation of the US beam is higher in stiffer and steatotic livers. Therefore measurements are more variable in patients with severe fibrosis or high degrees of steatosis.

An image of the recommended transducer positioning and placement of the measurement box is provided in Fig. 4.14. Table 4.1 summarizes the protocol recommended for accurate liver stiffness measurements.

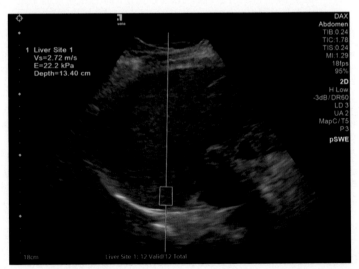

Fig. 4.13 Siemens has a deep abdominal transducer *(DAX)*, which has a lower frequency that allows for deeper penetration. The transducer is calibrated to provide similar stiffness measurements to the standard C5 transducer even though the acoustic radiation force imaging frequency is lower to allow measurements of liver stiffness up to 14 cm.

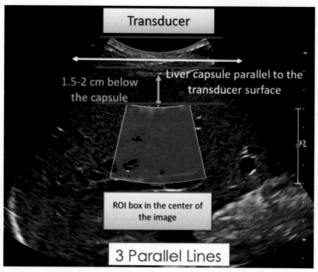

Fig. 4.14 Figure demonstrates the appropriate protocol for taking measurements. Note the *three parallel red lines:* the transducer, the liver capsule, and the measurement box. *ROI,* Region of interest.

TABLE 4.1 ■ **Strict protocol for acquiring accurate liver stiffness values**

Patient should fast for at least 4 hours.

Exam should be performed in the supine or slight left lateral position (30 degrees) with the arm extended above the head to increase the intercostal space.

Measurements should be taken through an intercostal approach at the location of the best acoustical window.

Measurements should be taken 1.5 to 2.0 cm below the liver capsule to avoid reverberation artifact. The optimal location for maximum shear wave generation is 4.0 to 4.5 cm from the transducer. In 2-dimensional shear wave elastography (2D-SWE) the region of interest (ROI)/filed of view box can be placed closer to the liver capsule because the reverberation artifact can be seen and avoided.

The transducer should be perpendicular to the liver capsule in both planes.

Placement of the ROI should avoid large blood vessels, bile ducts, masses, and artifacts.

10 measurements should be obtained from 10 independent images, in the same location, with the median value used for TE and pSWE techniques.

Three or five measurements may be appropriate for 2D-SWE when a quality assessment parameter is used.

The interquartile range/median (IQR/M) should be used as a measure of quality. For kilopascal measurements, the IQR/M should be ≤30%, and for meters per second, it should be ≤15% for an accurate data set.

For transient elastography the appropriate transducer should be selected based on the patient's body habitus.

Results Can Be Reported in Meters per Second or in Kilopascals

Every US system directly measures the SWS in meters per second. By assuming that the SWS does not change with the magnitude or frequency of the applied force or with the position and direction in the tissue, it can be converted to the Young modulus in kilopascals: $E = 3(vS^2 \rho)$, where E is the Young modulus, vS is the SWS, and ρ is the density of the tissue in homogeneous isotropic tissues. The assumption is made that the tissue density is 1 g/mL. It is worth mentioning that the Young modulus E (strain modulus) is the unit of measure used for all US SWE, whereas the shear modulus G, which is also reported in kilopascals but is approximately three times smaller than the Young modulus E, is used in MRE. Thus the values are not directly comparable. MRE measurements in kilopascals are approximately a third of the measurement obtained with US SWE in kilopascals.

The choice of whether to display the SWS in meters per second or the Young modulus in kilopascals is generally one of user preference. Theoretically, it is better to report results in units of meters per second rather than kilopascals. In fact, this is the unit of SWS, which is the quantity measured by all US systems. The conversion to kilopascals using a simple equation is based on many assumptions, including that the tissue has very simple behaviors (i.e., that is linear, isotropic, and homogeneous) and is incompressible, that may not be correct. Nonetheless, the measure of stiffness using the Young modulus in kilopascals has become quite common in clinical practice since the availability of the FibroScan and clinicians are more familiar with kilopascals than with the SWS measurement. Therefore the update to the Society of Radiologists in Ultrasound (SRU) consensus has allowed both possibilities.[4] Many systems provide the measurements in both meters per second and kilopascals, and reporting both is helpful so the referring physician can use whichever measurement they feel comfortable with.

Number of Measurements Required

Ten measurements should be obtained with pSWE, and the result should be expressed as the median together with the interquartile range/median (IQR/M). Fewer than 10 measurements with pSWE can be obtained if necessary (at least 5); however, the IQR/M should be within the recommended range. For 2D-SWE, five measurements should be obtained when the manufacturer's quality criteria are available, and the result should be expressed as the median together with the IQR/M.

When performing a measurement on biological tissues with a device, a technical or biological within-subject variability must be taken into consideration. The technical variability is associated with the analytical performance in terms of measurement errors; it can be strictly controlled but not completely removed. The within-subject biological variability represents the physiological changes that may occur in each individual due to biological factors. Therefore a single measurement is likely inaccurate because it will ignore the possibility of correlated variability.

For multiple measurements, the mean (average) is usually the best measure when the data distribution is continuous and symmetrical. This is not the case with SWE measurement in which the data set generally has a skewed distribution due to the presence of outliers (i.e., values that are unusual compared to the rest of the data set by being abnormally smaller or larger). The mean value will include the outliers in the computation, and therefore it may be misleading. The median value is preferred because it is a robust statistic of the central tendency, and the outliers have little effect on the result.

For pSWE, 10 measurements are usually recommended. However, studies have shown that acquiring 5 measurements does not decrease the accuracy if the IQR/M is within the recommended range.[26-28] It is recommended to take 10 measurements when starting a liver stiffness program. Only after mastery of the technique with good results should fewer measurements be taken.

When using 2D-SWE, artifacts can be visualized and avoided. Selection of an area of higher accuracy can be identified using confidence or quality maps. Therefore only five measurements are recommended. The IQR/M should be ≤30% in kilopascals and ≤15% in meters per second as in pSWE.

Another quality criterion that should be applied is that >60% of the measurements should be "good" measurements. A good measurement in pSWE is when a value is obtained, not 000 or xxx. When the result is 000 or xxx the system cannot calculate an estimate of the SWS due to poor quality. In 2D-SWE a bad measurement is usually not colored in the velocity/elasticity map. The expert opinion is that if 50% or more of the velocity/elasticity map in 2D-SWE is not colored, it should be considered a bad measurement. Note that a good measurement does not mean it is accurate. When <60% of the measurements are good, it is unlikely that any of the measurements are accurate. Taking more measurements to obtain the 5 or 10 suggested measurements is unlikely to produce accurate measurements. This often occurs in patients with high body mass indexes.

Reliability Criteria

The most important reliability criterion is an IQR/M ≤30% of the 10 measurements (pSWE) or 5 measurements (2D-SWE) for kilopascals and ≤15% for measurements in meters per second (SWS).

The interquartile range, also called the "middle fifty," is a measure of the statistical dispersion of the data being equal to the difference between the upper and lower quartiles. Several studies have reported that the level of variability between consecutive acquisitions, assessed by means of the IQR/M, is the most important quality criterion.[26-28] An IQR/M value ≤30% for measurements taken in kilopascals and ≤15% for measurements taken in meters per second suggest that a data set is good. The difference between IQR/M for kilopascals and meters per second is due to the conversion of meters per second to kilopascals, which is not linear. When the IQR/M is >30% for measurements given in kilopascals and >15% for measurements in meters per second, the accuracy of the technique decreases and values should be judged as unreliable (Fig. 4.15).[4] The IQR/M can be presented also as decimals (e.g., ≤0.30 or ≤0.15).

When IQR/M is above 30% (for values given in kilopascals) but all the values are in the normal range (e.g., up to 5 kPa), liver fibrosis can confidently be excluded. This exception to the

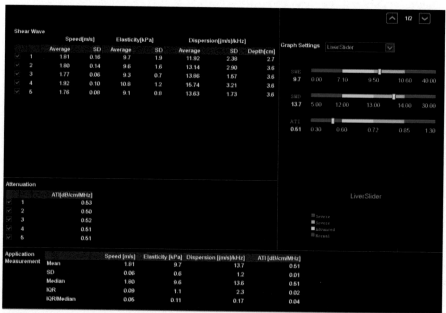

Fig. 4.15 Report of a multiparametric acquisition obtained with the Aplio i800 ultrasound system (Canon Medical Systems, Japan). The stiffness results are given both in meters per second and kilopascals. The interquartile range/median (IQR/M) reported in the last line is 0.05 for the median value of five measurements in meters per seccond (shear wave speed) and 0.11 for the median value of elasticity in kilopascals. The dispersion value in meters per second per kilohertz and the attenuation coefficient (ATI) in decibels per centimeter per megahertz are also shown. The graph on the right side gives a visual assessment of these values based on vendor's suggested cutoff values.

rule cannot be applied to patients with compensated advanced chronic liver disease because studies have shown that the accuracy of stiffness decreases when the IQR/M is above the recommended range.[29,30] Moreover, these patients need follow up the most. Therefore a reliable measurement must be obtained to detect changes in stiffness over time.

B-Mode Liver Imaging

Adequate B-mode liver imaging is a prerequisite for point and 2D-SWE as shear waves are tracked with B-mode.

With the ARFI techniques, the shear waves are generated by the ARFI push pulse and their propagation, which is transverse to ARFI pulse, is tracked by conventional B-mode. Therefore the quality of the B-mode image is of outmost importance.

The operator must identify the best acoustic window holding the transducer at 90 degrees (perpendicular) to the liver capsule both in the superior/inferior plane and the right to left plane; segment 7, 8, or 5 can be selected. At 90 degrees, the liver capsule should appear as a sharp white line. A study in a phantom indicated that the ROI angle may have a slight but significant influence on the values and therefore affects the diagnostic accuracy.[14] The lowest variation was found at a perpendicular ROI position in the center of the transducer surface (Figs. 4.4 and 4.14).

Several studies have shown that operators require only a short period of training to perform reliable liver stiffness measurements; however, the reproducibility over time of liver stiffness measurements with 2D-SWE is higher for expert operators than for novice operators.

Take Only One Measurement for Each Acquisition

With 2D-SWE, most vendors may allow the placement of multiple measurement boxes within the elastogram. This is discouraged because, if there is an error in that image, the error is reproduced in all the measurements from that image and reflected in the median.[5]

Size and Positioning of the Measurement Box

The measurement box should be placed in an area of high quality (discussed in vendor-specific information) and should avoid all artifacts (see Chapter 6). In pSWE, the size of the measurement box is fixed and cannot be changed. It is critical to understand where artifacts occur (reverberation artifact, artifact around blood vessels, etc.) in pSWE as these artifacts are not displayed as they are in 2D-SWE. In 2D-SWE the measurement box size can be varied. Generally, the default measurement box size by the vendors is usually appropriate. However, if one wants to average more liver tissue (while excluding artifacts) the measurement box can be enlarged. If there are artifacts around the area of highest quality, the measurement box can be decreased to avoid including the artifacts.

Measurements in Pediatric Patients with the ARFI Techniques

The procedure used for adults should be adopted.[4] A more complete discussion of pediatric liver stiffness measurements is presented in Chapter 7.

In children who are unable to hold their breath, the SRU consensus panel suggests recording a 2D-SWE cine loop for up to 30 seconds if real-time 2D-SWE is available, reviewing it, and choosing the image demonstrating the most stable pattern for the stiffness measurement.[4] No more than one image should be chosen in each recorded cine loop.

Some studies have suggested that measurements be performed with a free-breathing technique. However, it should be kept in mind that the value that is obtained is probably unreliable because the noise due to the movement can actually be measured as a stiffness value. A study performed in children has shown that the free-breathing technique revealed systematically lower liver stiffness values with a mean difference of −11.1% of the mean liver stiffness values.[31]

Major Potential Confounding Factors

Major potential confounding factors include acute hepatitis, severe liver inflammation indicated by aspartate aminotransferase (AST) and/or alanine aminotransferase (ALT) elevation greater than five times upper normal limits, obstructive cholestasis, liver congestion, and infiltrative liver disease (these all lead to overestimation of the stage of fibrosis).

US SWE techniques measure liver stiffness not fibrosis. Stiffness is influenced by fibrosis, inflammation, and congestion. Stiffness is directly related to liver fibrosis; however, other factors that may lead to an increase of stiffness values independently from fibrosis must be taken in consideration.

Acute Hepatitis

The overestimation of liver stiffness in cases of acute hepatitis was reported in two seminal studies.[32,33] Arena et al. analyzed the stiffness values in 18 patients with acute hepatitis at three different time points: (1) peak increase in aminotransferase, (2) aminotransferase 50% or less of the peak, and (3) aminotransferase levels less than two times the upper limit of normal.[32] In all patients, the degree of liver stiffness at the time of the peak increase in aminotransferases exceeded the cutoff values proposed for the prediction of significant fibrosis or cirrhosis, even though all patients did not have fibrosis. Sagir et al. analyzed 20 patients with acute liver damage of different etiologies and showed that the initial liver stiffness values measured by VCTE during the acute phase of the liver damage were suggestive of liver cirrhosis even though none of the patients showed any signs of liver cirrhosis during the physical or US examinations.[33] Parallel to the decrease in the ALT levels, as a marker for the inflammation, liver stiffness returned to values below the cirrhosis threshold. The authors suggested that the elevated stiffness values in acute liver damage could be related to hepatocyte swelling, cholestasis, or infiltrates of inflammatory cells in the acutely inflamed liver. This confounding factor has been analyzed in several other studies. The effect of inflammation on the increase of tissue stiffness values has been documented in other organs.[18,34]

Severe Inflammation Indicated by AST and/or ALT Elevation Greater than Five Times Upper Normal Limits

Severe acute exacerbation of hepatitis is mainly observed in patients with chronic hepatitis B. Moderate to severe liver fibrosis superimposed on the acute inflammation may lead to a misdiagnosis of liver cirrhosis. The seminal study that demonstrated. ALT values were independently associated with liver stiffness in patients with chronic hepatitis was published by Coco and coworkers.[35] In their study, the liver stiffness profile over time paralleled that of ALT, increasing 1.3- to 3-fold during ALT flares in 10 patients with hepatitis exacerbations.

The interval of time needed for reliable liver stiffness measurement in patients with chronic hepatitis B experiencing acute exacerbation has been assessed in small cohorts. Using VCTE in 21 patients with ALT values higher than five times the upper limit of normal, it was determined that stiffness assessment must be postponed for at least 3 months after stabilization of ALT below two times the upper limit of normal.[36] Similar results were reported in a study of 29 patients with severe hepatitis B flares (ALT >10 times the upper limit of normal) who were followed up for 1 year. They demonstrated a liver stiffness increase in the acute phase, which returned to near normal levels by 6 months. Therefore the authors recommended that, for a correct assessment of liver fibrosis, stiffness measurement should be performed at least 6 months after flares.[37]

It is important to note that an alcohol binge may lead to an overestimation of liver stiffness, likely due to acute inflammation of the liver. In this regard, a short-term impact of alcohol withdrawal on liver stiffness values has been reported.[38] In a series of 137 patients hospitalized for alcohol withdrawal, liver stiffness decreased significantly in nearly half of heavy drinkers after only 7 days of abstinence. Moreover, an individual patient data metaanalysis on the cutoff values of VCTE for the staging of fibrosis in alcohol-related liver disease found that the cutoffs were highly correlated with transaminases value and bilirubin values: for AST and bilirubin concentrations that were in the low level, the cutoffs were similar to those reported in chronic hepatitis C, whereas for AST and bilirubin concentrations that were elevated, the cutoffs were the highest reported in a liver disease to date.[39]

Obstructive Cholestasis
The increased hydrostatic pressure alone seems to contribute to increased liver stiffness. In fact, there is a rapid decrease of liver stiffness after biliary drainage.[40]

Liver Congestion
Any pathology affecting the right heart may lead to an increase in the pressure of the right atrium, inferior vena cava, and hepatic veins. The liver capsule is minimally distensible, therefore hepatic congestion will lead to an increase of liver stiffness. The first report of an increase in liver stiffness due to liver congestion was of a heart transplant patient with heart failure: the patient had a very stiff liver and cardiac hepatopathy but did not have liver cirrhosis at histology. One year after another heart transplant, a liver biopsy showed that there was a significant improvement of the cardiac hepatopathy, and the liver stiffness value was within the normal range.[41] Several other reports/studies have since been published.

It must be emphasized, however, that SWE can play a role in cases of liver congestion due to right-sided heart failure, congenital heart diseases, or valvular diseases that goes beyond the staging of liver fibrosis.[42-44] These are discussed in Chapter 9.

Infiltrative Liver Disease
Amyloidosis, lymphomas, and extramedullary hemopoiesis may lead to an overestimation of liver fibrosis assessed with SWE techniques.[45-47]

Intense Physical Exercise
During physical exercise, there is a redistribution of blood flow mainly to skeletal muscles. A study in seven healthy volunteers demonstrated that liver stiffness significantly increased during an episode of intense physical activity and returned to normal within 10 minutes after the completion of the activity.[48]

VIBRATION CONTROLLED TRANSIENT ELASTOGRAPHY

Three different probes are available on the FibroScan unit: a pediatric S probe, a standard M probe, and an XL probe. The S probe is used in children with a thoracic circumference <75 cm, the M probe when the thoracic circumference is >75 cm and the skin-to-liver capsule distance ≤25 mm, and the XL probe when the skin-to-liver capsule distance is ≥25 mm. This latter is dedicated to overweight/obese subjects with more reliable results as compared with the M probe. The software of the system automatically suggests the correct choice of the probe.

Measurements are taken in fasting conditions, with the patient lying supine and with the right arm elevated to facilitate access to the right liver lobe. The tip of the probe is positioned in the ninth to eleventh intercostal space. The best examination site is the median axillary line on the first intercostal space under the liver percussion dullness upper limit. The operator, assisted by an A-mode image and a time-motion image, locates a liver portion at least 6 cm thick and free of large vessels. The operator then presses the probe button to start the measurement; no breath hold is required. The liver stiffness is assessed in a fixed area in a volume that approximates a cylinder 1 cm wide and 4 cm long, between 25 and 65 mm below the skin surface with the M probe, and

35–75 mm with the XL probe. The software determines whether each "shot" is successful or not. When a shot is unsuccessful, the value is not shown. The entire procedure is considered to have failed when no values are obtained after 10 shots. Successful measurements are validated using the following criteria: (1) 10 valid shots and (2) IQR/M ≤30%. Results are given in Young modulus units (i.e., kilopascals).

According to a study, VCTE results should be classified as "very reliable" if IQR/M ≤10%, regardless of liver stiffness measurement; "reliable" if IQR/M ≤30%, or IQR/M >30% with the Young modulus <7.1 kPa and "poorly reliable" if IQR/M >30% with the Young modulus ≥7.1 kPa.[30]

The confounding factors described in the ARFI-based techniques paragraph were mostly reported with VCTE. The confounding factors are valid with all the SWE techniques.

Quality Assessment

VENDOR-SPECIFIC QUALITY ASSESSMENT

Measurements should be obtained in areas of highest quality as determined by a high amplitude of the shear waves, a normal shear-wave propagation, and a linear slope of the time-to-peak and distance from ARFI pulse from the displacement curves (Fig. 4.16). Each vendor provides a confidence or quality number or map that combines these factors into one number for easy clinical use.

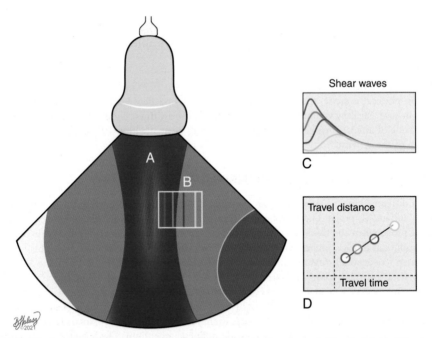

Fig. 4.16 Most confidence maps evaluate the quality of the shear waves by evaluating the height of the shear waves (A), signal-to-noise of the shear waves (B), that the displacement curves (C) follow a regular pattern, and that the slope of the distance from the acoustic radiation force imaging pulse to the time of the maximum displacement curve peak is a straight line (D). The combination of the quality of each of these factors is summarized into one number usually from 0 (no confidence) to 100 (high confidence).

However, none of the quality maps depicts all artifacts, and knowledge of artifacts is crucial for obtaining accurate liver stiffness values. Therefore it is very important to evaluate both the quality map and the elasticity/velocity map.

Canon Medical Systems

The quality factor of the Canon ARFI technology is the propagation map. It indicates the propagation of the SWS using lines. The elastogram and the propagation map of the shear waves are displayed within a sample box over the conventional B-mode image, side-by-side. A proper propagation is displayed by parallel lines, and the intervals between lines are constant. The distance between the lines corresponds to the SWS, with a larger distance between the lines correlating to faster SWSs. When the lines are not parallel to each other and at the same distance, the reliability of the obtained data is low (Fig. 4.17).

Philips Medical Systems

Philips has both pSWE (ElastPQ) and 2D-SWE (ElastQ) techniques. Each single ElastPQ measurement is the mean value obtained with a sequence of several push pulses; it is displayed on the monitor of the US system together with the standard deviation. When the standard deviation is higher than 30% of the reported value, the quality of the measurement is poor (Fig. 4.18). If the acquisition has a very low signal-to-noise ratio, a value is not shown.

The quality factor of ElastQ is the confidence map, which is a color-coded representation of the effectiveness of the ARFI push pulses and the quality of the resultant shear waves. The map is based on three colors, as for a traffic light: green is Go (high quality), yellow is a Caution (less than optimal quality), and red means Stop (poor quality). There is also a confidence threshold (CT) that can be set by the operator and is expressed in percent. At a CT of 60% or higher, only high-quality signals are displayed in colors on the elasticity/velocity map, whereas areas with the confidence value lower than the threshold are left blank (Fig. 4.19). In difficult patients, the CT

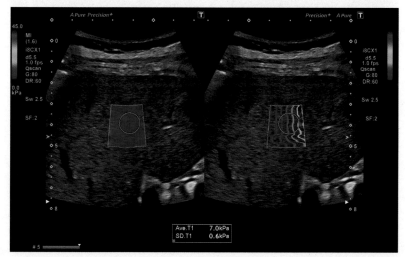

Fig. 4.17 Two-dimensional shear wave elastography technique (Canon Medical Systems, Japan). Image obtained with an Aplio i800 series ultrasound system. The system filters out values with a low signal-to-noise ratio, and these areas are left blank. The propagation map, which is a quality assessment map, and the elasticity map are shown side-by-side on the monitor. A good acquisition has a propagation map with parallel lines, and the intervals between the lines have the same distance. When these criteria are not fulfilled, the reliability of the obtained data is low. The propagation map is the guidance for placing the measurement box *(round circle)*.

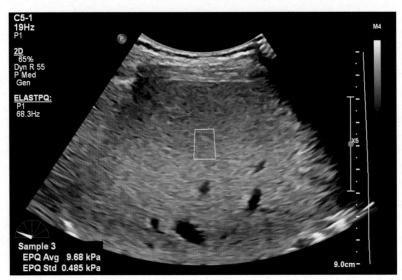

Fig. 4.18 Point shear wave elastography technique (ElastPQ, Philips Healthcare, The Netherlands). Image obtained with the Epiq Elite ultrasound system. The region of interest *(yellow rectangle)* has a fixed size. The mean value of the push-track sequences is given together with the standard deviation (Std). An Std ≤30% of the mean value indicates an acquisition of good quality. When the signal-to-noise ratio of an acquisition is very low, a value is not shown.

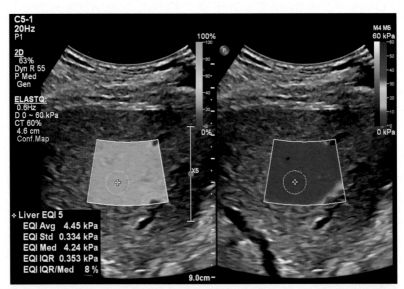

Fig. 4.19 Two-dimensional shear wave elastography technique (EQI, Philips Healthcare, The Netherlands). Image obtained with the Epiq Elite ultrasound system. Color-coded elasticity map *(right side)* and confidence map *(left side)* are shown side-by-side. The color-coded confidence map is an evaluation of the quality of the acquired signals. The confidence map is set with colors like a traffic light for quality assessment: *green color* means that the signals in the corresponding areas of the elasticity map are of good quality, *yellow color* is a warning, and *red color* indicates areas with low quality of the acquisition. With a confidence threshold set at 60%, as in this case, the low and some medium quality signals are filtered out in the elasticity map.

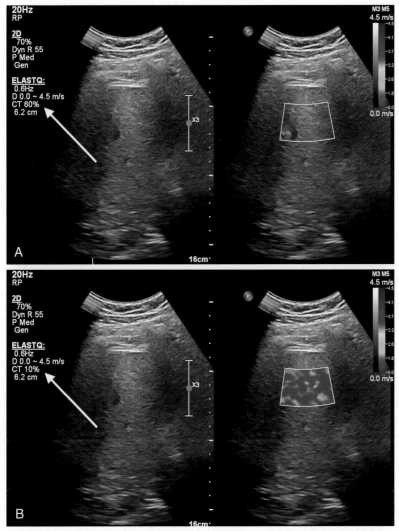

Fig. 4.20 (A) A velocity map has minimal coloring. Note that in this image the confidence map *(arrow)* is 60%. (B) If the confidence level is decreased to 10% *(arrow)*, the velocity map is fully colored and measurements can be taken. However, with a confidence threshold of less than 60%, the measurements are less accurate and below 30%, thus they should not be used.

can be lower to have more coloring in the velocity map and to allow for a measurement to be taken, but the operator should be aware that those measurements are less accurate and should be reported as such. A measurement with the CT of 30% or less should not be taken (Fig. 4.20).

Hologic

The quality factor available on the MACH 40 system is the stability index (SI), which is derived from the spatial and temporal stiffness stability of the circular quantitation box (Qbox) used to perform the measurement. The SI appears into the measurement box, and its value may change

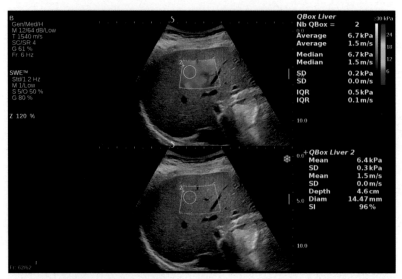

Fig. 4.21 Two-dimensional shear wave elastography technique (SSI, Hologic, USA). Image obtained with the Aixplorer ultrasound system. The system filters out values with a low signal-to-noise ratio, and these areas are left blank. Stability index *(SI)* is an indicator of temporal stability, and it is displayed while positioning the measurement box *(Qbox)*. An acquisition of good quality should have an SI >90%.

when moving the measurement box inside the velocity/elasticity map. The vendor recommends an SI >90% (Fig. 4.21).

Fujifilm Healthcare, Previously Hitachi Ltd.

The shear wave measurement (SWM) method is a pSWE technique. Each measurement is the median value of the effective shear wave velocity measured from multiple points in the ROI's depth direction from several push-track sequences after subtraction of noisy values. The percentage of effective measurements is a reliability index termed *VsN*. A reliable measurement should have a VsN ≥50% (Fig. 4.22). When the signal-to-noise ratio of an acquisition is very low, the mean value is not shown. As of July 2021, a 2D-SWE technique is also available (Fig. 4.23), but a quality factor has not been implemented yet with it.

Samsung Medical Systems

Samsung has both a pSWE and a 2D-SWE technique. The quality of each measurement is assessed with the performance index, "Reliability Measurement Index" (RMI), which is calculated by the weighted sum of the residual of the wave equation and the magnitude of the shear wave. RMI is on both the pSWE and 2D-SWE techniques. An RMI of >90% indicates a high-quality measurement (Fig. 4.24).

Mindray Medical Systems

Mindray Sound Touch Elastography (STE) comes with two quality criteria: the motion stability (M-STB) index and the reliability (RLB) map. M-STB index monitors interferences due to motion, either induced by patient respiration or movement of the transducer, and is visualized by stars on the right upper corner of the image. The highest stability of the acquired elasticity image is indicated by five green stars, whereas red stars indicate motion. The RLB map is color-coded

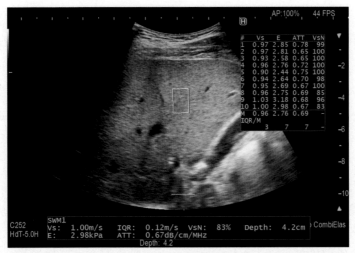

Fig. 4.22 Point shear wave elastography (pSWE) technique (SWM, Fujifilm Healthcare, previously Hitachi Ltd., Japan). Image obtained with the Arietta 850 ultrasound (US) system. SWM is a pSWE technique, thus the region of interest *(the yellow rectangle)* has a fixed size. All measurements and the final report with median value and interquartile range/median *(IQR/M)* of the parameters are shown directly on the image (or on a separate report). *VsN* is a reliability index that indicates the percentage of effective push-track sequences. A measurement of good quality should have a VsN ≥50%. When the signal-to-noise ratio of an acquisition is very low, the mean value is not shown. The system simultaneously quantifies the attenuation of the US beam in decibels per centimeter per megahertz with a proprietary algorithm (attenuation measurement function *[ATT]*).

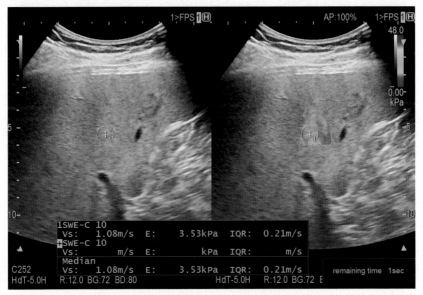

Fig. 4.23 Two-dimensional shear wave elastography technique (Fujifilm Healthcare, previously Hitachi Ltd., Japan). The system filters out values with a low signal-to-noise ratio, and these areas are left blank in the elasticity map.

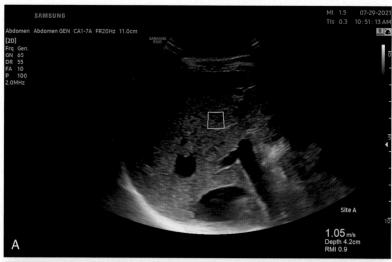

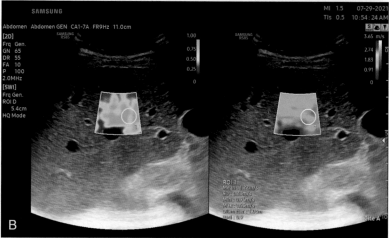

Fig. 4.24   (A) Point shear wave elastography technique (S-Shearwave, Samsung Healthcare, South Korea). The quality of each measurement is assessed with the performance index, "Reliability Measurement Index" *(RMI)*, which is calculated by the weighted sum of the residual of the wave equation and the magnitude of the shear wave. The RMI is also used in the 2-dimensional shear wave elastogram technique (B). An RMI of greater than 90% indicates a high-quality measurement. *ROI,* Region of interest.

and shown together with the elasticity map side-by-side. The color goes from purple, which indicates poor reliability, to green, which indicates the highest reliability (Fig. 4.25).

Siemens Healthineers

Both pSWE technology (VTQ) and 2D-SWE (VTQI) are available. With VTQ, the system automatically filters out the measurements that are not good. In these cases, the numeric value of SWS is replaced by an "XXX" sequence (Fig. 4.26). On newer software versions, the system will obtain 15 individual pSWE measurements, assess the quality of each measurement, accept only those of good quality, and report the mean and IQR/M with a single button push. (Fig. 4.27).

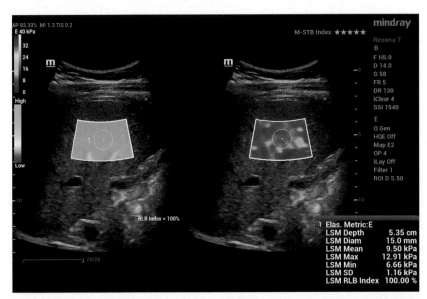

Fig. 4.25 Two-dimensional shear wave elastography *(2D-SWE)* technique (STE, Mindray Medical Systems, China). Image obtained with the Resona 7 ultrasound system. STE is a 2D-SWE technique. Two quality criteria are provided: motion stability *(M-STB; green stars)* index (right upper part of the image) and reliability *(RLB)* map (left side of the image). The M-STB index is indicated by stars: the highest stability of the acquired elasticity image is indicated by five green stars, whereas red stars indicate motion. It guides in choosing the most stable image in a cine loop. The RLB map ranges in color from purple, which indicates poor reliability, to green, which indicates the highest reliability. The RLB is a guide for the placement of the measurement box.

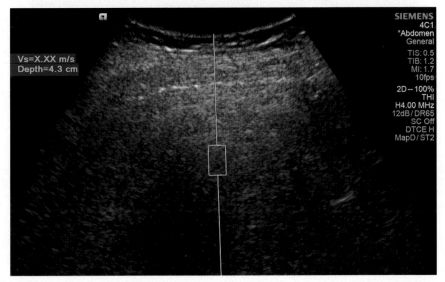

Fig. 4.26 Point shear wave elastography technique (VTQ, Siemens Healthineers, Germany). The system automatically filters out the measurements that are not good. In these cases, the numeric value of shear wave speed is replaced by an *XXX* sequence.

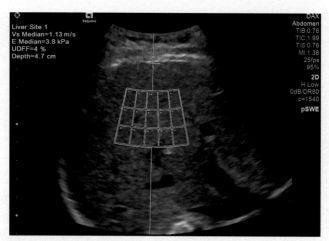

Fig. 4.27 A one-button push point shear wave elastography *(pSWE)* method is available on the Siemens system. The system takes 15 pSWE measurements with the single button push, evaluates the quality of the shear waves, deletes the measurements felt to be unreliable, and provides the median and interquartile range/median. For this method the line above the measurement area is placed at the liver capsule to standardize the depth of the measurement.

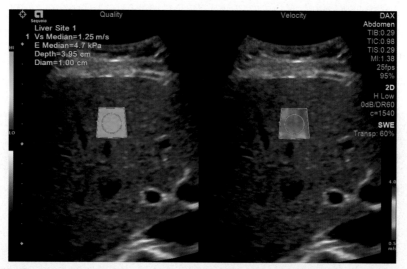

Fig. 4.28 Two-dimensional shear wave elastography technique (Siemens Healthineers, Germany). Image obtained with the Acuson Sequoia ultrasound system. The system filters out values with a low signal-to-noise ratio, and these areas are left blank in the velocity map (not shown). The quality map *(left)* is color-coded from green (highest quality) to red (poor quality). Areas colored green or yellow are of acceptable quality.

With 2D-SWE (VTQI), areas of poor quality are not colored on the velocity/elasticity map. A confidence map is available in which green and yellow are acceptable quality and red is poor quality and should not be used. (Fig. 4.28).

General Electric (GE)

The system performs 2D-SWE using the comb-push excitation technique with time-interleaved shear wave tracking.[49] A confidence map ranging from 0 (no confidence) to 100 (high confidence)

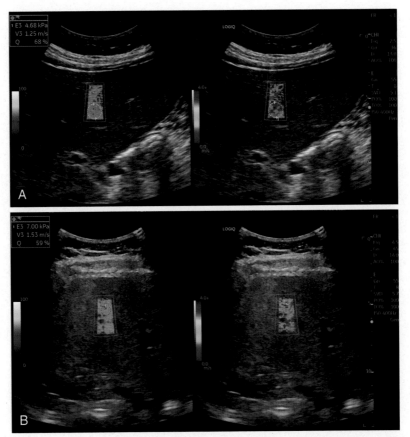

Fig. 4.29 (A) Two-dimensional shear wave elastography (2D-SWE) technique (GE Healthcare, USA). The image on the right is the velocity map and the image on the left is the confidence map. The confidence map ranges from 0 (no confidence, red) to 100 (high confidence, white). (B) The 2D-SWE technique color codes the measurement box *red* if the measurement is of low quality.

is provided. The confidence map is color-coded with red as poor quality and yellow and white as good quality (Fig. 4.29). The size of the measurement box within the ROI can be varied. When the measurement box is placed in an area of poor quality, it changes from white to red, flagging the measurement as not accurate.

Vibration-Controlled Transient Elastography

The system does not generate a B-mode image; however, the portion of the liver being studied is shown both in TM-mode and A-mode whereas the elastogram is graphically displayed as a function of depth (y-axis) and time (x-axis). The TM-mode and A-mode should be evaluated to confirm that no masses or vessels are present in the area of measurement. The system automatically filters out invalid measurements, and their number, if any, is shown on the monitor (Fig. 4.30).

Reproducibility, Failures, and Unreliable Results

REPRODUCIBILITY

US imaging techniques are subject to user dependency, therefore the reproducibility of measurements with US SWE is an important issue. Reproducibility has been assessed by several studies

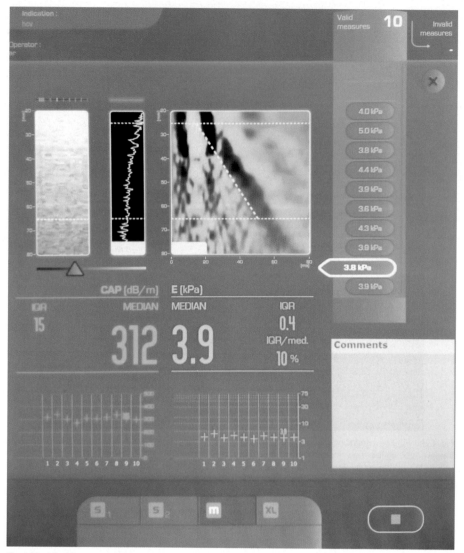

Fig. 4.30 Vibration-controlled transient elastography (VCTE; Echosens, France). The system automatically filters out invalid measurements, and their number, if any, is shown on the monitor.

that have reported a high interobserver reproducibility and an excellent agreement between measurements performed by different operators.

Factors that affect the reproducibility of the measurement are similar across the different techniques and are related to the operator's experience and to factors dependent on the subject being examined.

For both the ARFI-based techniques and VCTE, a learning curve should be considered. For pSWE and 2D-SWE, experience in B-mode US is mandatory. The learning curve for pSWE is as low as one day for operators already trained in B-mode US. For 2D-SWE, the learning curve is longer. It has been suggested that at least 50 supervised scans and measurements should be performed by a novice operator to obtain consistent measurements.[50] For VCTE, a study has reported that an experience of fewer than 500 examinations was associated with a higher rate of failures or unreliable results.[51]

The time required for the measurement with VCTE, pSWE, and 2D-SWE is usually less than 5 minutes.[6,52]

Point Shear Wave Elastography

In a study performed in 166 individuals (47 consecutive patients with chronic hepatitis C undergoing liver biopsy and 69 healthy volunteers) two expert operators performed the pSWE measurements of liver stiffness and the agreement was assessed by means of the concordance correlation coefficient, which ranges from 0 (no agreement) to 1 (perfect agreement).[53] The intraobserver and interobserver agreement were assessed by comparing the median values of all 10 measurements and by comparing several combinations of 5 measurements or a single measurement. Both operators had an intraobserver agreement of 0.96 for the median value of 10 measurements, and it ranged from 0.83 to 0.93 for only one measurement. Interobserver agreement was 0.93 for the median value of 10 measurements, and it ranged from 0.91 to 0.93 for the combination of measurements and from 0.83 to 0.89 for only one measurement. Moreover, the reproducibility of the technique was similar in healthy subjects and in patients with chronic viral hepatitis.

In a series of 91 subjects in which almost 65% had decompensated liver cirrhosis, the intraobserver reproducibility, assessed in 33 subjects, was 0.90 and the interobserver reproducibility, assessed in 58 subjects, was 0.81.[54] The intraoperator reproducibility was lower in patients with ascites (0.80).

A study on 50 healthy volunteers reported that the interobserver reproducibility of shear wave velocity measurements performed by two observers with different levels of experience and assessed with an intraclass correlation coefficient (ICC) was 0.86. Of note, prior training on a group of 10 patients was given to establish an adequate consensus between the two observers.[55]

Two-Dimensional Shear Wave Elastography

Intraobserver agreement was assessed in a study that included 42 healthy volunteers.[50] Measurements were performed by two operators, an expert and a novice. Additionally, in a subset of volunteers (n = 18) measurements were performed twice on two different days. Intraobserver and interobserver agreement were assessed by ICC. The intraobserver agreement was 0.95 for the expert and 0.93 for the novice and it decreased to 0.84 and 0.65 for the expert and the novice, respectively, for measurements in different days. The interobserver agreement was 0.88. The results of this study show that an expert operator has higher reproducibility of measurements over time than a novice operator. This finding is likely due to several causes. Physiological differences over time could be one factor. In fact, lower values of liver elasticity were obtained in the second day by both operators. The lower intraobserver agreement obtained in different days by the novice could be explained by the operator's expertise, which plays a more relevant role in 2D-SWE because the sample box has a larger FOV.

Vibration Controlled Transient Elastography

In a series of 200 patients with chronic liver disease of mixed etiology who underwent liver biopsy, the overall intraobserver and interobserver agreement of liver stiffness measurement with VCTE were both 0.98. The agreement decreased for measurements taken in patients with steatosis (ICC: 0.90), in patients who were overweight (ICC: 0.94), or in patients who had an early stage of liver fibrosis (ICC: 0.60).[56] Gender, patient age, etiology, or severity of liver disease did not affect the agreement. These results were confirmed in a subsequent independent study that also showed that the highest agreement was obtained at the site usually used for liver biopsy.[57]

In a North American multicenter cohort of patients with hepatitis B or C, the intraobserver and interobserver ICC were 0.95 and 0.98, respectively.[58]

FAILURES AND UNRELIABLE RESULTS

With the ARFI techniques, failure is defined as the inability to acquire any reliable acquisition following the manufacturer's quality criteria for each single measurement. An unreliable result is when the IQR/M is higher than 30% for values in kilopascals or higher than 15% for values in meters per second or when the success rate is less than 60%.[4] Generally, the rate of failures or unreliable results increases in cases of obesity, liver steatosis, or narrow intercostal spaces.

With VCTE, failure is defined as zero valid shots, and unreliable examinations are defined as fewer than 10 valid shots, an IQR/M greater than 30%, or a success rate less than 60%. Based on some published studies, this latter criterion is not recommended by the vendor anymore; however, it has been used in the majority of published studies.

Using VCTE in a very large series of patients, failure occurred in 3.1% of all examinations and was independently associated with obesity, operator experience fewer than 500 examinations, age ≥52 years, and type 2 diabetes. Unreliable results were obtained in a further 15.8% of cases and were independently associated with the same factors responsible for failures plus female sex and hypertension. Waist circumference was the most important factor determining failure and unreliable results in the subgroup of patients with this parameter available.[51] It should be highlighted, however, that in this study only the M probe was available. In a more recent study in which both the probes (M and XL) were used, the failure rate was 3.2% (55/1696) and unreliable measurements, 3.9%. The proportion of unreliable scans was significantly lower for the operator with more experience.[59]

Intersystem Variability

It is well known when staging liver fibrosis with the SWE techniques, the cutoff values based on histology cannot interchangeably be applied across different US systems because different systems may give different stiffness values in the same subject. These differences occur due to the difference in bandwidth and mean frequency of the transducer, assumptions made on the propagation direction, and algorithm biases and ability to reject artifacts. Because of these differences, the same US system must be used to follow up the liver stiffness changes in any given patient.

The Radiological Society of North America (RSNA) Quantitative Imaging Biomarker Alliance (QIBA) US SWS committee has developed elastic and viscoelastic phantoms to evaluate system dependencies of SWS estimates used to noninvasively stage liver fibrosis. Previous elastic phantom studies demonstrated intersystem variability ranging from 6%–12% in phantoms with nominal SWS of 1.0 and 2.0 m/s.[60] In viscoelastic phantoms that more accurately simulate liver, the median SWS estimates for the greatest outliers' system in each phantom/focal depth combination ranged from 12.7%–17.6%, which included both system and site differences (variability of those performing the examination).[61]

It should be underscored that *in vivo* there are several factors that affect the measurement of liver stiffness, including but not limited to the amount of subcutaneous fat, liver depth, breathing, motion from heartbeat, reverberation from the liver capsule, and fasting. Also, bile ducts and blood vessels in the liver should be avoided when obtaining measurements. All these factors cannot be assessed in phantoms.

A study has evaluated the intersystem and interobserver variability of stiffness measurements in patients with varying degrees of liver stiffness using six US systems, four with pSWE and two with 2D-SWE.[62] VCTE was used as the reference standard. The variability was assessed in "ideal conditions" (i.e., following the protocol for acquisitions described in this chapter). The agreement was above 0.80 for all the pairs of systems. The mean difference between the values of the two systems with 2D-SWE technique was 1.54 kPa, whereas the maximum mean difference between the values of three out of four systems with pSWE technique was 0.79 kPa. Of note, limits of agreement were above 2 kPa for all pairs of systems. The variability between measurements obtained with different systems was higher in stiffer liver. The range of values obtained with the two 2D-SWE systems paralleled that of VCTE in cases of very stiff liver (>15 kPa), whereas the four systems with a pSWE technology gave lower values in the higher range of liver stiffness. The intrapatient concordance for all systems was 0.89 and the interobserver agreement was above 0.90. The results of this study show that the agreement between measurements of liver stiffness performed with different US systems is excellent. However, an excellent agreement does not necessarily mean that the values are the same; it mainly shows that there is a concordance between values because they follow the same direction.

The differences between the different systems were smaller in patients with liver stiffness values less than 15 kPa, which is the more clinically relevant range of values for the staging of liver fibrosis.

Another study compared liver stiffness values obtained with several US systems with VCTE values in a series of patients with chronic hepatitis C and showed only a moderate concordance between the results obtained with the ARFI techniques and those obtained with VCTE.[63]

KEY POINTS

1. A very strict protocol must be followed for accurate liver stiffness measurements.
2. An IQR/M of ≤30% in measurements taken in kilopascals and ≤15% in measurements taken in meters per second is the best quality assessment of the results.
3. The use of quality features provided by US vendors should be well understood and utilized to increase accuracy of the measurements.
4. There are multiple confounding factors that should be recognized and taken into consideration when using the results for clinical management.
5. For the ARFI techniques there can be a depth dependance of the measurement and follow-up studies should be taken at the same depth.
6. The recognition of artifacts is critical in performing liver stiffness measurements to obtain accurate values.
7. Optimization of the B-mode image is required as B-mode tracks the shear waves to provide the estimate of the SWS. The B-mode image should be free of artifacts especially shadowing.

References

1. Barr RG, Ferraioli G, Palmeri ML, et al. Elastography assessment of liver fibrosis: Society of Radiologists in Ultrasound Consensus Conference Statement. *Radiology.* 2015;276:845-861.
2. Ferraioli G, Filice C, Castera L, et al. WFUMB guidelines and recommendations for clinical use of ultrasound elastography: part 3: liver. *Ultrasound Med Biol.* 2015;41:1161-1179.
3. Barr RG, Ferraioli G, Palmeri ML, et al. Elastography assessment of liver fibrosis: Society of Radiologists in Ultrasound Consensus Conference Statement. *Ultrasound Q.* 2016;32:94-107.
4. Barr RG, Wilson SR, Rubens D, Garcia-Tsao G, Ferraioli G. Update to the Society of Radiologists in Ultrasound Liver Elastography Consensus Statement. *Radiology.* 2020;296:263-274.
5. Ferraioli G, Wong VW, Castera L, et al. Liver ultrasound elastography: an update to the World Federation for Ultrasound in Medicine and Biology Guidelines and Recommendations. *Ultrasound Med Biol.* 2018;44:2419-2440.

6. Dietrich CF, Bamber J, Berzigotti A, et al. EFSUMB guidelines and recommendations on the clinical use of liver ultrasound elastography, update 2017 (long version). *Ultraschall Med.* 2017;38:e16-e47.

7. Ferraioli G, Parekh P, Levitov AB, Filice C. Shear wave elastography for evaluation of liver fibrosis. *J Ultrasound Med.* 2014;33:197-203.

8. Barr RG. Shear wave liver elastography. *Abdom Radiol (NY).* 2018;43:800-807.

9. Ferraioli G. Review of liver elastography guidelines. *J Ultrasound Med.* 2019;38:9-14.

10. Mederacke I, Wursthorn K, Kirschner J, et al. Food intake increases liver stiffness in patients with chronic or resolved hepatitis C virus infection. *Liver Int.* 2009;29:1500-1506.

11. Arena U, Lupsor Platon M, Stasi C, et al. Liver stiffness is influenced by a standardized meal in patients with chronic hepatitis C virus at different stages of fibrotic evolution. *Hepatology.* 2013;58:65-72.

12. Berzigotti A, De Gottardi A, Vukotic R, et al. Effect of meal ingestion on liver stiffness in patients with cirrhosis and portal hypertension. *PLoS One.* 2013;8:e58742.

13. Ferraioli G, Tinelli C, Lissandrin R, et al. Ultrasound point shear wave elastography assessment of liver and spleen stiffness: effect of training on repeatability of measurements. *Eur Radiol.* 2014;24:1283-1289.

14. Karlas T, Pfrepper C, Wiegand J, et al. Acoustic radiation force impulse imaging (ARFI) for non-invasive detection of liver fibrosis: examination standards and evaluation of interlobe differences in healthy subjects and chronic liver disease. *Scand J Gastroenterol.* 2011;46:1458-1467.

15. Horster S, Mandel P, Zachoval R, Clevert DA. Comparing acoustic radiation force impulse imaging to transient elastography to assess liver stiffness in healthy volunteers with and without Valsalva manoeuvre. *Clin Hemorheol Microcirc.* 2010;46:159-168.

16. Grgurevic I, Cikara I, Horvat J, et al. Noninvasive assessment of liver fibrosis with acoustic radiation force impulse imaging: increased liver and splenic stiffness in patients with liver fibrosis and cirrhosis. *Ultraschall Med.* 2011;32:160-166.

17. Toshima T, Shirabe K, Takeishi K, et al. New method for assessing liver fibrosis based on acoustic radiation force impulse: a special reference to the difference between right and left liver. *J Gastroenterol.* 2011;46:705-711.

18. Barr RG, Zhang Z. Effects of precompression on elasticity imaging of the breast: development of a clinically useful semiquantitative method of precompression assessment. *J Ultrasound Med.* 2012;31:895-902.

19. Wegner M, Iskender E, Azzarok A, Sagir A. Comparison of acoustic radiation force impulse imaging with the convex probe 6C1 and linear probe 9L4. *Medicine (Baltimore).* 2020;99:e19701.

20. Boursier J, Isselin G, Fouchard-Hubert I, et al. Acoustic radiation force impulse: a new ultrasonographic technology for the widespread noninvasive diagnosis of liver fibrosis. *Eur J Gastroenterol Hepatol.* 2010;22:1074-1084.

21. Yamashita H, Hachisuka Y, Kotegawa H, Fukuhara T, Kobayashi N. Effects of posture change on the hemodynamics of the liver. *Hepatogastroenterology.* 2004;51:1797-1800.

22. D'Onofrio M, Gallotti A, Mucelli RP. Tissue quantification with acoustic radiation force impulse imaging: measurement repeatability and normal values in the healthy liver. *AJR Am J Roentgenol.* 2010;195:132-136.

23. Hall TJ, Milkowski A, Garra B, et al. RSNA/QIBA:Shear wave speed as a biomarker for liver fibrosis staging. *Proc IEEE Int Ultrason Symp.* 2013;397-400.

24. Palmeri M, Nightingale K, Fielding S, et al. RSNA QIBA ultrasound shear wave speed Phase II phantom study in viscoelastic media. *Proc IEEE Int Ultrason Symp.* 2015;1-4.

25. Selzo MR, Rosenzweig SJ, Milkowski A. Obtaining equivalent liver shear wave speed measurements with multiple transducers. In: IEEE International Ultrasonics Symposium (IUS) 2018. 2018:1-4.

26. Ferraioli G, Maiocchi L, Lissandrin R, et al. Accuracy of the ElastPQ technique for the assessment of liver fibrosis in patients with chronic hepatitis C: a "real life" single center study. *J Gastrointestin Liver Dis.* 2016;25:331-335.

27. Ferraioli G, De Silvestri A, Reiberger T, et al. Adherence to quality criteria improves concordance between transient elastography and ElastPQ for liver stiffness assessment—a multicenter retrospective study. *Dig Liver Dis.* 2018;50:1056-1061.

28. Roccarina D, Iogna Prat L, Buzzetti E, et al. Establishing reliability criteria for liver ElastPQ shear wave elastography (ElastPQ-SWE): comparison between 10, 5 and 3 measurements. *Ultraschall Med.* 2021;42:204-213.

29. Boursier J, Cassinotto C, Hunault G, et al. Criteria to determine reliability of noninvasive assessment of liver fibrosis with virtual touch quantification. *Clin Gastroenterol Hepatol.* 2019;17:164-171.

30. Boursier J, Zarski JP, de Ledinghen V, et al. Determination of reliability criteria for liver stiffness evaluation by transient elastography. *Hepatology*. 2013;57:1182-1191.
31. Yoon HM, Cho YA, Kim JR, et al. Real-time two-dimensional shear-wave elastography for liver stiffness in children: interobserver variation and effect of breathing technique. *Eur J Radiol*. 2017;97:53-58.
32. Arena U, Vizzutti F, Corti G, et al. Acute viral hepatitis increases liver stiffness values measured by transient elastography. *Hepatology*. 2008;47:380-384.
33. Sagir A, Erhardt A, Schmitt M, et al. Transient elastography is unreliable for detection of cirrhosis in patients with acute liver damage. *Hepatology*. 2008;47:592-595.
34. Sousaris N, Barr RG. Sonographic elastography of mastitis. *J Ultrasound Med*. 2016;35:1791-1797.
35. Coco B, Oliveri F, Maina AM, et al. Transient elastography: a new surrogate marker of liver fibrosis influenced by major changes of transaminases. *J Viral Hepat*. 2006;14:360-369.
36. Park H, Kim SU, Kim D, et al. Optimal time for restoring the reliability of liver stiffness measurement in patients with chronic hepatitis B experiencing acute exacerbation. *J Clin Gastroenterol*. 2012;46:602-607.
37. Fung J, Lai CL, But D, et al. Reduction of liver stiffness following resolution of acute flares of chronic hepatitis B. *Hepatol Int*. 2010;4:716-722.
38. Trabut JB, Thépot V, Nalpas B, et al. Rapid decline of liver stiffness following alcohol withdrawal in heavy drinkers. *Alcohol Clin Exp Res*. 2012;36:1407-1411.
39. Nguyen-Khac E, Thiele M, Voican C, et al. Non-invasive diagnosis of liver fibrosis in patients with alcohol-related liver disease by transient elastography: an individual patient data meta-analysis. *Lancet Gastroenterol Hepatol*. 2018;3:614-625.
40. Millonig G, Reimann FM, Friedrich S, et al. Extrahepatic cholestasis increases liver stiffness (FibroScan) irrespective of fibrosis. *Hepatology*. 2008;48:1718-1723.
41. Lebray P, Varnous S, Charlotte F, Varaut A, Poynard T, Ratziu V. Liver stiffness is an unreliable marker of liver fibrosis in patients with cardiac insufficiency. *Hepatology*. 2008;48:2089.
42. Millonig G, Friedrich S, Adolf S, et al. Liver stiffness is directly influenced by central venous pressure. *J Hepatol*. 2010;52:206-210.
43. Colli A, Pozzoni P, Berzuini A, et al. Decompensated chronic heart failure: increased liver stiffness measured by means of transient elastography. *Radiology*. 2010;257:872-878.
44. Ferraioli G, Barr RG. Ultrasound liver elastography beyond liver fibrosis assessment. *World J Gastroenterol*. 2020;26:3413-3420.
45. Lanzi A, Gianstefani A, Mirarchi MG, Pini P, Conti F, Bolondi L. Liver AL amyloidosis as a possible cause of high liver stiffness values. *Eur J Gastroenterol Hepatol*. 2010;22:895-897.
46. Trifanov DS, Dhyani M, Bledsoe JR, et al. Amyloidosis of the liver on shear wave elastography: case report and review of literature. *Abdom Imaging*. 2015;40:3078-3083.
47. Ichikawa K, Narita Y, Ota Y, Komatsu N, Koike M. Transient elastography-derived liver stiffness measurements were found to be useful for predicting liver infiltration in a case of mature T-cell neoplasm involving liver dysfunction. *Int J Clin Exp Pathol*. 2015;8:4220-4226.
48. Gersak MM, Sorantin E, Windhaber J, Dudea SM, Riccabona M. The influence of acute physical effort on liver stiffness estimation using Virtual Touch Quantification (VTQ). Preliminary results. *Med Ultrason*. 2016;18:151-156.
49. Song P, Macdonald M, Behler R, et al. Two-dimensional shear-wave elastography on conventional ultrasound scanners with time-aligned sequential tracking (TAST) and comb-push ultrasound shear elastography (CUSE). *IEEE Trans Ultrason Ferroelectr Freq Control*. 2015;62:290-302.
50. Ferraioli G, Tinelli C, Zicchetti M, et al. Reproducibility of real-time shear wave elastography in the evaluation of liver elasticity. *Eur J Radiol*. 2012;81:3102-3106.
51. Castéra L, Foucher J, Bernard PH, et al. Pitfalls of liver stiffness measurement: a 5-year prospective study of 13,369 examinations. *Hepatology*. 2010;51:828-835.
52. Aitharaju V, De Silvestri A, Barr RG. Assessment of chronic liver disease by multiparametric ultrasound: results from a private practice outpatient facility. *Abdom Radiol (NY)*. 2021;46(11):5152-5161.
53. Ferraioli G, Tinelli C, Lissandrin R, et al. Point shear wave elastography method for assessing liver stiffness. *World J Gastroenterol*. 2014;20:4787-4796.
54. Bota S, Sporea I, Sirli R, Popescu A, Danila M, Costachescu D. Intra- and interoperator reproducibility of acoustic radiation force impulse (ARFI) elastography–preliminary results. *Ultrasound Med Biol*. 2012;38:1103-1108.

55. Guzmán-Aroca F, Reus M, Berná-Serna JD, et al. Reproducibility of shear wave velocity measurements by acoustic radiation force impulse imaging of the liver: a study in healthy volunteers. *J Ultrasound Med*. 2011;30:975-979.

56. Fraquelli M, Rigamonti C, Casazza G, et al. Reproducibility of transient elastography in the evaluation of liver fibrosis in patients with chronic liver disease. *Gut*. 2007;56:968-973.

57. Boursier J, Konate A, Gorea G, et al. Reproducibility of liver stiffness measurement by ultrasonographic elastometry. *Clin Gastroenterol Hepatol*. 2008;6:1263-1269.

58. Afdhal NH, Bacon BR, Patel K, et al. Accuracy of FibroScan, compared with histology, in analysis of liver fibrosis in patients with hepatitis B or C: a United States multicenter study. *Clin Gastroenterol Hepatol*. 2015;13:772-779.

59. Vuppalanchi R, Siddiqui MS, Van Natta ML, et al. Performance characteristics of vibration-controlled transient elastography for evaluation of nonalcoholic fatty liver disease. *Hepatology*. 2018;67:134-144.

60. Hall TJ, Milkowski A, Garra B, et al. RSNA/QIBA: shear wave speed as a biomarker for liver fibrosis staging. In: Ultrasonics Symposium (IUS), 2013 I.E. International 2013. 2013:397-400.

61. Palmeri M, Nightingale K, Fielding S, et al. RSNA QIBA ultrasound shear wave speed Phase II phantom study in viscoelastic media. In: Proceedings of the 2015 IEEE Ultrasonics Symposium, 2015. 2015:397-400.

62. Ferraioli G, De Silvestri A, Lissandrin R, et al. Evaluation of inter-system variability in liver stiffness measurements. *Ultraschall Med*. 2019;40:64-75.

63. Piscaglia F, Salvatore V, Mulazzani L, et al. Differences in liver stiffness values obtained with new ultrasound elastography machines and FibroScan: a comparative study. *Dig Liver Dis*. 2017;49:802-808.

CHAPTER 5

Tips and Tricks for Liver Stiffness Evaluation

Giovanna Ferraioli ■ Richard G. Barr

Before Scanning the Patient

It is important to remember that liver stiffness is measured, not liver fibrosis. Liver stiffness is influenced by fibrosis, inflammation, and congestion. Therefore obtaining clinical information before starting the examination is helpful. Important patient factors that can influence liver stiffness include elevated transaminase values, acute hepatitis, infiltrative diseases, alcohol ingestion, increased right heart pressure, deep inspiration, and recent ingestion of food. These factors all increase liver stiffness and would therefore overestimate the degree of liver fibrosis if cutoff tables are used.

It is also important to know the reason why the patient is undergoing ultrasound (US) examination and to know the etiology of liver disease (rule of 4 or 5 presented in Chapter 7 applicable only to viral hepatitis and nonalcoholic fatty liver disease [NAFLD]).[1,2] In patients with viral hepatitis under treatment or successfully treated, the liver stiffness values may be lower than expected even though the fibrosis stage is not changed (due to the resolution of inflammation). Knowing when the treatment was completed is helpful in analyzing the results. Always ask if the patient is under treatment or has been treated for any liver disease. The etiology is important, for example, in cases of amyloidosis or other diffuse infiltrating liver diseases because there could be an increase of stiffness not related to fibrosis. B-mode findings are important in patients with suspected or known liver disease. All focal liver lesions should be evaluated and included in the report. As discussed in Chapter 13, focal liver lesions in patients with chronic liver disease are concerning for possible hepatocellular carcinoma.

There is evidence that exercise increases liver stiffness, thus having the patient resting for 5–10 minutes before starting the examination is recommended. Eating can increase the liver stiffness value by increasing the blood flow through the portal vein, so asking the patient when they last ate is important. Ingestion of food can only elevate the liver stiffness, so it may not be necessary to cancel the examination if the patient ate and the liver stiffness is normal: in this case nothing else needs to be done. If the liver stiffness is elevated, a comment can be added to the report stating that the patient ate, and the liver stiffness value may be artificially elevated. This lets the referring doctor decide if a repeat study is needed.

If this is a follow-up examination, review of the previous study(ies) is important. The same US system, transducer, software, depth of measurement, and location will make comparison more accurate. In general, the error of measurement of all US elastography systems is +/– 10%. As discussed in other chapters of this book, there is variability between US systems, transducer frequency, and the depth of measurement.

During the Acquisition

PATIENT POSITIONING

Patient positioning is important especially in patients with high body mass index (BMI). A high-quality B-mode image is required for accurate liver stiffness measurements. Having the patient raise their right arm above their head to increase the intercostal space can be very helpful in acquiring accurate liver stiffness measurements. The B-mode image in the location of the measurement should be free of artifacts before turning on elastography. The signal intensity of the liver should be uniform to confirm there is no partial shadowing. Many of the US techniques to optimize B-mode imaging, such as compounding and harmonic imaging, are not compatible with shear wave imaging and are automatically turned off when in elastography mode. Therefore there will be a decrease in the imaging quality of the liver in the elastography mode. Confirming that the B-mode image is free of artifacts BEFORE turning on elastography is important because, in the elastography mode, some B-mode artifacts may not be as apparent. Scanning the liver at several intercostal locations should be performed to find a location with fewer large vessels and bile ducts. This can be done during a limited or complete US examination if performed before the elastography. Generally, the supine position is used. However, in obese subjects, a slight left side decubitus, not more than 30 degrees, can be helpful. To achieve this position, a pillow can be placed under the upper right side of the patient. If greater decubitus positions are used, there can be an increase of the pressure in the inferior vena cava, which is transmitted to the hepatic veins and therefore increases the liver stiffness value.

PLACEMENT OF THE MEASUREMENT BOX

Using the penetration setting (if available on the system) can help by increasing the energy deposition of the push-pulse as well as improving the B-mode tracking of the shear waves. On most systems the area of maximum energy deposition and therefore the best shear wave generation is at 4.0–4.5 cm from the transducer. Every attempt to take the measurement in this location should be made. In point shear wave elastography (pSWE) the region of interest (ROI) must be placed 1.5–2.0 cm from the liver capsule to avoid the reverberation artifact. In two-dimensional shear wave elastography (2D-SWE), if a confidence or quality map is available, the reverberation artifact can be seen and avoided. However, it must be highlighted that, since reverberation artifacts may give rise to signals that appear as good quality also because they are stable over time, the confidence or quality map may not recognize them. Therefore it is critical to look also at the velocity/elasticity map that will depict areas of increased stiffness in the upper part of the field of view (FOV) due to the reverberation artifact to avoid measurements in that area. If the reverberation artifact is less than 1.5–2.0 cm when seen on 2D-SWE, the measurement box can be placed closer to the liver capsule, avoiding the artifact. This cannot be done on pSWE as the artifact is not seen. This is extremely helpful in patients with a large thickness of subcutaneous tissue, allowing the measurement box to be placed closer to the optimal area. To maximize the push energy, the transducer must be parallel to the liver capsule both in the superior and inferior planes and the right to left plane (see Fig. 4.4). With correct positioning of the transducer, the liver capsule should be a sharp bright line and visualized in most of the image, especially where the measurements will be taken. Some vendors recommend applying pressure with the transducer to compress the subcutaneous tissue to place the measurement box closer to the optimal 4.0–4.5 cm from the transducer and to avoid the reverberation artifact. With the intercostal approach this maneuver does not compress the liver.

LIMITING MOTION

The shear waves only travel over a few millimeters before being attenuated, especially in steatotic or fibrotic livers. So motion during the acquisition both by the patient or the examiner leads to inaccurate measurements. With deep inspiration there is a change in the right atrial pressure, which is transmitted to the liver, affecting the stiffness measurement. Measurements should be taken in a neutral (mid) breathing breath hold. In pediatric patients or patients with pulmonary disease in whom a breath hold may not be possible, the use of a real-time 2D-SWE technique can be helpful. By obtaining a clip of approximately 30 seconds in shallow breathing, a review of the cine clip can identify frames where motion is limited and a neutral breathing position is present. Measurement can then be obtained on one of these frames, choosing it from a short sequence of the images with stable signals. It is recommended to perform only one measurement for each cine clip, otherwise a possible error made during that acquisition will be multiplied. Using pSWE in patients unable to hold their breath, the measurement could be taken at the end of the expiratory phase, taking advantage of the little delay between each respiratory phase. However, this requires a lot of experience and absolute absence of transducer movements.

NUMBER OF MEASUREMENTS

For pSWE, 10 independent measurements should be obtained. In difficult patients, a smaller number can be obtained; however, at least five measurements are required as long as the quality measures are maintained. For 2D-SWE, five independent measurements (one from each cine clip with real-time 2D-SWE) should be obtained. A review of the measurements and deleting those that are discrepant is not appropriate. If the measurement was obtained improperly (motion, angling transducer, etc.), it should not be placed in the report page. The median value is used as two single extreme measurements (very high and very low) and do not affect the median whereas they can significantly affect the mean (average). If measurements at different locations in the liver are of interest, a complete set of measurements for each location should be obtained. As there is a depth dependance of the acoustic radiation force impulse (ARFI) techniques, acquisitions in different locations for one measurement will add variability into the results.

PLACEMENT OF THE ROI BOX

Placement of the measurement box is critical. It should be placed in a region where the quality measures are of highest quality. Both the confidence/quality map and velocity/elasticity map should be assessed for artifacts. Although the confidence/quality maps are good, they are not perfect and areas of color map differences in the velocity/elasticity map should be considered possible artifact (Fig. 5.1). As reported in Chapter 6, artifacts are generated also around blood vessels (Fig. 5.2). Therefore, because in pSWE the visualization of artifacts is not possible, it is critical that the ROI be placed in a region at least 5 mm from vessels and bile ducts. Remember that the generation of shear waves is a three-dimensional process (same as throwing a stone in water), and artifacts can be generated from vessels and bile ducts adjacent to the plane being imaged. The size of the measurement box in pSWE is fixed by all vendors and cannot be changed. In 2D-SWE the size of the measurement box can be adjusted to limit taking a measurement in a region with artifacts or enlarged to average more liver tissue (if free of artifacts).

2D-SWE: SIZE OF THE FIELD OF VIEW/ROI AND OF THE MEASUREMENT BOX

In some US systems the FOV/ROI may be fixed. In others it may be adjustable within a defined range. In general, having the FOV/ROI at the vendor default is most appropriate in the majority of cases. Making the box too large may limit the accuracy of the shear wave estimate as the ARFI pulses are spread farther apart. It is critical the FOV/ROI be parallel to the transducer as well as the liver capsule.

HOW TO USE THE MANUFACTURER QUALITY PARAMETERS

All vendors have some form of quality parameters (see Chapter 4). Some have more than one, and all should be used in assessing the quality of the data.

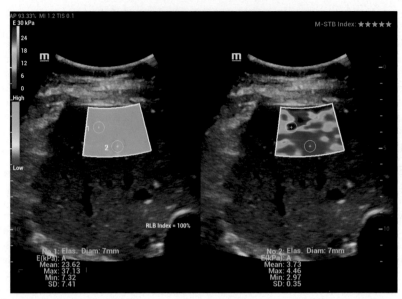

Fig. 5.1 Although the quality measures are good, they are not perfect. Evaluation of both the quality/confidence map *(left)* and the velocity/elasticity map *(right)* is required for accurate measurements. In this image, there are *five green stars* confirming no motion, and the confidence map is all green, suggesting no artifacts. However, on the velocity/elasticity map, it is clear that there is reverberation artifact near the liver capsule *(red)*, as shown by the high stiffness value on the bottom left side of the image, and other artifacts present.

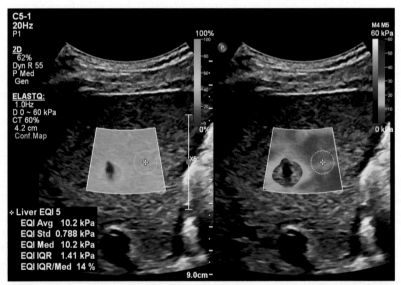

Fig. 5.2 This figure demonstrates the artifact that is seen adjacent to vessels. On the velocity/elasticity map *(right)* a blood vessel is seen near the center of the image. Note that the area around the vessel does not color as the system detects this as an artifact. But in addition, the *yellow and teal areas* around the vessel are also artifacts and should be avoided. The quality map *(left)* demonstrates the majority of the artifact as poor quality *(yellow and red)*; however, some of the artifact *(the yellow and teal on the velocity/elasticity map)* is listed as high quality.

Assessing Motion Artifact with Real-Time 2D-SWE

Although motion is somewhat included in all quality maps, there are some systems that have quality assessment specific for motion (Fig. 5.3). Also, when using a real-time 2D-SWE, collecting a cine clip of multiple frames can be used to evaluate for motion. After collecting the clip, images without motion can be found by reviewing the B-mode images from the clip.

Assessing Shear Wave Quality

Many vendors have a quality index or confidence map that grades the quality of the shear waves either on a color or numerical scale. This map or index usually evaluates the height of the displacement curves, the noise in the displacement curves, the linearity of the time-to-peak to distance from ARFI pulse curve, and the signal-to-noise of the shear waves. It is recommended to use the vendor's specific instruction on how to use their index/map. Chapter 4 gives a detailed presentation of the vendors quality criteria. Examples of evaluation of quality are presented in Figs. 5.4–5.10.

Standard Deviation of a Given Measurement

Some systems provide a standard deviation of an individual acquisition (different than the interquartile range/median [IQR/M]) (Fig. 5.11). As a general rule, when the standard deviation is greater than 30% of the reported value, the measurement is poor.

Interquartile Range/Median

As discussed in Chapter 4, the IQR/M is a quality measure that assesses the sum of the measurements taken. When the IQR/M is >30% in kilopascals or >15% in meters per second, the quality of the data set is unreliable.

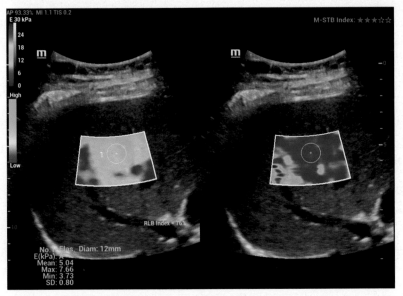

Fig. 5.3 Some vendors have a quality measure that evaluates motion as well as a quality/confidence map. In this image the *three red stars* in the upper right (M-STB) inform that there is motion in the image and the image is not acceptable for measurement. Also, the confidence map has an *area of purple,* depicting areas of poor quality. The reliability index (RLB) in the measurement box is 76%: it should be 100% for an accurate measurement.

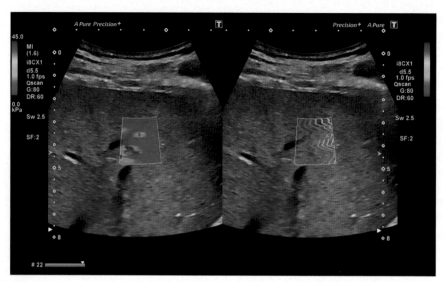

Fig. 5.4 In the Canon systems, the propagation map can be used to identify artifacts. In the liver where the tissue stiffness should be similar, the propagation lines should be parallel and at the same distance. If there are artifacts, the shear wave velocity will change and the lines will not be parallel. In this image note that propagation lines *(right image)* are not parallel due to the artifact from the hepatic vein located on the left side of the region of interest. Note the artifactually high *(red)* velocities in the velocity/elasticity map *(left)* due to the artifact.

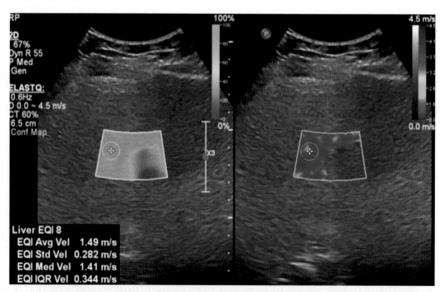

Fig. 5.5 In this image there is a large area of *red/yellow* in the confidence map. It corresponds to an *area of shadowing* in the velocity map. Note that the echogenicity of the liver is not uniform. In the area of poor quality, the liver is hypoechoic to the rest of the liver representing shadowing. Also note that in this case the liver capsule is not identified as a bright white line suggesting poor technique.

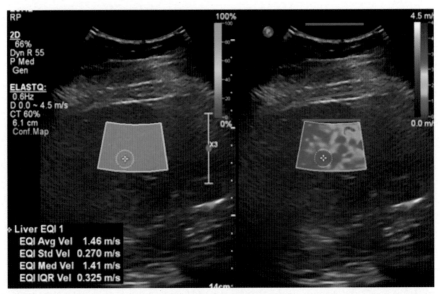

Fig. 5.6 In this case the liver capsule is a bright, sharp line; however, it is not parallel to the liver capsule of the region of interest *(red lines)*. This results in a velocity map *(right)* with many artifacts *(teal, yellow and red areas)*, but the confidence map *(left)* does not recognize these as areas of low confidence.

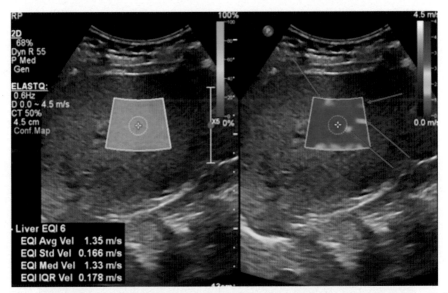

Fig. 5.7 It is important to remember that shear waves are generated in 3D (like throwing a stone in the water). Therefore, if vessels are immediately out of plane, reverberation artifact from them can occur. In the velocity map there are several teal areas *(red arrows)* that do not match the rest of the velocity map and are artifacts from vessels just outside the imaging plane. Note they are not identified as artifacts in the confidence map *(left image)*. The teal area in the bottom of the velocity map is due to poor signal-to-noise of the shear waves because of attenuation of the acoustic radiation force imaging pulse at that depth.

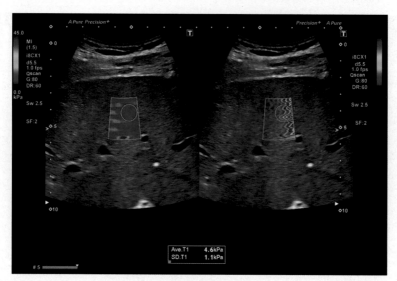

Fig. 5.8 The measurement is correctly taken at 4 cm in the center of the image and with the liver capsule parallel to the transducer. However, the propagation map *(right image)* (which is an indicator of the quality of shear waves) warns that the measurement has a poor quality because the lines are not parallel and at the same distance. Moreover, the elasticity map *(right image)* has a heterogenous distribution of colors.

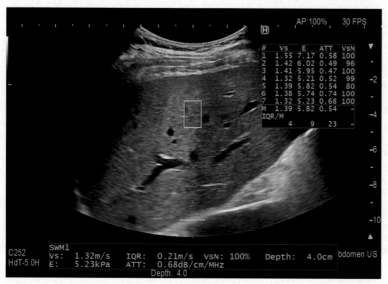

Fig. 5.9 The vendor's quality factor (VsN: ≥50%, in the last column on the upper right side of the image) indicates that these seven acquisitions are of a good quality. However, there are several mistakes that were made: the region of interest is too close to the liver capsule, a vessel is nearby the region of interest, and the liver capsule is not parallel to the transducer.

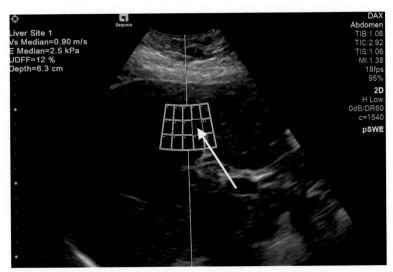

Fig. 5.10   In the Siemens one push point shear wave elastography *(pSWE)*, the technique acquires 15 pSWE measurements. If a measurement is of poor quality (same as xxx for single measurement pSWE) the poor-quality measurement is depicted by not having a box with dots *(arrow)*.

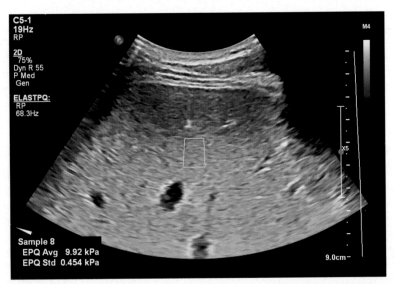

Fig. 5.11   In point shear wave elastography the standard deviation *(Std)* of the measurements taken within the measurement box can be used as a quality measure. A Std of >30% suggests a poor measurement because it suggests substantial variability of the stiffness in the measurement box. That variability is most likely due to other structures such as blood vessels in the measurement box. In this case the Std is 5% (0.454/9.92 kPa), suggesting a good measurement.

CONFOUNDERS AND THE ROLE OF B-MODE ULTRASOUND

There are several confounding factors that can affect the liver stiffness measurement. Trying to eliminate them or at least documenting them is important. Although questioning of the patient can help, they often can give incorrect information. Tricks that may be helpful in detecting confounding factors include:

- Eating: sometimes the patient does not give the correct information. Check for a contracted gallbladder suggesting a recent meal.
- Check the inferior vena cava/hepatic veins for dilation, suggesting increased right heart pressure.
- Confirm the inferior vena cava contracts to >50% with respiration to confirm increased right heart pressure is unlikely.
- Ask patient about their recent alcohol intake. Look for signs of alcohol abuse including a review of the patient's chart.
- Review the chart for recent transaminase levels.

Most confounding factors increase the liver stiffness, therefore liver stiffness values in the normal range may confidently exclude the presence of liver fibrosis.

When a definite diagnosis of liver cirrhosis on B-mode US is made but stiffness value is lower than expected, it should be reported that the patient has cirrhosis and that some patients with cirrhosis can have lower than expected liver stiffness values. As explained in Chaper 7, in patients with chronic viral hepatitis undergoing antiviral treatment or after treatment the rule of 4 with ARFI techniques or rule of 5 with vibration controlled transient elastography (VCTE) are no longer applicable. A baseline measurement after treatment should be obtained and the delta change be used to determine if there is progression or regression of disease.

LIVER STEATOSIS

There are conflicting results in the literature about the effect of liver steatosis on the measurement of liver stiffness. With steatosis there is attenuation of both the ARFI pulse and the shear waves, which makes measurements less accurate due to the decrease in signal-to-noise. Therefore measurements are more variable in these patients, and this may account for the conflicting results in the literature.

TRANSDUCER FREQUENCY

In the ARFI techniques the shear wave speed is related to the mean ARFI frequency. Therefore, with a higher frequency transducer, the ARFI frequency is most likely higher and will estimate higher stiffness values. The guidelines assume the use of a standard abdominal transducer in the range of 3–5 MHz. So, for example, when a linear higher frequency transducer is used in pediatric patients, the cutoff values will be different, and it is recommended that vendor-specific cutoffs in this case be used. One vendor (Siemens Healthineers) has adjusted all their transducers that can be used for liver stiffness measurement to provide the same value (calibrated to their C5 transducer).[3] When vendors upgrade the system with newer software or hardware, there may be a change in the stiffness values; therefore be aware that this may lead to more variability on repeat studies.

WHAT TO DO IF ACCURATE MEASUREMENTS CANNOT BE OBTAINED

There are a small number of patients whose accurate liver stiffness values cannot be obtained. This is reported to be about 5% of patients but will vary depending on your locality.[4] In patients with high BMI, with a very steatotic liver, or who are unable to cooperate with the study, it may not be possible to make an accurate assessment of liver stiffness despite using all the tips and tricks listed above. If less than 60% of the measurements attempted (assuming done correctly) are bad measurements (no value on pSWE, no coloring, or all low confidence on the quality/confidence map for 2D-SWE), additional measurements should not be attempted. These patients should be reported that accurate liver stiffness could not be obtained.

After Data Acquisition, Before the Patient Is Discharged

After completion of data acquisition, the results should be reviewed before discharging the patient. Confirmation that an IQR/M of ≤30% for measurements in kilopascals or ≤15% for measurement in meters per second was obtained should be made. If this quality measure is not achieved, it is important to determine the reason. If the patient is not a difficult patient, consider repeating the study at a different acoustic window. The overall quality of the facility and individuals performing the examination can be monitored by the IQR/M over time and suggest if additional training may be needed.

If the results are different than expected, such as the patient has a normal-appearing liver, but the results suggest compensated advanced chronic liver disease (cACLD), question the patient for possible confounding factors.

Reporting Results

In reporting results, the system and transducer used should be reported so repeat studies can be done on the same system (and software) if possible. The technique used (VCTE, pSWE, or 2D-SWE) should be documented. The number of valid measurements taken along with the median value and IQR/M should be included. A statement should be included if the IQR/M suggests a high-quality data set (≤30% for measurements taken in kilopascals or ≤15% for measurements taken in meters per second) or poor-quality data set. The liver stiffness value can be reported either in kilopascals or in meters per second; however, providing both is helpful, as the preference varies depending on the referring physician. Most systems provide the results in both kilopascals and meters per second in their report page. The report should suggest the degree of liver fibrosis based on the rule of 4 (pSWE and 2D-SWE) or rule of 5 (VCTE) for patients with viral hepatitis or NAFLD. It is preferred to give a likelihood of normal/probability of cACLD instead of using cutoff values based on histology.

The report should also include a list of possible confounding factors and their possible effect on the assessment of liver fibrosis. If appropriate, the following should be added: in the setting of elevated transaminase levels; nonfasting, vascular congestion; etc., the stage of liver fibrosis may be overestimated. A discussion considering other factors should be included such as the type of liver disease, if the patient is being treated or has been treated for a liver disease, and if any other liver disease is present (e.g., amyloidosis) that may complicate interpretation of the liver stiffness measurement. All focal lesions should be documented with size and image characterization and commented on as benign, indeterminate, or high suspicion for malignancy.

Although guidelines now recommend reporting results as probability of cACLD, for those who would like a value to rule out significant fibrosis, most studies that used ARFI techniques (pSWE and 2D-SWE) suggest that a liver stiffness value of less than 7 kPa (1.5 m/s) can help rule out significant fibrosis.[1]

Alanine aminotransferase adopted cutoff values of liver stiffness that have been reported as improving liver fibrosis assessment in patients with chronic hepatitis B[5]; however, the use of these cutoffs is not recommended.[1]

For patients with NAFLD, liver stiffness values of >9 kPa (1.7 m/s) are suggestive of cACLD. However, in some patients with NAFLD and cACLD, the stiffness value may be between 7 and 9 kPa, and additional testing or follow-up should be recommended in these patients.[1]

KEY POINTS

1. Asking appropriate questions before the examination is started is important.
2. For follow-up studies use the same system, transducer, and software if possible. Make measurements at the same depth and similar location.
3. Use B-mode findings to identify possible confounding factors (elevated right atrial pressure, nonfasting state).
4. Spend time to find the best acoustical window free of artifacts to perform the examination.
5. Always follow the protocol, and use tips and tricks listed above, particularly in difficult patients to maximize the probability of getting accurate results.
6. Placement of the measurement box in both 2D-SWE and pSWE is critical for accurate measurements.
7. Perform the examination with the liver capsule and ROI/measurement box parallel to the transducer (i.e., three parallel lines).
8. Use the IQR/M as a quality measure of the study. It can also be used to evaluate the quality of the laboratory and persons performing the examination to determine if further training could be helpful.
9. The report should be complete with all the information needed for someone else to repeat the study if done at a different facility.
10. The report should include a statement if the results are of good or poor quality (IQR/M).
11. The conclusion should provide the probability of cACLD and recommend additional testing if needed.
12. The report should note if confounding factors were present and how they could affect the liver stiffness estimate.
13. The report should also include if any focal liver lesion is present and provide an indication if the lesion(s) are benign, indeterminate, or suggestive of malignancy.

References

1. Barr RG, Wilson SR, Rubens D, Garcia-Tsao G, Ferraioli G. Update to the Society of Radiologists in Ultrasound Liver Elastography Consensus Statement. *Radiology.* 2020;296:263-274.
2. de Franchis R, Baveno VI Faculty. Expanding consensus in portal hypertension: report of the Baveno VI Consensus Workshop: stratifying risk and individualizing care for portal hypertension. *J Hepatol.* 2015;63:743-752.
3. Selzo MR, Rosenzweig SJ, Milkowski A. Obtaining equivalent liver shear wave speed measurements with multiple transducers. In: *2018 IEEE International Ultrasonics Symposium (IUS).* IEEE; 2018.
4. Aitharaju V, De Silvestri A, Barr RG. Assessment of chronic liver disease by multiparametric ultrasound: results from a private practice outpatient facility. *Abdom Radiol (NY).* 2021;46:5152-5161.
5. Zeng J, Zheng J, Jin JY, et al. Shear wave elastography for liver fibrosis in chronic hepatitis B: adapting the cut-offs to alanine aminotransferase levels improves accuracy. *Eur Radiol.* 2019;29:857-865.

CHAPTER 6

Artifacts in Liver Stiffness Evaluation

Spencer Moavenzadeh ■ Mark L. Palmeri ■ Giovanna Ferraioli ■
Richard G. Barr

Overview of Artifacts in Liver Shear Wave Elastography

The use of shear wave elastography techniques proves valuable in providing qualitative and quantitative elasticity maps of the liver. There are, however, common disturbances that can affect the tissue measurements of stiffness. Image artifacts, signals that appear present on the image but are not present in the body, can result in overestimation, underestimation, and highly variable calculations of tissue stiffness maps.[1] Several artifacts can influence stiffness measurements for most techniques, most notably ultrasound-based techniques. These include:

- Poor acoustic windows that result in both limited push and tracking penetration and cause high variability in elasticity measurement and rib or lung shadowing, which produce further instabilities in elasticity values.[2] Poor signal-to-noise ratio in the shear wave data or the resultant shear wave speed reconstructions is commonly reported on commercial systems through quality metrics and images.[3]
- Cardiac pulsatility artifacts that result from both the creation of natural shear waves from a high heart rate and the presence of pulsating vessels near the region of interest.[2]
- Liver boundary, or Glisson capsule, artifacts due to interactions with portal vessels and the distortion of shear wave motion around the liver capsule.[4]
- Tissue viscosity that causes both vibration-frequency dependent shear wave speeds, especially when comparing measurements between modalities, and overestimation bias due to reconstruction assumptions of pure elasticity.[5-7]
- Tissue nonlinearity such that stiffness changes nonlinearly with strain due to extracellular matrix heterogeneity and is underestimated when calculated with linear assumptions.[8]
- Motion artifacts due to patient motion and natural motion from breathing.[4]
- Shear wave reflection artifacts due to stiffness gradients within the liver.[9]
- Nonperpendicular probe placement that results in nonlinear signal decay and liver stiffness overestimation.[4]
- Compression with the probe/nonlinear tissue response.

VIBRATION CONTROLLED TRANSIENT ELASTOGRAPHY

Vibration controlled transient elastography (VCTE) relies upon external, mechanical vibration to induce shear waves within tissue. The shear waves are tracked via Doppler-like ultrasound techniques from which Young's modulus can be calculated, assuming homogenous, isotropic, and elastic behavior.[4] There are, however, limitations with VCTE and difficulties in interpretation. For example, without controlled probe compression force, the excitation can distort and decrease in center-frequency, resulting in lower stiffness measurements.[10] Excessive compression can also lead to nonlinear stiffening of the compressed tissues. Similarly, without proper damping of the mechanical vibration, duplicate shear waves may be induced, and regression algorithms may misrepresent actual tissue elasticity. These artifacts that were observed with the first version of the FibroScan are less evident in the subsequent versions by controlling the vibration.

ACOUSTIC RADIATION FORCE IMPULSE TECHNIQUES ARTIFACTS

Both general ultrasound limitations and limitations of acoustic radiation force impulse (ARFI) techniques result in tissue stiffness variability estimations. The most common sources of artifacts in ARFI are a poor acoustic window (Fig. 6.1), limited penetration (Fig. 6.2), organ shadows (Fig. 6.3), vessel pulsation (Fig. 6.4), loss of signal (Fig. 6.5), reverberations within the liver

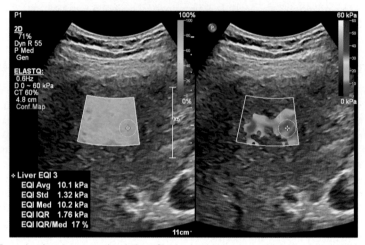

Fig. 6.1 Example of a poor acoustic window. Shadowing is present on both the right and left side of the B-mode image. Of the elasticity map *(on the right),* 50% has no coloring due to the shadowing. Note that the liver capsule is not a bright white line, suggesting that the transducer is also not parallel to the liver capsule. The confidence map on the left confirms poor quality of the elasticity map. The measurement box was placed in an area with medium-high confidence on the confidence map. However, with the poor acoustic window, the measurement should not be used.

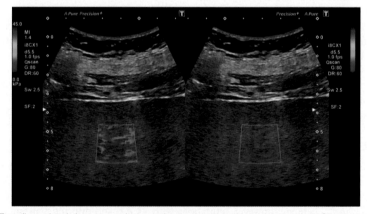

Fig. 6.2 Two-dimensional shear wave elastography measurement in an obese patient. Signal dropout due to limited penetration. There is a thick subcutaneous tissue (>3 cm) that decreases the strength of the push-pulse, leading to a low signal-to-noise in the estimate of tissue stiffness. For this reason, a large part of the elasticity map is void of color. Note that the region of interest (ROI) has been positioned 1.5 cm below the Glisson capsule, as per guidelines; however, the center of the ROI is already at 5.5 cm from the transducer: this is not an optimal location because the maximum strength of the ultrasound is at 4–4.5 cm from the transducer. Tips: in cases like this one, the ROI can be moved closer to the liver capsule, making sure that reverberation artifacts are not present in the proximal portion of the ROI. However, it should be acknowledged that there is a rate of failures in the liver stiffness measurement.

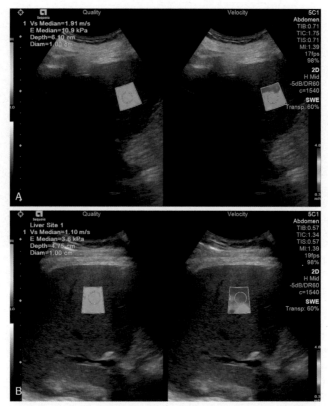

Fig. 6.3 Image taken in the supine position at rib level where lung artifact and rib artifact are present (A). Stiffness measurement in the same patient position but moving down two rib levels (B). Note that, when correctly taken, the liver stiffness is 3.6 kPa (B), whereas, taken incorrectly (A), the liver stiffness is 10.9 kPa.

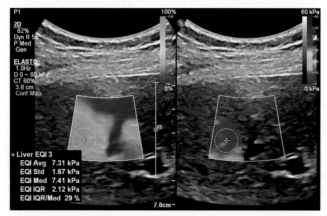

Fig. 6.4 In this image the liver capsule is a bright white line and almost parallel to the top of the elasticity map. Note that there is no coloring around the portal vessel, which was included in the field of view. This is due to both vessel pulsations and reverberation of the shear waves off the vessel wall. The small color-coded *(blue and green)* area on the left side of the elasticity map is mainly due to artifacts generated by the vessel pulsation. The confidence map *(on the left side)* detects the majority of artifacts, showing them in *red* and *yellow*, except the one due to vessel pulsation on the bottom left side of the field of view *(green)*. The measurement in this area is incorrect and leads to an overestimation of liver stiffness.

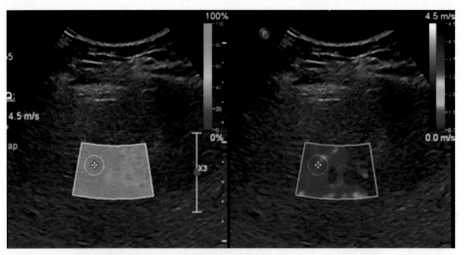

Fig. 6.5 Although the acoustic radiation force impulse pulse generates the shear waves, it is the B-mode imaging that tracks the displacements caused by the shear waves and uses that information to estimate the shear wave speed. In this case the B-mode image is of poor quality with low signal intensity leading to poor quality liver stiffness measurement.

(Figs. 6.6 and 6.7), and motion artifacts (Fig. 6.8).[2] Proper placement of the region of interest within the liver can reduce many potential artifacts. Additionally, ARFI is more susceptible to shear wave dispersion effects than fixed excitation frequency methods such as VCTE and magnetic resonance elastography (MRE); in a viscoelastic medium, shear wave velocity is dispersive, meaning velocities vary with frequency, and ARFI shear wave speed estimations can be biased based on the specific imaging system used.[5]

Shear waves propagating across tissue stiffness gradients both in and out of the imaging plane can cause image artifacts in shear wave reconstruction in the ARFI techniques (Fig. 6.9).[9] The magnitude of the reflected shear wave is a function of mechanical contrast between adjacent tissues, with greater shear impedance mismatches causing higher energy reflected waves. Two-dimensional shear wave elastography (2D-SWE) techniques track shear waves in a small, two-dimensional region of interest following a series of push-pulses to create plane shear waves. 2D-SWE reconstruction algorithms often assume homogeneity and that the propagation of shear waves is unidirectionally outwards from the focal zone. Reconstructing images while assuming tissue homogeneity in presence of reflections from tissue stiffness gradients can cause reconstruction artifacts and underestimation of tissue stiffness. Directional filters can be used to help reduce the influence of reflected shear waves that are propagating in directions not consistent with what the shear wave sources could generate (Fig. 6.10).[9]

There are two common types of vessel-ARFI technique artifacts impacting tissue elasticity measurements (Figs. 6.11 and 6.12). Pulsations around the branches of the portal vein can cause motion-pulsatility artifacts.[2] The increased stiffness of the portal vessel wall also biases estimates toward elevated elasticity near the liver capsule. Similarly, signal dropout within other vessels due to the nonviscous nature of blood that prevents shear wave propagation can cause signal dropout.

Cardiac reverberations are a significant source of variability in stiffness measurement on the left lobe of the liver (Fig. 6.13). Shadowing from the ribs and lungs on the left lobe of the liver also reduces the intensity of the detection beams in this region, yielding highly variable elasticity values (Fig. 6.14).

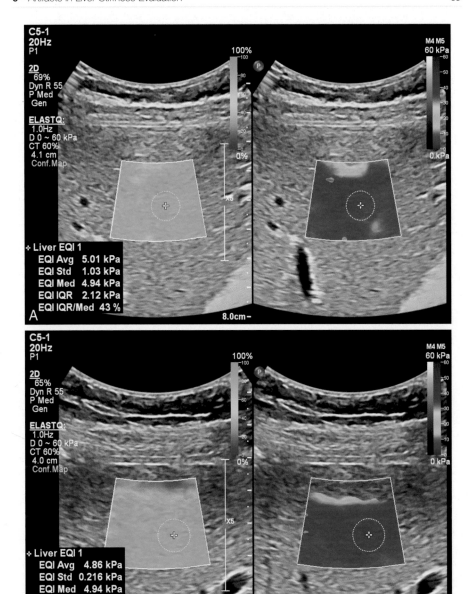

Fig. 6.6 Reverberation artifact below the liver capsule. (A) The elasticity map helps in identifying the artifact, which appears as an area of increased stiffness in the upper part of the image. Note that the confidence map, even though set at a high threshold (60%), is not able to identify the artifact because it is stable over time. Another area of increased stiffness is also seen in far field *(right side)*: it is due to a vessel crossing the region of interest just out of the plane. (B) In this other case, the confidence map detects the artifact below the liver capsule, and most of the area is left blank in the elasticity map.

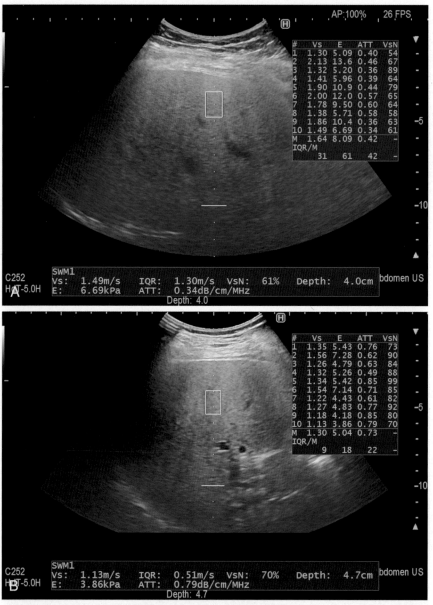

Fig. 6.7 A 57-year-old woman with liver steatosis. (A) The region of interest for liver stiffness measurement is placed at 4.0 cm from the transducer; kk, it is too close to the liver capsule (<1 cm). Moreover, the liver capsule is not parallel to the transducer. Even though the quality criterion of the manufacturer is fulfilled (i.e., VsN >50%), there is a high variability of the stiffness values that range from 5.09 kPa (1.30 m/s) to 13.6 kPa (2.13 m/s), leading to an interquartile range/median *(IQR/M)* of 61% for measurements in kilopascals and 31% for measurements in meters per second. (B) Acquisitions made in another intercostal space and correctly holding the transducer. The median stiffness value is within the normal range, and the IQR/M is within the recommended range. The high stiffness values observed in (A) are likely due to reverberation artifacts.

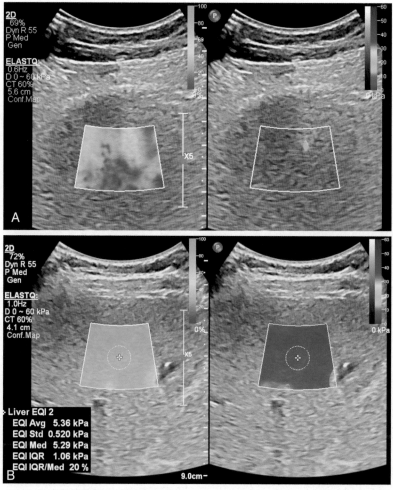

Fig. 6.8 When there is motion, the field of view will not fill with color due to an inability to accurately estimate liver stiffness value (A). (B) Image obtained in the same patient with suspended breathing and limited motion.

Compression of the tissues with the transducer can cause increased stiffness.[11] Protocol stress measurements must be made by an intercostal approach, which limits the ability to compress the liver with the transducer. If an intercostal approach is not used (e.g., a substernal approach), the liver can be compressed with the transducer, leading to over estimation of the liver stiffness (Fig. 6.15).

Additional reviews of ARFI artifacts are available.[12-14]

MAGNETIC RESONANCE ELASTOGRAPHY ARTIFACTS

MRE, as a phase-contrast magnetic resonance imaging (MRI) technique, is subject to unique artifacts specific to MRI. Most directly, paramagnetic materials, such as embolization coils, transjugular intrahepatic shunts, or metallic clips in or adjacent to the liver, can all cause interference, loss of signal intensity, and underestimation of tissue stiffness.[15] The large impact of these

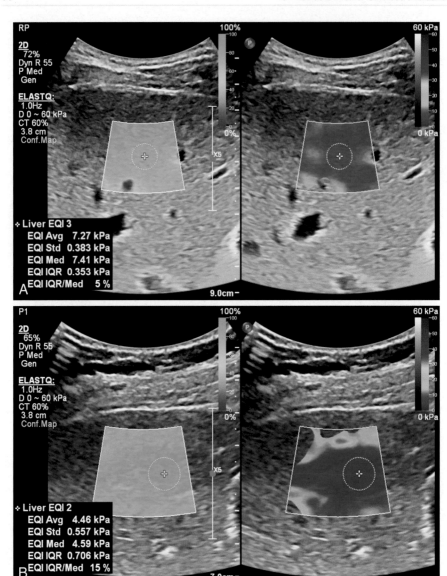

Fig. 6.9 Shear waves are generated in three dimensions just like tossing a stone in water where the ripples are the shear waves. (A) In this case, artifacts from vessels just outside the imaging plane can be seen on the left edge of the elasticity map *(light blue areas)*. Note that the confidence map *(green)* suggests that these artifacts are signals of high quality. These artifacts were not included in the measurement box. A similar artifact showing a false increase of stiffness can be seen around the vessels that appear in the left side and at bottom of the elasticity map: they were detected by the confidence map *(red and yellow colors)*. It is important to always evaluate BOTH the confidence map and the elasticity map to assess for artifacts. (B) Artifacts due to a vessel just outside the imaging plane can be seen in the lower part of the elasticity map, both on the right and the left side. Note the reverberation artifacts below the Glisson capsule.

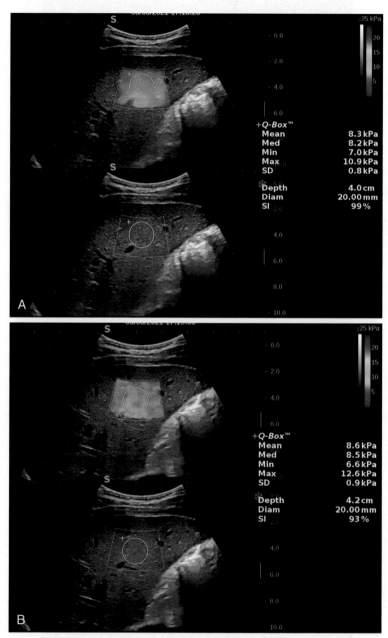

Fig. 6.10   The use of filters applied by the vendor helps eliminate some artifacts by detecting and/or eliminating reverberation and other artifacts. Note the difference in (A) filters applied and (B) filters not applied. Note the small areas of *red* and more *yellow* at the bottom of the image in (B) that are filtered out when the filters are applied. Note that there is a small change in the liver stiffness between A and B.

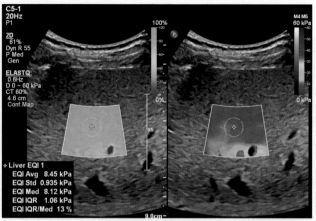

Fig. 6.11 Artifact due to vessel pulsation. There is a false increase of liver stiffness around a branch of the portal vein that crosses the region of interest in the far field *(right side)*. This artifact is due to the pulsation induced by the hepatic artery that accompanies the portal vein. The confidence map detects the artifact highlighting it with the *red* color.

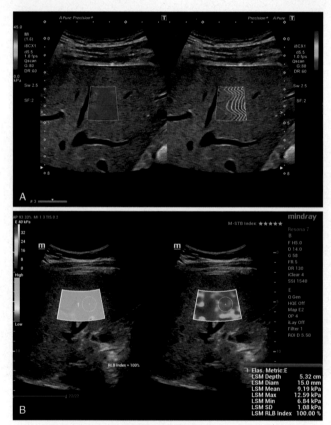

Fig. 6.12 Signal dropout artifact due to vessels. (A) This image shows that there is loss of color signal around the hepatic vein (on the *left side* of the elasticity map). The propagation map shows that the front of the lines is interrupted, and the lines are distorted and unevenly spaced. This artifact is due to the lack of propagation of the shear waves in the fluids. (B) Branches of the hepatic vein have been included in the elasticity map *(on the right side)*: note that around the vessels there is a false decrease of liver stiffness coded with *dark blue* color. The reliability map *(on the left side)* fails in detecting this artifact. The measurement box is correctly positioned away from this artifact.

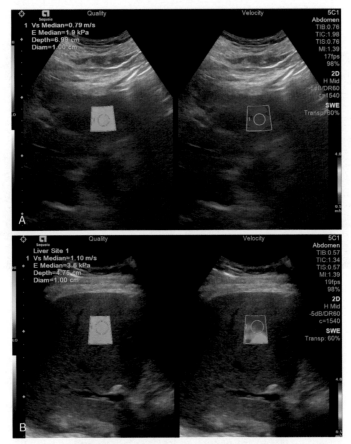

Fig. 6.13 Attempt at taking a liver stiffness measurement in the left lobe of the liver via a substernal approach (A). Although a measurement showing good confidence is obtained, the liver stiffness value of 1.9 kPa is significantly different than (B) the measurement obtained using the recommended protocol in the right lobe of the liver, which has a liver stiffness value of 3.6 kPa.

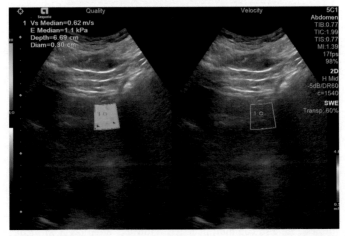

Fig. 6.14 An attempt of obtaining liver stiffness measurement via a left intercostal approach demonstrates the problems of rib shadowing and other artifacts when trying to use this window. Note that the stiffness value of 1.1 kPa is different than the value obtained using the recommended protocol in the right lobe of the liver 3.6 kPa (same patient as in Fig. 6.13).

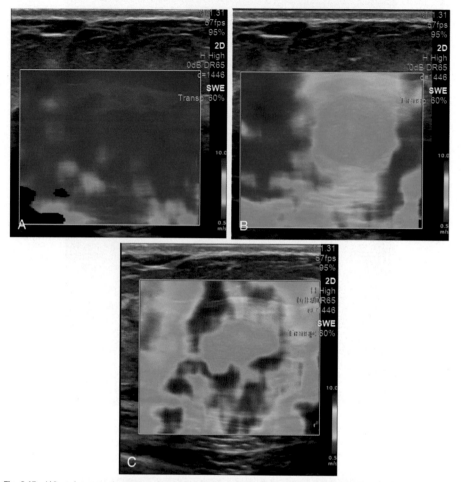

Fig. 6.15 When increased pressure is applied to tissues by the transducer, the stiffness of the tissue increases. This is best seen in superficial organs such as the breast. In this series of images of a benign breast cyst, (A) shear wave elastography is performed without precompression, (B) with moderate increased precompression, and (C) with marked increase in precompression. Note how the lesion stiffness increases with the increase in precompression.

materials on MRE is due to the long pulse-duration sequences, about 20 ms, used during MRE. Similarly, conditions such as hemochromatosis or hepatic steatosis can also cause slight phase-shifts in the MRI signal and alter elasticity measurements.

Motion artifacts also play a large role in MRE. The relatively long duration of pulse sequences allows any motion to influence image reconstruction. Although most MRE protocols use breath-hold sequences, breathing can cause variations in elasticity measurements. Cardiac pulsations can also cause motion artifacts throughout the duration of MRE.

Liver hotspots, which are regions of elevated liver stiffness that do not reflect actual regions of increased stiffness, are also common in MRE. Hotspots often occur in predictable regions nearest the mechanical driver or along the surface of the liver. On the anterior aspect of the liver nearest the mechanical driver, the mechanical vibrations cause excessive, distorted vibrations in the tissue, resulting in perceived increases in stiffness from slow net propagation. Along the surface of the liver, shear waves can reorient and progress across the liver dome. These waves appear thicker than shear waves and result in elevated stiffness values. Other uncommon hotspots may also result from random areas of wave distortion.

KEY POINTS

1. Recognizing artifacts and knowing how to avoid them is critical to obtain accurate shear wave speed measurements.
2. B-mode tracking of shear waves is used in the ultrasound techniques. If the B-mode image is poor or has artifacts, the resultant shear wave estimate will be inaccurate.
3. Avoiding artifacts is critical to obtaining accurate liver stiffness measurements.
4. Artifacts can lead to overestimation or underestimation of the liver stiffness.
5. 2D-SWE quality/confidence maps and the velocity/elasticity map should be evaluated for artifacts, and these areas should be avoided when placing the measurement box.
6. In point shear wave elastography a quality/confidence map and velocity/elasticity map are not present, therefore careful placement of the measurement box away from areas know to create artifacts (liver capsule, blood vessels, areas of shadowing) is critical.
7. The placement of the measurement box should never contain artifacts.
8. Liver shear wave elastography artifacts are common, and some of them cannot be avoided because they are due to the technique itself.
9. Following a standardized protocol in the acquisition of measurement helps in decreasing the artifacts, at least those due to the operator techniques.

References

1. Rouze NC, Wang MH, Palmeri ML, Nightingale KR. Parameters affecting the resolution and accuracy of 2-D quantitative shear wave images. *IEEE Trans Ultrason Ferroelectr Freq Control.* 2012;59:1729-1740.
2. Bruce M, Kolokythas O, Ferraioli G, Filice C, O'Donnell M. Limitations and artifacts in shear wave elastography of the liver. *Biomed Eng Lett.* 2017;7:81-89.
3. Deng Y, Palmeri ML, Rouze NC, Haystead CM, Nightingale KR. Evaluating the benefit of elevated acoustic output in harmonic motion estimation in ultrasonic shear wave elasticity imaging. *Ultrasound Med Biol.* 2018;44:303-310.
4. Mueller S, Mueller J, Elshaarawy O. Interpretation of shear wave propagation maps (elastogram) using transient elastography. In: Mueller S, ed. *Liver Elastography.* 1st ed. Switzerland: Springer Nature; 2020:495-508.
5. Palmeri ML, Milkowski A, Barr R, et al. Radiological Society of North America/Quantitative imaging biomarker alliance shear wave speed bias quantification in elastic and viscoelastic phantoms. *J Ultrasound Med.* 2021;40(3):569-581.
6. Rouze NC, Deng Y, Trutna CA, Palmeri ML, Nightingale KR. Characterization of viscoelastic materials using group shear wave speeds. *IEEE Trans Ultrason Ferroelectr Freq Control.* 2018;65:780-794.
7. Nightingale K, Rouze N, Rosenzweig S, et al. Derivation and analysis of viscoelastic properties in human liver: impact of frequency on fibrosis and steatosis staging. *IEEE Trans Ultrason Ferroelectr Freq Control.* 2015;62:165-175.
8. Wells RG. Liver mechanics and the profibrotic response at the cellular level. In: Mueller S, ed. *Liver Elastography.* 1st ed. Switzerland: Springer Nature; 2020:495-508.
9. Lipman SL, Rouze NC, Palmeri ML, Nightingale KR. Evaluating the improvement in shear wave speed image quality using multidimensional directional filters in the presence of reflection artifacts. *IEEE Trans Ultrason Ferroelectr Freq Control.* 2016;63:1049-1063.
10. Sandrin L, Cassereau D, Fink M. The role of the coupling term in transient elastography. *J Acoust Soc Am.* 2004;115:73-83.
11. Barr RG, Zhang Z. Effects of precompression on elasticity imaging of the breast: development of a clinically useful semiquantitative method of precompression assessment. *J Ultrasound Med.* 2012;31:895-902.

12. Bouchet P, Gennisson JL, Podda A, Alilet M, Carrié M, Aubry S. Artifacts and technical restrictions in 2D shear wave elastography. *Ultraschall Med.* 2020;41:267-277.
13. Dubinsky TJ, Shah HU, Erpelding TN, Sannananja B, Sonneborn R. Propagation imaging in the demonstration of common shear wave artifacts. *J Ultrasound Med.* 2019;38:1611-1616.
14. O'Hara S, Zelesco M, Rocke K, Stevenson G, Sun Z. Reliability indicators for 2-dimensional shear wave elastography. *J Ultrasound Med.* 2019;38:3065-3071.
15. Guglielmo FF, Venkatesh SK, Mitchell DG. Liver MR elastography technique and image interpretation: pearls and pitfalls. *Radiographics.* 2019;39:1983-2002.

CHAPTER 7

Staging Liver Fibrosis with Shear Wave Elastography

Giovanna Ferraioli ■ Davide Roccarina ■ Jonathan R. Dillman ■ Richard G. Barr

Introduction

Chronic liver disease is a major worldwide health problem. It may be due to several etiological factors that lead to necroinflammation with subsequent fibrosis (i.e., formation of scar tissue). Fibrosis, which is the consequence and not the cause of liver injury, may progress to cirrhosis and its complications if the cause of liver injury is left untreated. The prevalence of cirrhosis is probably underestimated as most patients remain asymptomatic with symptoms developing at a late stage.[1] A recent study based on the National Health and Nutrition Examination Survey data source estimated that the prevalence of cirrhosis was 0.27% of the general U.S. population, with hepatitis C, alcohol, and diabetes mellitus playing a significant role.[2] Furthermore, it found that nearly 70% of the participants with cirrhosis replied that they were never informed that they had liver disease.

With the availability of effective treatments for viral hepatitis, the rate of virus-induced chronic liver disease will significantly decrease, whereas the proportion of nonalcoholic fatty liver disease (NAFLD)/nonalcoholic steatohepatitis (NASH) will increase due to the obesity epidemic and sedentary lifestyles.

The stage of liver fibrosis is important to determine the prognosis, for surveillance, for prioritization for treatment, and even to determine the potential for reversibility.[3] Therefore it is important to diagnose liver fibrosis and assess its severity to provide appropriate management and to prevent further liver damage.[4]

With the availability of shear wave elastography (SWE) techniques, the number of liver biopsies performed for staging liver fibrosis in several clinical settings has drastically decreased, and liver biopsy is now seldom required outside the research setting.

SWE techniques were validated using liver histology as the reference standard. However, it should be kept in mind that elastography measures the stiffness, not the fibrosis, and therefore it is inappropriate to report and interpret the values using a histological classification. Moreover, stiffness is a quantitative estimate, whereas the histological scoring systems for liver fibrosis are based on categorical scales. Therefore even in the "ideal" conditions, an overlap between consecutive stages of liver fibrosis is inevitable when using liver stiffness as a surrogate marker of liver fibrosis.

The spectrum of advanced fibrosis (METAVIR F3 stage) and cirrhosis (METAVIR F4 stage) is a continuum in asymptomatic patients, and distinguishing between the two is often not possible on clinical grounds.[3] The Baveno VI consensus on portal hypertension considered these uncertainties, and has proposed the term *compensated advanced chronic liver disease* (cACLD), which includes F3 and F4 stages.[5]

Before performing elastography, the patient should be evaluated clinically. As highlighted by guidelines/consensus on liver SWE, the interpretation of liver stiffness measurement (LSM) depends on the specific clinical scenario, the prevalence of disease in the population under investigation, the current patient's comorbidities, and the etiology of the liver disease.[3,6,7] Therefore anamnesis, clinical examination, and abdominal ultrasound examination are suggested prior to the elastography evaluation, and elastography should not be performed without information on the patient's current complaints, past medical history, and laboratory tests.

The operator performing the examinations must acquire appropriate knowledge and training in ultrasound elastography. Moreover, for the acoustic radiation force impulse (ARFI) techniques (point shear wave elastography [pSWE] and two-dimensional SWE [2D-SWE]), experience in B-mode ultrasound is mandatory.

Chronic Viral Hepatitis and Nonalcoholic Fatty Liver Disease

STAGING LIVER FIBROSIS

There are differences among elastography modalities, therefore the cutoff values for fibrosis staging are not the same for every ultrasound system. However, the differences between the different systems are smaller in patients with LSMs up to 15 kPa, which is the most clinically relevant range of values for the staging of liver fibrosis.[8] From a clinical point of view it is more important to rule in or rule out advanced disease (cACLD) than it is to provide an exact stage of liver fibrosis by using a histological scoring system.

Differences in cutoffs among published studies may also be due to differences in cirrhosis prevalence and severity in the studied populations (i.e., the spectrum effect). For patients chronically infected with hepatitis C virus (HCV), it is recommended to start treatment with direct-acting antiviral (DAA) drugs no matter the stage of liver fibrosis. Considering all these points, the use of clinical categories based on low/high likelihood of disease is suggested.

In patients with virus-related chronic hepatitis or with NAFLD, guidelines have been suggested to interpret LSMs by VCTE by using the rule of 5: LSM ≤ 5 kPa has a high probability of being normal; LSM < 10 kPa in the absence of other known clinical signs rules out cACLD; LSM between 10 and 15 kPa is suggestive of cACLD but needs further tests for confirmation; LSM > 15 kPa is highly suggestive of cACLD, whereas LSM ≥ 20–25 kPa indicates clinically significant portal hypertension.[5,7]

ARFI-based techniques give different values with different ultrasound systems. However, the update to the Society of Radiologists in Ultrasound (SRU) consensus has highlighted that the overlap of LSMs between METAVIR stages is as large if not larger than the difference between vendor's techniques.[3] The SRU consensus recommends using a low cutoff value below which there is a high probability of no or mild fibrosis and a high cutoff value above which there is a high probability of cACLD.

It also suggests, based on published studies, to use a "rule of 4" for fibrosis staging with ARFI-based techniques in patients with chronic viral hepatitis or NAFLD: LSM ≤ 5 kPa (1.3 m/s) has high probability of being normal; LSM < 9 kPa [1.7 m/s] in the absence of other clinical signs of chronic liver disease rules out cACLD; LSM between 9 and 13 kPa (2.1 m/s) is suggestive of cACLD but may need further tests for confirmation; and LSM > 13 kPa is highly suggestive of cACLD. There is a high risk of clinically significant portal hypertension with LSMs > 17 kPa (2.4 m/s), but additional tests may be required (Table 7.1). In patients with NAFLD, the cutoff values for cACLD may be lower, and follow-up or additional testing even among those with LSMs between 7 and 9 kPa is recommended.[3] Each vendor's technique has its own sensitivity and specificity using these cutoffs.

The SRU consensus has highlighted that most studies that used ARFI-based techniques (pSWE and 2D-SWE) suggest that a liver stiffness value of less than 7 kPa (1.5 m/s) can help rule out significant fibrosis.

TABLE 7.1 ■ Recommendation for Interpretation of Liver Stiffness Values Obtained with ARFI Techniques in Patients with Viral Hepatitis and NAFLD[3]

Liver Stiffness Value	Recommendations
≤ 5 kPa (1.3 m/s)	High probability of being normal
< 9 kPa (1.7 m/s)	In the absence of other known clinical signs, rules out cACLD. If there are known clinical signs, may need further test for confirmation
9–13 kPa (1.7–2.1 m/s)	Suggestive of cACLD but need further test for confirmation
> 13 kPa (2.1 m/s)	Rules in cACLD
> 17 kPa (2.4 m/s)	Suggestive of CSPH

ARFI, Acoustic radiation force impulse; *cACLD,* compensated advanced chronic liver disease; *CSPH,* clinically significant portal hypertension; *NAFLD,* nonalcoholic fatty liver disease.

Figs. 7.1–7.6 show some cases of liver stiffness assessment in patients with chronic liver disease.

Due to the rapid decline of liver stiffness in patients with chronic viral hepatitis who achieve sustained virologic response (SVR) after treatment, the "rule of 4" (ARFI techniques) or the "rule of 5" (VCTE) cannot by applied to stage liver fibrosis in these cases (Fig. 7.7).

Given the NAFLD disease burden, the use of noninvasive tests is a cost-saving measure and can decrease the risk related to performing a liver biopsy. A recent individual-patient-data meta-analysis (37 studies with 5735 subjects) that evaluated noninvasive tests versus liver histology has reported that sequential combinations of noninvasive markers with a lower cutoff to rule out advanced fibrosis and a higher cutoff to rule in cirrhosis can reduce the need for liver biopsy in

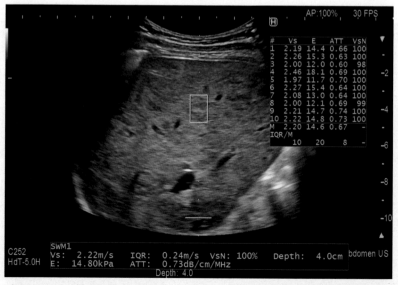

Fig. 7.1 Asymptomatic 48-year-old woman with chronic hepatitis B and normal laboratory tests. A point shear wave elastography technique (SWM, Arietta 850 ultrasound system, Fujifilm Healthcare previously Hitachi Ltd) shows that the median liver stiffness value is 14.6 kPa, which indicates compensated advanced chronic liver disease. The measurement is of good quality (IQR/M: 20%), and the quality criterion provided by the manufacturer for each acquisition, VsN, is fulfilled for all acquisitions (range: 98%–100%). *IQR/M,* Interquartile range/median.

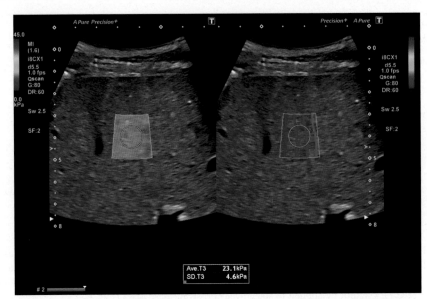

Fig. 7.2 Treatment-naïve 64-year-old man with chronic hepatitis C. The patient had had an episode of liver decompensation a month before the examination. The stiffness value obtained with a two-dimensional shear wave elastography technique (Aplio i800 ultrasound system, Canon Medical Systems) is 23.1 kPa, indicating a high likelihood of clinically significant portal hypertension. The measurement was taken following the quality criterion given by the manufacturer (i.e., the lines were parallel and equally spaced in the propagation map *[right]*).

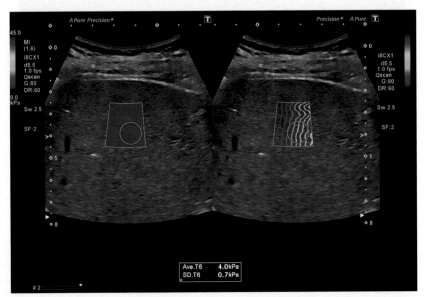

Fig. 7.3 Treatment-naïve 55-year-old woman with chronic hepatitis C. The stiffness value, obtained with the Canon two-dimensional shear wave elastography technique, is below 5 kPa. Therefore there is a high likelihood of absence of liver fibrosis.

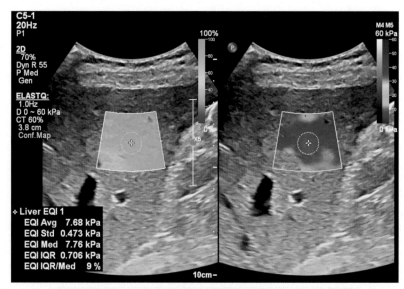

Fig. 7.4 A 35-year-old woman with chronic hepatitis B under antiviral treatment and with laboratory tests in the normal range. The liver stiffness obtained with a two-dimensional shear wave elastography technique (ElastQ, Epiq7 ultrasound system, Philips Medical Systems) is 7.68 kPa, a value that indicates significant fibrosis. The confidence map on the *left side* is used for positioning the measurement box in the best quality area, which is highlighted with the *green* color.

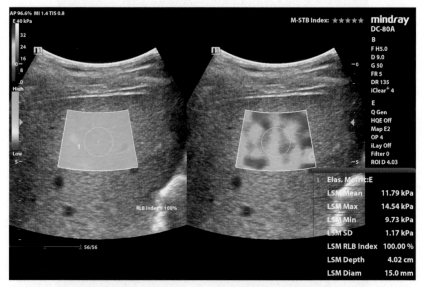

Fig. 7.5 Treatment-naïve 35-year-old man with chronic hepatitis C and normal laboratory tests. The liver stiffness obtained with a two-dimensional shear wave elastography technique (STE, DC-80A ultrasound system, Mindray Medical Systems) is 11.79 kPa, a value that is suggestive of compensated advanced chronic liver disease. The measurement was made in a reliable area, as indicated by the reliability map on the *left,* and no motion was detected, as indicated by the *five green stars* on the *right top* side of the image. Both reliability map and motion stability index are manufacturer's quality criteria.

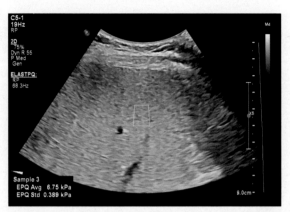

Fig. 7.6 Asymptomatic 42-year-old woman with nonalcoholic fatty liver disease and alanine aminotransferase value of 52 IU/L. The liver stiffness obtained with a point shear wave elastography technique (ElastPQ, Epiq7 ultrasound system, Philips Medical Systems) is 6.75 kPa, a value that may exclude significant fibrosis. The manufacturer quality criterion is the standard deviation of each measurement shown below the average value on the *left bottom* side of the image. It must be up to 30% of the average value.

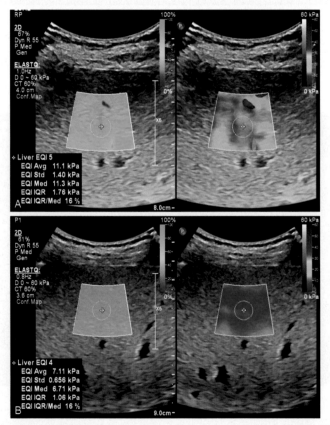

Fig. 7.7 A 67-year-old man with compensated advanced chronic liver disease due to hepatitis C virus infection. (A) Baseline two-dimensional shear wave elastography technique (ElastQ, Epiq7 ultrasound system, Philips Medical Systems) performed a few days before starting direct-acting antiviral treatment shows a liver stiffness value of 11.1 kPa, which indicates advanced fibrosis. (B) The assessment of liver stiffness after 1 month of treatment showed that liver stiffness had decreased by 3.99 kPa. This rapid decrease is likely due to resolution of inflammation.

patients with NAFLD.[9] This algorithm can identify patients with low-risk NAFLD who can be managed in primary care and evaluate the severity of NAFLD without the need for liver biopsy in secondary care settings. The combinations were: Fibrosis-4 Index (FIB-4) < 1.3 followed by LSM by VCTE < 8 kPa to rule out advanced fibrosis, and FIB-4 ≥ 2.67 followed by LSM ≥ 10 kPa to rule in advanced fibrosis (66% sensitivity and 86% specificity). With cutoffs of FIB-4 and LSM, respectively, ≥ 3.48 and ≥ 20 kPa, the specificity increased to 90%.

MONITORING FIBROSIS: HEPATITIS C AND ANTIVIRAL TREATMENT

In patients with chronic hepatitis C who have been successfully treated with DDAs, a rapid decline of liver stiffness has been reported by several studies.[3,6,7]

A metaanalysis has estimated the decrease in liver stiffness by VCTE in patients with HCV who achieved SVR either after DAAs or interferon-based therapies. Twenty-four studies on 2934 patients with HCV and with paired VCTE before and after antiviral therapy were included.[10] SVR was achieved in 75.5% of patients. With respect to baseline values, the decrease in liver stiffness was 2.4 kPa at the end of treatment, 3.1 kPa 1–6 months after therapy, 3.2 kPa 6–12 months after therapy, and 4.1 kPa 1 year or more after treatment. The median decrease at 6–12 months after end of treatment was 28.2%. No significant changes were observed in patients who did not achieve SVR, and the decreases in liver stiffness were significantly greater in patients treated with DAAs than with interferon-based therapy (4.5 kPa vs. 2.6 kPa). The decline in LSMs was higher in patients with higher alanine aminotransferase (ALT) baseline values (i.e., a marker of hepatic inflammation). The early decline in LSM observed at the end of treatment is likely due to resolution of hepatic inflammation, whereas the slow and continued decline beyond 1 year after end of treatment may be related to fibrosis regression.[10]

By using liver histology as the reference standard, a study using a pSWE technique determined that the optimal cutoff values of shear wave speed for the staging of liver fibrosis in patients with chronic hepatitis C were significantly higher in untreated patients than in patients who had achieved SVR after treatment: 1.49 m/s vs. 1.26 m/s for ≥ F2; 1.51 m/s vs. 1.31 m/s for ≥ F3; and 1.51 m/s vs. 1.49 m/s for F4.[11]

Therefore the use of liver stiffness cutoff values obtained in treatment-naïve patients can underestimate liver fibrosis in patients who have achieved SVR with DAAs.

To overcome this limitation, the SRU consensus has proposed to use the delta change of LSM over time instead of the absolute value as the best method to assess progression or regression of chronic liver disease. Due to the rapid decline of stiffness values after viral eradication observed in patients with HCV who were treated with DAAs, the baseline stiffness value for follow up must be the one obtained at the end of the treatment.[3] It must be emphasized that guidelines have recommended that changes of liver stiffness values after successful anti-HCV treatment should not affect the management strategy (e.g., monitoring for hepatocellular carcinoma [HCC] and portal hypertension in patients at risk).[6,7]

A study in which 84 HCV infected liver transplant recipients with at least METAVIR stage F1 had paired liver biopsy at baseline and at 12 months post-SVR (achieved either with interferon-based therapies or DAAs) showed that 67% presented a decrease of at least 1 stage in the METAVIR stage at follow-up biopsy.[12] However, of the 37 patients with cirrhosis, 92% remained at F4 fibrosis or decreased to F3 fibrosis; that is, most remained with advanced fibrosis. Hepatic venous pressure gradient > 10 mmHg and liver stiffness by VCTE > 21 kPa, as well as liver decompensations before treatment, identified patients with a lower likelihood of fibrosis regression. Of note, posttreatment LSMs below 10 kPa were observed in some patients who remained with advanced fibrosis. Because complications such as HCC may occur in patients with regression to METAVIR F3 fibrosis and normalization of liver stiffness values after successful antiviral therapies, liver stiffness cutoffs obtained in treatment-naïve patients cannot rule out the presence of advanced fibrosis and guide screening strategies in patients who achieve SVR (Fig. 7.8).[13]

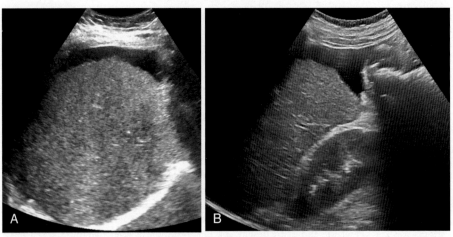

Fig. 7.8 Pretreatment image of a 66-year-old man with decompensated cirrhosis from chronic hepatitis C virus (A). At that time the patient's liver stiffness was 25 kPa. On follow-up 11 months post–direct-acting antiviral treatment, his liver stiffness decreased to 15 kPa, 16 months posttreatment it decreased to 11.5 kPa, and 2 years posttreatment it decreased to 7.4 kPa. However, despite the good liver stiffness response to treatment, the patient still remained in decompensated cirrhosis (B).

MONITORING FIBROSIS: HEPATITIS B AND ANTIVIRAL TREATMENT

VCTE has been largely used for evaluating the longitudinal changes in LSMs in patients with chronic hepatitis undergoing antiviral treatment. All the studies have shown a significant decline of liver stiffness in the long-term follow-up.[14] However, without histological confirmation with paired liver biopsies, whether the decrease in LSMs is associated with regression of liver fibrosis, improvement in necroinflammation, or both, is unclear.[14] In fact, in patients with chronic infection with hepatitis B virus (HBV), transaminases flares may occur. High ALT level is one of the major confounding factors for LSM, and even patients with HBV with mild to moderate ALT elevation (1–5 times the upper limit of normal) seem to have higher LSM than those with normal ALT levels.[7]

Whether the decline in liver stiffness value results from regression of fibrosis, stabilization of activity, or both, it can be regarded as a beneficial effect of antiviral treatment.[14]

Only a few studies have used paired liver biopsies. A multicenter study in which paired liver biopsies at baseline and after 2 years were available for some 30% of the patients showed a rapid to slow decline of liver stiffness values, and the decline continued even after the normalization of ALT values.[15] The pattern of decline in liver stiffness likely reflected the remission of both liver inflammation and fibrosis during the first 24 weeks and fibrosis regression during long-term antiviral therapy, in particular, after ALT normalization. The LSM decline was greater in patients with higher baseline necroinflammatory activity and with a higher baseline fibrosis stage. After 2 years of treatment, regression of fibrosis was documented in 59.8% (98/164) of patients, with 64.3% (63/98) having at least a one-point decrease in Ishak fibrosis stage scores.

Another multicenter study with a large series of patients with paired liver biopsy results at baseline and at week 72 demonstrated that the regression of fibrosis and the improvement of inflammation were obtained in 51.2% and 74.4% of cases, respectively, and a liver stiffness decrease of ≥ 30% was associated with regression of fibrosis, significant histological response, and ALT normalization.[16]

CLINICAL OUTCOMES

Elastography has been proposed as a tool to predict the risk of death or complications in patients with chronic liver disease. LSM by VCTE combined with platelet count is a validated noninvasive method for varices screening, with very good results in terms of invasive procedures being spared. ARFI-based techniques also show promising results in this setting. This topic is presented in detail in Chapter 8.

In patients with cACLD, the risk of liver decompensation increases with increasing LSM. A study that followed patients up to 4 years found that there were no events in the population with an LSM by VCTE < 21 kPa. An LSM of more than 35 kPa was associated with a decompensation risk of 39% at 4 years. For each unit increase in the LSM above 20 kPa, the risk of liver-related outcome increased by 6% after adjusting for age, sex, the model for end stage liver disease (MELD) score, cohort source, and etiology of liver disease.[17]

A metaanalysis that included studies performed with VCTE or magnetic resonance elastography (MRE) found that each kilopascal unit increase in LSM was associated with a 7% higher risk of developing decompensated cirrhosis and with an 11% higher risk of HCC.[18] In another metaanalysis, for each unit increment of liver stiffness by VCTE, the summary relative risk was 1.06 for all-cause mortality and liver-related events (i.e., hepatic decompensation, HCC, and/or liver-related mortality).[19]

Using VCTE, a study in a small cohort of patients with cACLD as defined by an LSM ≥ 10 kPa reported that a combination of baseline LSM and its change over time was more useful in predicting the risk of presenting the endpoint (composite outcome that included death, liver decompensation, and impairment of at least one point in the Child-Pugh score) than either of the two parameters alone. In addition, patients with baseline LSM ≥ 21 kPa and an increase in delta-LSM ≥ 10% had a twofold risk of presenting the endpoint as compared with those with baseline LSM ≥ 21 kPa and delta-LSM < 10%.[20] Of note, patients with LSM < 21 kPa and delta-LSM < 10% had zero risk of presenting the endpoint over a period of 43.6 months.

A study in a large series of U.S. veterans who initiated HCV treatment and had at least one liver stiffness before (n = 492) or after (n = 877) HCV therapy reported that posttreatment liver stiffness > 20 kPa by VCTE, but not pretreatment liver stiffness, was independently associated with the development of decompensated cirrhosis and the composite outcome of death, liver transplant, decompensated cirrhosis, or HCC.[21]

A recent multicenter study has investigated the value of LSM to predict clinical outcomes in patients with ACLD due to several etiologies.[22,23] The patients were followed for a median period of 33.1 months. The best performance was obtained by combining the MELD score and LSMs. A MELD score of 10 points and an LSM of 20 kPa by 2D-SWE were the optimal cutoffs for stratifying the 2-year risk of mortality, and the authors named this algorithm M10LS20. By using the M10LS20 algorithm, the patients were stratified in three different risk groups: good prognosis (patients with both MELD score and LSM below the cutoffs), intermediate prognosis (patients with one parameter above and the other one below the cutoff), and poor prognosis (patients with both parameters above the cutoffs). The three groups had significantly different survival rates both at short-term (90 days) and long-term follow-up (2 years) and different risk of decompensation or further decompensation. The M10LS20 algorithm was tested also using LSMs obtained with pSWE and VCTE and showed a similar performance.

In patients with chronic hepatitis B, a score that includes age, albumin, HBV-DNA, and LSM has been proposed for predicting the risk of hepatocellular carcinoma (LSM-HCC).[24]

The LSM-HCC score was obtained in a large cohort study of some 1500 consecutive patients. The cutoff values of 8.0 kPa and 12.0 kPa by VCTE were chosen to define three strata of LSM because these values had the highest sum of sensitivity and specificity, and specificity above

90% for HCC, respectively. By applying the cutoff value of 11.0, the score excluded future HCC with high negative predictive value (99.4%–100%) at 5 years.

PREDICTION OF LIVER-RELATED EVENTS OR HEPATOCELLULAR CARCINOMA AFTER TREATMENT

In patients with chronic viral hepatitis, the risk of developing liver-related events cannot be completely eliminated even in those who achieve complete virological response; this risk is mainly related to the degree of liver fibrosis before starting the treatment.

Some models that include LSM have been developed to predict the risk of HCC in patients with chronic hepatitis B treated with antivirals. The most used are modified risk estimation for hepatocellular carcinoma in chronic hepatitis B (mREACH-B) based on gender, age, ALT, hepatitis B e-antigen, and LSM[25] and derived from the REACH-B score[26]; the cirrhosis and age (CAGE-B) score based on age at year 5 and cirrhosis in relation to LSM at year 5 of follow-up under therapy; and the stiffness and age (SAGE-B) score based on age and LSM at year 5 of follow-up under therapy.[27]

In the study that developed the mREACH-B score, the incidence of development of liver-related events was 1.3% in patients with an LSM by VCTE after complete virologic response < 8.0 kPa, 14.8% in patients with an LSM between 8.0 and 13.0 kPa, and 28.8% in patients with an LSM > 13.0 kPa. Therefore these three different categories of liver stiffness values had an increasing weight in the score.[25]

The mREACH-B score was obtained in an Asian cohort, whereas the CAGE-B and SAGE-B scores were developed in a White cohort of some 1500 patients. Both SAGE-B and CAGE-B have shown acceptable performance in predicting HCC after 5 years of antiviral therapy in Asian patients with chronic hepatitis B.[28]

Successful treatment with DAAs in patients with compensated or decompensated cirrhosis is associated with reduced risk for HCC.[29] The relative risk reduction is similar in patients with and without cirrhosis.[30] Nonetheless, another study has demonstrated that patients with cirrhosis before SVR to treatment for HCV infection continue to have a high risk for HCC (>2% per year) for several years and should continue surveillance.[31]

In a study that included more than 500 patients with HCV who achieved SVR after DAA therapy, at a median follow-up of 2.8 years the incidence of liver-related events was relatively low, and de novo HCC was the most frequent complication.[32] The main predictors of HCC risk in the study were albumin level and follow-up LSM by VCTE. Two main risk groups were identified: (1) patients with LSM at follow-up < 10 kPa or patients with LSM between 10 and 20 kPa with albumin ≥ 4.4 g/dL at follow-up in whom the incidence of HCC was 0.6/100 patient-years and (2) patients with LSM ≥ 20 kPa at follow-up or those with LSM between 10 and 20 kPa but albumin < 4.4 g/dL at follow-up in whom the incidence was 2.9/100 patient-years.[32] Of note, in contrast to what was reported in other studies, when patients were stratified for the risk of HCC according to LSM at baseline, there were no differences in HCC incidence among patients with LSM ≥ 20 kPa and those with LSM < 20 kPa.

Another study reported that a 30% decrease in LSM after DAAs was one of the predictors inversely associated with the risk of presenting with HCC.[33]

Alcohol-Related Liver Disease

Alcohol-related liver disease (ALD) is a major cause of severe liver disease worldwide; however, most patients with ALD are often unaware of their underlying condition. Therefore it can progress without patients seeking medical advice until a first sign of clinical decompensation such as jaundice, ascites, or variceal bleeding presents.[34] Besides being diagnosed at a late stage, patients with ALD are more likely to die at a younger age and to experience liver-related events than patients with liver disease of any other etiology.[35]

A population-based cohort study in Sweden reported that individuals with biopsy-proven ALD have a near fivefold increased risk of death compared with the general population. Individuals with ALD without cirrhosis were also at increased risk of death, which was highest in the first year after baseline but persisted after 10 or more years of follow-up.[36]

Screening for ALD in at-risk patients should be routinely implemented because it is vital to allow an early intervention.[37] In fact, cessation of drinking at any point in the natural history of the disease reduces the risks of disease progression and occurrence of complications from cirrhosis.[38] It has been shown that the 5-year survival rate for people with cirrhosis who stop drinking is about 90% compared with 70% for those who continue to drink and that, even after the development of complications from cirrhosis, abstinence is essential because the survival rate is approximately 60% for those who stop drinking and 35% for those who do not.[39,40]

ALD includes a wide spectrum of lesions ranging from steatosis, which is present in almost all heavy drinkers, to steatohepatitis, progressive liver fibrosis, and cirrhosis and its complications.

Similar to other chronic liver diseases, the severity of liver fibrosis correlates with patient outcomes: patients with stage F0–F2 fibrosis have 100% 10-year survival compared with only around 50% in patients with stage F3–F4.[41,42]

cACLD is the main predictor of long-term survival, therefore it is of outmost importance to diagnose patients with advanced fibrosis before decompensation occurs to promote abstinence and improve survival.[34]

A study performed in two cohorts of patients, one with a high pretest probability of alcohol-related cirrhosis and the other one with a low pretest risk, reported that VCTE and 2D-SWE had a high diagnostic accuracy for advanced fibrosis and cirrhosis in heavy drinkers and the performance of the two techniques was comparable. Both methods had a very high negative predictive value.[43] The optimal cutoff values of VCTE and 2D-SWE were 9.6 and 10.2 kPa for significant fibrosis and 19.7 and 16.4 kPa for cirrhosis. Negative predictive values were high for both groups, but the positive predictive value for cirrhosis was > 66% in the high-risk group vs. approximately 50% in the low-risk group.

Several other studies have demonstrated that stiffness cutoff values are almost twofold higher in patients with ALD than in patients with HCV. An individual-patient-data metaanalysis that included 10 studies in 1026 patients who had undergone liver biopsy and were assessed with VCTE, reported that the cutoffs were 7 kPa for $F \geq 1$ fibrosis, 9 kPa for $F \geq 2$, 12.1 kPa for $F \geq 3$, and 18.6 kPa for $F = 4$ with the areas under the receiver operating characteristic curve (AUROCs) of 0.83, 0.86, 0.90, 0.91, respectively. Aspartate aminotransferase (AST) and bilirubin concentrations had a significant effect on liver stiffness, and higher concentrations were associated with higher liver stiffness values and with significantly higher cutoff values for diagnosis of all fibrosis stages except $F \geq 1$.[44] Of note, this metaanalysis reported that for concentrations of AST and bilirubin within the normal range the liver stiffness cutoffs were similar to those reported in chronic hepatitis C for all fibrosis stages. It also showed that the increased liver stiffness was associated with nonsevere histological signs of alcoholic hepatitis. The median liver stiffness value was almost twice as high in patients with asymptomatic and nonsevere histological signs of alcoholic hepatitis than in patients without.[44]

Therefore in patients with ALD, liver stiffness is markedly influenced by liver inflammation, and even minor increases in AST concentrations that would be considered indicative of mild inflammation in patients with HCV definitely affect liver stiffness values and might lead to overestimation of the severity of liver fibrosis.[41] It has been suggested that AST and bilirubin concentrations should be taken into account when using liver stiffness cutoffs in clinical practice for the diagnosis of liver fibrosis in patients with chronic and excessive alcohol consumption.[44]

An increase of liver stiffness associated with histological signs of alcoholic hepatitis has also been reported in studies performed using a pSWE technique.[45,46]

Active drinking has also been shown to increase liver stiffness, and a rapid decrease in liver stiffness has been observed after alcohol withdrawal (0.5 to 4 weeks of abstinence).[47-49] The decrease is associated with a normalization of transaminases, bilirubin, alkaline phosphatase, and/or gammaglutamyltransferase.

A study has suggested that AST levels should be considered when assessing fibrosis through liver stiffness values in patients with ALD and that elevated stiffness values observed at AST > 100 IU/L should be interpreted cautiously due to the possibility of false-positive results for the presence of steatohepatitis.[50] The authors also underscore that even modest signs of liver inflammation become relevant for fibrosis stages lower than F4.

A recent multicenter study has addressed the issue of the ideal timing for liver stiffness assessment about the influence of alcohol consumption.[51] VCTE and biochemistry data were obtained on the same day as the liver biopsy after a median of 6 days of abstinence in 259 patients hospitalized for alcohol detoxification. The cutoffs for ruling out and ruling in cACLD, respectively, were 10 and 25 kPa. The ruling-out cutoff remained very accurate regardless of alcohol consumption during 1- and 2-month follow-up. Of note, among patients with initial liver stiffness of 10 to 25 kPa (i.e., in the gray area), more than half of those with an absence of cACLD at histology had liver stiffness below 10 kPa during the same follow-up period.

Cholestatic and Autoimmune Liver Disease

Studies for assessing liver fibrosis in primary biliary cholangitis (PBC), primary sclerosing cholangitis (PSC), and autoimmune hepatitis are very few and have been performed in a small number of subjects, mostly using VCTE.

It must be underlined that liver biopsy is no longer necessary in the diagnostic work up of PBC because of the diagnostic value of specific autoantibodies in the context of cholestatic liver biochemistry, unless there is suspicion of coexistence of autoimmune hepatitis, NASH, or other comorbidities or in cases unresponsive to the therapy.[35,52]

In a diagnostic cohort of 103 patients with PBC, a liver stiffness cutoff of 10.7 kPa by VCTE was identified for advanced fibrosis, and an increase of stiffness of 2.1 kPa/yr or higher was associated with an 8.4-fold increased risk of liver decompensations, liver transplantations, or deaths in the monitoring cohort of 150 patients who were followed up with for up to 5 years.[53] Of note, during the follow-up, liver stiffness was stable in the majority of patients with noncirrhotic PBC who were on treatment.

In patients with PSC, studies performed using VCTE have shown that LSM has a good accuracy in predicting advanced fibrosis and cirrhosis. In a series of 73 patients with PSC the threshold of liver stiffness by VCTE to identify patients with cACLD was 9.6 kPa with sensitivity, specificity, and accuracy above 80% and an AUROC > 0.90.[54]

In patients with autoimmune hepatitis, hepatic inflammation is a confounding factor that can lead to overestimation of liver stiffness independently from fibrosis stage. Therefore guidelines have recommended to stage liver fibrosis after at least 6 months of immunosuppressive therapy.[35]

Screening for Liver Fibrosis in the General Population

The diagnosis of a chronic liver disease is seldom made in the precirrhotic stage or in early cirrhosis because generally the patients are asymptomatic and thus they do not seek medical advice. Sometimes the diagnosis is made when the disease has already reached the later stages with decompensation of cirrhosis or development of HCC.[55] Fibrosis is the most important driver in determining the progression to cirrhosis, therefore the assessment of a patient with chronic liver disease is based on the assessment of fibrosis.[55] Due to the high prevalence of chronic liver diseases and the role of cirrhosis and HCC as major causes of death worldwide, the possibility of screening the general population for liver fibrosis could be of interest.[55]

Few studies have reported results on screening for liver fibrosis in the general population. A study on subjects from the general population who were older than 45 years old, without previously known liver disease, and attending a primary care center for a medical check-up found that 89 out of 1190 (7.5%) subjects had LSM > 8 kPa including nine patients with LSM > 13 kPa.[56] Even though the liver tests were normal in 43% of them, a specific cause of chronic liver disease was found in all subjects, and the most frequent etiologies were NAFLD and ALD. Among the patients undergoing liver biopsy, cirrhosis was confirmed in all subjects with LSM > 13 kPa (100% positive predictive value).

In another study, subjects from an Asian population were randomly selected from the government census database and were invited for a check-up. Subjects with positive hepatitis B surface antigen or antibody against HCV, secondary causes of fatty liver, and decompensated liver disease were excluded. The final analysis included 922 subjects[57]; of those, 264 (28.6%) had fatty liver detected by magnetic resonance spectroscopy, with a prevalence higher in men than in women. Eight (3.7%) patients with fatty liver and seven (1.3%) controls had liver stiffness by VCTE ≥ 9.6 kPa, a level suggestive of advanced fibrosis. Of note, fatty liver was found in 14.3% of subjects with normal ALT according to the updated lower cutoff values (< 30 IU/L in men and < 19 IU/L in women). Therefore the diagnosis of chronic liver disease would have been missed if patients had been evaluated with the standard diagnostic algorithms used in primary care.[58]

In a European population-based study among individuals 45 years of age and older, 5.6% of the 3041 participants had LSM ≥ 8.0 kPa, which was the cutoff used to define clinically relevant fibrosis.[59] The adjusted predicted probability of LSM ≥ 8.0 kPa increased per age decade, with probabilities ranging from 1.4% in participants ages 50–60 years old to 9.9% in participants older than 80 years old. Participants with both diabetes and steatosis had the highest probabilities of LSM ≥ 8.0 kPa.

A study that included 1918 diabetic patients from primary care and hospital clinics reported that some 18% had increased liver stiffness as assessed by VCTE (≥ 9.6 kPa by M probe or ≥ 9.3 kPa by XL probe).[60] Patients with high body mass index, dyslipidaemia, and increased ALT were at highest risk of increased liver stiffness. Patients with suspected advanced fibrosis or cirrhosis based on LSMs were invited to undergo liver biopsy. Among patients with liver biopsy, 56% had steatohepatitis, 21% had advanced fibrosis, and 29% had cirrhosis.

In a study on patients with type 2 diabetes or excessive alcohol consumption and with abnormal blood biomarkers attending primary care practice, a liver stiffness > 8 kPa was found in 27% of cases.[61]

Altogether the rate of undiagnosed chronic liver disease in apparently healthy subjects is not negligible. Considering the healthcare costs linked to treating patients with advanced liver disease, screening programs for liver fibrosis with noninvasive tests in categories of subjects at risk could be cost-effective. However, it must be emphasized that the interpretation of liver stiffness results should always take into consideration patient demographics, disease etiology, key laboratory findings, and confounding factors.[3,6,7,62,63]

Pediatrics

Chronic liver diseases are increasingly prevalent in the pediatric population worldwide. This increase in frequency is, in part, driven by the increasing prevalence of NAFLD in more developed countries, including the United States.[64] There are numerous other causes of chronic liver disease in children, some of which are unique to the pediatric population and others that are also common in adults. Such causes may be congenital (e.g., biliary atresia, Alagille syndrome), metabolic/genetic (e.g., progressive familial intrahepatic cholestasis), inflammatory (e.g., autoimmune hepatitis, PSC), and infectious (HBV and HCV infections), among others. All of these disorders can cause progressive liver injury over time, leading to repeated attempts at healing and the deposition of scar tissue, or liver fibrosis.

As in adults, histologic evaluation is the current reference standard for detecting and staging liver fibrosis. However, liver biopsy has numerous disadvantages. These include poor patient acceptance, its invasive nature that can result in procedure-related complications (e.g., internal bleeding), its relatively high cost (children are commonly admitted to the hospital for observation following such procedures), the need for sedation or general anesthesia that also adds to procedural cost, and sampling error. Sampling error is a particularly clinically important concern, as liver biopsy procedures sample only very tiny fractions of the liver and as a result can both underestimate and overestimate the overall extent of liver fibrosis.[65]

In part, due to the limitations previously mentioned, clinicians are increasingly turning to noninvasive quantitative diagnostic tools to detect and stage liver fibrosis, including SWE techniques.

SHEAR WAVE ELASTOGRAPHY IN CHILDREN: CHALLENGES

There are several unique challenges when performing ultrasound SWE in children compared with adults. First, adult patients are typically requested to abstain from eating for at least 4 hours prior to imaging. In very young children (e.g., neonates and infants) this could potentially be harmful. Other children simply may be unable or unwilling to fast for 4 hours. In these situations, a fast of at least 2 hours is attempted. If fasting cannot be achieved, elastography is performed as it can still provide useful information. If the results are normal, there is no substantial liver fibrosis; if the results are markedly abnormal, there is likely substantial liver fibrosis. If the LSM is borderline or only mildly elevated, then repeat imaging should be considered as this apparent stiffening could be the result of increased blood flow to the liver. Another potential solution to this problem is to try to schedule these examinations early in the morning, soon after the patient has awoken from sleep.

Another challenge in the pediatric population relates to breath holding, typically required for ARFI techniques. Despite this potential challenge, 2D-SWE has high technical success rates in children. 2D-SWE demonstrated a 95% technical success rate in a mostly pediatric study containing 573 examinations.[66] A few studies have assessed the feasibility of free breathing ultrasound SWE in children (Figs. 7.9–7.11). No significant difference in LSMs using 2D-SWE during breath held and free breathing conditions (7.21 kPa vs. 7.22 kPa) has been reported in a series of 57 children.[67] However, it was found that 2D-SWE values were 11% lower when measured during free breathing conditions in 45 children with liver disease.[68]

Challenges related to liver size also can arise in very young children. If a region of interest is placed too close to the liver surface (e.g., within 1–2 cm of the capsular surface), reflection of shear waves can occur, resulting in erroneous measurements.[3] Furthermore, linear high-frequency transducers are commonly used to image very small children due to improved overall image quality, including superior spatial resolution. In some instances, high-frequency linear and low-frequency curved transducers might yield slightly different stiffness measurements.[69] However, studies have demonstrated no or minimal (and unlikely to be clinically relevant) differences in LSMs when comparing linear and curved transducers in the same pediatric patients.[70,71]

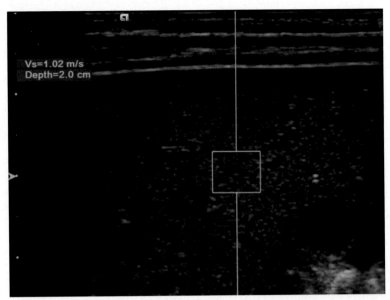

Fig. 7.9 A 2-month-old infant with persistent jaundice and neonatal hepatitis. Point shear wave elastography image shows normal liver stiffness (1.02 m/s, 3.12 kPa). The examination was performed free breathing using a linear transducer. Note that the transducer is oriented parallel to the liver capsule.

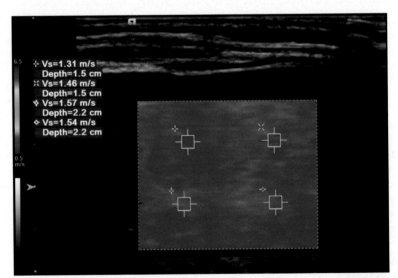

Fig. 7.10 A 2-month-old infant with persistent jaundice and neonatal hepatitis (same patient as in Fig. 7.9). Two-dimensional shear wave elastography image shows a homogeneous liver with liver stiffness measurements ranging from 1.31 to 1.57 m/s (5.15–7.39 kPa) (four regions of interest were placed as part of a research protocol). The examination was performed free breathing using a linear transducer. Note that the transducer is parallel to the liver capsule. Two-dimensional liver stiffness measurements were slightly higher than point liver stiffness measurements obtained using the same ultrasound system and transducer.

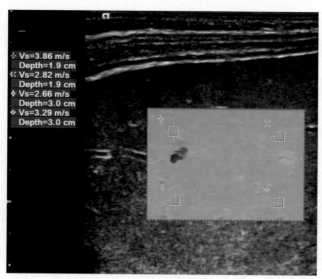

Fig. 7.11 A 6-week-old boy with persistent jaundice and surgically proven biliary atresia. Preoperative two-dimensional shear wave elastography image shows a heterogeneous liver with marked stiffening. Liver stiffness measurements range from 2.66 to 3.86 m/s (21.23–44.70 kPa) (four measurement boxes were placed as part of a research protocol). The examination was performed with the patient awake and free breathing in the neonatal intensive care unit.

ULTRASOUND VERSUS MAGNETIC RESONANCE ELASTOGRAPHY

Ultrasound SWE and MRE both have distinct advantages and disadvantages when compared with one another. Advantages of ultrasound SWE compared with MRE include its faster examination time from start to finish on average, lower cost, and potential to allow more frequent serial monitoring. Ultrasound also does not require sedation or anesthesia, and it can be performed with the patient's parent or guardian at the bedside. Advantages of MRE compared with ultrasound SWE include larger elastograms that allow a greater volume of tissue to be sampled and its ability to accurately detect and measure liver fat and iron. In particular, MRE may be preferred in children with NAFLD due to MR imaging's ability to obtain robust measurements of proton density fat fraction, a surrogate marker of hepatic steatosis.

Unfortunately, there is a paucity of published studies comparing ultrasound SWE methods and MRE head-to-head in the same pediatric patients. A study demonstrated substantial correlation between measurements when the spread of ultrasound measurements is minimal, whereas correlation is poor when the spread is substantial.[72] The same study found that the spread of ultrasound SWE measurements, based on shear wave speed interquartile range/median, was significantly associated with body mass index.

SHEAR WAVE ELASTOGRAPHY TECHNIQUES: INTEROPERATOR AGREEMENT

In a study that included 51 children with NAFLD, VCTE failure rates were 10%–12% and had a positive association with increasing obesity.[73] Intraoperator agreement for LSMs was near-perfect (concordance correlation coefficient [CCC] = 0.85), and interoperator agreement was substantial (CCC = 0.76). Interoperator agreement was inversely associated with body mass index.

In a study on 63 pediatric patients with various liver diseases, the interobserver agreement of a 2D-SWE technique was excellent (intraclass correlation coefficient [ICC] = 0.95) with no relationships between agreement and patient age or liver stiffness.[68]

NORMATIVE LIVER STIFFNESS VALUES

Vibration Controlled Transient Elastography

Multiple studies have described the use of VCTE in healthy children to acquire normative liver stiffness data. In a metaanalysis that included healthy individual participant data from 10 pediatric studies (652 nonobese, nondiabetic children), mean liver stiffness was 4.45 kPa in children ≥ 3 years of age.[74] The normal liver stiffness reference range in healthy children ranged from 2.45 to 5.56 kPa.

Point Shear Wave Elastography

Multiple studies have performed point SWE in healthy children to obtain normative liver stiffness data. In a series of 103 children (2 weeks to 17 years of age) the mean liver stiffness was 1.12 m/s (3.76 kPa) (VTQ, Siemens Healthineers, Germany).[75] Using a similar ultrasound system in 150 healthy children (2 months to 17 years of age), a mean liver stiffness of 1.07 m/s (3.43 kPa) was identified.[76] By using a Samsung ultrasound system in 243 healthy children (4 to 17 years of age), a median liver stiffness of 4.1 kPa (interquartile range, 3.6–4.7 kPa) was obtained.[77]

Two-Dimensional Shear Wave Elastography

There is a general paucity of normative liver stiffness data in children for 2D-SWE. Using a Canon system in a series of 128 healthy children less than 18 years of age, the mean liver stiffness was 1.29 m/s (4.99 kPa), and 1.55 m/s (7.20 kPa) was the upper limit of normal.[78] Using the Aixplorer system (Hologic) in 51 healthy children (0 to 15 years of age), mean liver stiffness was 6.94 kPa when using an SC6-1 curved transducer and slightly lower when using a SL15-4 linear transducer (5.96 kPa).[79] Using the 2D-SWE technique implemented in a GE Healthcare ultrasound system in 243 healthy children between the ages of 4 and 17 years old, the median liver stiffness was 3.3 kPa, with an interquartile range of 2.7–4.3 kPa.[77] Using the same technology in 202 healthy children without liver disease (newborn to 16 years of age), the mean liver stiffness was 4.29 kPa.[70]

It is worth noting that multiple studies have assessed the impact of patient age on LSMs in the pediatric population, with a small positive correlation commonly identified for VCTE, pSWE, and 2D-SWE.[76,77,80,81]

Normative pediatric liver stiffness publications and major results are provided in Table 7.2.

STAGING OF LIVER FIBROSIS

The majority of studies have been performed in a small number of children with mixed etiologies of liver disease, often including patients with Fontan disease, which causes liver congestion in addition to fibrosis. This limits the applicability of the results in the clinical practice.

A metaanalysis identified 69 pediatric studies using some form of ultrasound SWE technique to evaluate the liver.[83] Of these publications, 40 addressed technical feasibility and measurement reliability. There was no significant difference in the pooled proportions of technical failure between pSWE and 2D-SWE (4.1% and 2.2%, respectively). A systematic review and metaanalysis evaluated the diagnostic performance of ultrasound SWE in children for staging liver fibrosis.[84] Based on 12 eligible studies and 550 patients, ultrasound elastographic methods had a pooled sensitivity of 81% and a pooled specificity of 91% for predicting significant (≥ F2) histologic liver fibrosis, with an AUROC of 0.91.

TABLE 7.2 ■ Published Ultrasound Shear Wave Elastography Liver Stiffness Normal Values in Healthy Children[a]

Study	Number of Children	Ultrasound (US) System	Mean/Median Liver Stiffness[b]	Upper Limits of Normal
Engelmann et al.[80]	240	VCTE (FibroScan)	4.7 kPa (1.25 m/s)	6.47 kPa (1.47 m/s)
Hanquinet et al.[82]	103	pSWE (Siemens US system)	1.12 m/s (3.76 kPa)	1.37 m/s (5.63 kPa)
Matos et al.[76]	150	pSWE (Siemens US system)	1.05 m/s (3.31 kPa)	1.27 m/s (4.84 kPa)
Mjelle et al.[77]	243	pSWE (Samsung US system)	1.14–1.24 m/s (3.90–4.61 kPa) (depending on age)	1.30–1.46 m/s (5.07–6.39 kPa) (depending on age)
Trout et al.[78]	128	2D-SWE (Canon US system)	1.29 m/s (4.99 kPa)	1.54 m/s (7.11 kPa)
Mjelle et al.[77]	243	2D-SWE (GE US system)	0.98–1.15 m/s (2.88–3.97 kPa) (depending on age)	1.15–1.45 m/s (3.97–6.31 kPa) (depending on age)
Galina et al.[70]	202	2D-SWE (GE US system)	4.29 kPa (1.20 m/s)	5.45 kPa (1.35 m/s)
Franchi-Abella et al.[79]	51	2D-SWE (Hologic US system)	6.94 kPa (1.52 m/s) (SC6-1 transducer) 5.96 kPa (1.41 m/s) (SL15-4 transducer)	9.72 kPa (1.80 m/s) (SC6-1 transducer) 8.53 kPa (1.69 m/s) (SL15-4 transducer)

[a]Upper limits of normal as described in publication or calculated *ad hoc* using mean liver stiffness + 1.96 (standard deviation).

[b]Values obtained in meters per second (shear wave speed) were converted to kilopascals or vice versa using Young's modulus: LSM (kPa) = [shear wave speed (m/s)]^2 × 3, where LSM = liver stiffness measurement.

It is worth noting that ultrasound elastographic methods likely have comparable diagnostic accuracy to MRE for staging liver fibrosis. In a study of 86 children and young adults with a median age of 14.2 years, MRE's AUROC for discriminating Ludwig liver fibrosis stages 0–1 from stage 2 or higher was only 0.70 (95% confidence interval, 0.59–0.81), with performance slightly improving to 0.82 when excluding patients with hepatic steatosis.[85] Using a shear modulus cutoff value of 2.27 kPa, MRE demonstrated a sensitivity of 68.6% and specificity of 74.3%. It must be highlighted that the MRE measurement of liver stiffness is given in shear modulus units that are approximately three times smaller than the Young's modulus units used for ultrasound SWE.

Examples of publications assessing the diagnostic performance of ultrasound SWE for staging histologic liver fibrosis in children are presented in Table 7.3.

Vibration Controlled Transient Elastography

Multiple pediatric studies have assessed the ability of VCTE to stage histologic liver fibrosis with reasonable success. A study in 33 children (2 months to 20 years of age) with mixed etiologies of liver disease and with available histologic data showed an AUROC of 0.88 for distinguishing F0–F3 from F4 liver fibrosis.[86] In a series of 104 children undergoing liver biopsy, the AUROCs were 0.79 and 0.96 for ≥ F3 and F4 liver fibrosis, respectively.[87] The optimal cutoff for significant fibrosis was 6.9 kPa (68% sensitivity, 78% specificity). A cutoff of 14.1 kPa for cirrhosis had a

TABLE 7.3 ■ **Diagnostic Performance of Ultrasound Shear Wave Elastography for Staging Histologic Liver Fibrosis in Children**

Study	Number of Children	Ultrasound System	Fibrosis Stages Differentiated	Area under the ROC Curve
de Lédinghen et al.[86]	33	VCTE (FibroScan)	F0–F3 vs. F4	0.88
Fitzpatrick et al.[87]	104	VCTE (FibroScan)	F0–F2 vs. F3–F4 F0–F3 vs. F4	0.79 0.96
Dillman et al.[88]	62	pSWE (Siemens US system)	0–2 vs. 3–6[a]	0.84
Alhashmi et al.[89]	46	2D-SWE (Canon US system)	F0–F1 vs. F2–F4	0.75
Farmakis et al.[90]	70	2D-SWE (GE US system)	F0–F1 vs. F2–F4	0.89
Franchi-Abella et al.[79]	45	2D-SWE (Hologic US system)	F0–F1 vs. F2–F4	0.98
Garcovich et al.[91]	68[b]	2D-SWE (Hologic US system)	F0–F1 vs. F2–F4	0.97
Dardanelli et al.[92]	213	2D-SWE (Hologic US system)	0–2 vs. 3–6[a]	0.89
Tutar et al.[93]	76	2D-SWE (Hologic US system)	F0 vs. F1–F4	0.95

[a]Ishak histologic liver fibrosis staging system.
[b]All individuals with nonalcoholic steatohepatitis.

sensitivity of 100% and specificity of 92%. In this series, 63.4% of children were affected by NAFLD or autoimmune hepatitis, whereas the remaining had viral hepatitis, Wilson disease, or miscellaneous conditions such as familial cholestasis or metabolic liver disease. VCTE performed best in children with autoimmune liver disease and in posttransplant children.

In a systematic review and metaanalysis that included 11 pediatric publications, summary sensitivity and specificity were 95% and 90% for detecting significant liver fibrosis ($\geq$ F2 histologic stage), with a hierarchic summary AUROC of 0.96.[94]

Point Shear Wave Elastography

Using pSWE (VTQ, Siemens Healthineers), 39 children (1 month to 14 years of age) were evaluated with correlative histologic data.[82] A cutoff value of 1.34 m/s (5.39 kPa) had 82% sensitivity and 45% specificity for detecting any degree of liver fibrosis (F > 0). In the same study, a cutoff value of 2.0 m/s (12 kPa) yielded a sensitivity of 100% and specificity of 32.1%. The same technology demonstrated an AUROC of 0.84 for distinguishing patients with no or mild (Ishak 0–2) liver fibrosis from those with moderate or severe (Ishak 3–6) liver fibrosis.[88]

Two-Dimensional Shear Wave Elastography

A small number of pediatric studies have looked at the association between LSMs acquired using 2D-SWE and liver histologic staging. For some ultrasound systems and 2D-SWE methods no published data exist. Examples of using ARFI techniques in clinical practice to assess liver fibrosis are provided in Figs. 7.12–7.14.

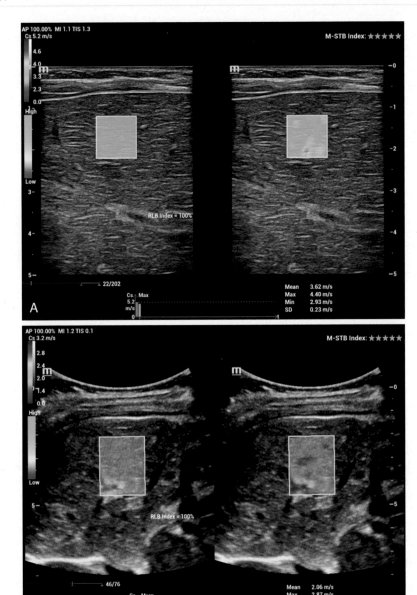

Fig. 7.12 Two different children with biliary atresia and substantial liver stiffening following Kasai portoenterostomy palliation presumably due to fibrosis. (A) Two-dimensional shear wave elastography (2D-SWE) performed using a linear transducer in a 2-year-old child shows a liver stiffness measurement of 3.62 m/s (39.31 kPa). (B) 2D-SWE performed using a curved transducer in a 3-year-old child shows a liver stiffness measurement of 2.06 m/s (12.73 kPa). Both acquisitions are of high quality, with motion stability indices *(M-STB)* showing five green stars and reliability indices *(RLB)* of 100%.

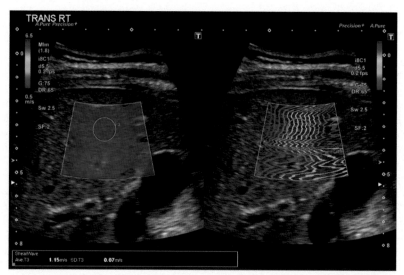

Fig. 7.13 A 9-year-old girl with treated hepatitis C virus. Two-dimensional shear wave elastography image shows a normal liver stiffness of 1.15 m/s (3.97 kPa), suggesting no liver fibrosis. The propagation image on the *right* shows many parallel lines located close together, indicative of normal shear wave speed.

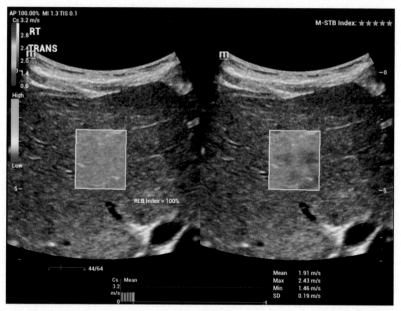

Fig. 7.14 A 14-year-old boy with Alagille syndrome. Two-dimensional shear wave elastography demonstrates increased liver stiffness (1.91 m/s, 10.94 kPa) likely due to fibrosis. The liver surface has a macronodular contour. The image is of high quality with a motion stability index *(M-STB)* of five green stars and a reliability index *(RLB)* of 100%.

Using a 2D-SWE technique (GE Healthcare, USA), 70 children (0 to 18 years of age) undergoing liver biopsy were evaluated.[90] The AUROC for differentiating F0–F1 from F2–F4 was 0.89, with a sensitivity of 94.6% and specificity of 78.6%. Using another 2D-SWE technique (Canon Medical Systems, Japan) in 46 children (0 to 18 years of age) with correlative liver histologic data, a cutoff value of 1.89 m/s (10.72 kPa) yielded an AUROC of 0.75 for separating patients with F0–F1 from F2–F4 histologic liver fibrosis, with a sensitivity of 73.7% and specificity of 77.8%.[89] The AUROC increased to 0.86 upon exclusion of children with histologic hepatic steatosis, suggesting that the presence of fat may confound LSMs.

Multiple studies have evaluated the relationship between LSMs obtained using the Aixplorer ultrasound system (Hologic, USA) and histologic liver fibrosis. A study in 45 children (1 month to 17 years of age) demonstrated an AUROC of 0.98 for distinguishing F0–F1 from F2–F4 liver fibrosis, with a sensitivity of 86.0% and specificity of 97.1% using a cutoff value of 12.1 kPa.[79] A study in 68 children (8 to 17 years of age) with NAFLD showed an AUROC of 0.97 for separating F0–F1 from F2–F4 liver fibrosis, with a sensitivity of 87% and specificity of 96% using a cutoff value of 6.7 kPa.[91] In a study on 213 children (2 months to 18 years of age), the AUROC for distinguishing Ishak 0–2 from Ishak 3–6 histologic liver fibrosis stages was 0.89, with a sensitivity of 89% and specificity of 80% using a cutoff value of 12 kPa.[92] Finally, LSMs were correlated with liver histologic data in 76 children (4 months to 17 years old).[93] A cutoff value of 10.6 kPa yielded an AUROC of 0.95, with a sensitivity of 91.5% and specificity of 94.0%.

CYSTIC FIBROSIS

Cystic fibrosis (CF) is a multiorgan autosomal recessive disease that affects mostly the lungs, pancreas, sweat glands, intestine, and liver.[95] Liver manifestations include hepatobiliary involvement, obliterative portal venopathy, steatosis, and other liver abnormalities due to infections, long-term antibiotic therapy, diabetes, nutritional deficiencies, hypoxemia, and hepatic congestion from right-side heart failure. Cirrhosis can significantly contribute to morbidity and mortality.

It has been reported that the incidence of CF-related liver disease (CFLD) increases by approximately 1% every year, reaching 32.2% by age 25.[96] The incidence of severe CFLD is 10% by age 30. Due to the improved survival of patients with CF, CFLD has become a more frequent complication of CF.

In a series of 160 consecutive children with CF, a liver stiffness of 5.55 kPa identified children with CFLD with 70% sensitivity and 82% specificity (AUROC: 0.82).[97] Furthermore, a 1-kPa liver stiffness increase was associated with a 2.4-fold increased odds ratio of having CFLD. A VCTE cutoff of 8.7 kPa differentiated patients with severe fibrosis (F3–F4 stages) from patients with mild to moderate fibrosis (F1–F2 stages). The combination of liver stiffness with serum blood tests improved the accuracy for the detection of severe fibrosis. This result confirms that of a previous metaanalysis that reported the accuracy of liver stiffness and AST to platelet ratio index (APRI) in detecting CFLD increased when they were combined: an LSM ≥ 5.95 kPa and an APRI score ≥ 0.329 had high positive and negative predictive values.[98]

Using a 2D-SWE technique, the optimal cutoff for identifying patients with CFLD was 6.85 kPa with 75% sensitivity and 71% specificity (AUROC: 0.79), and the cutoff of 9.05 kPa identified severe fibrosis with 0.95 AUROC.[99] In this study, advanced fibrosis/cirrhosis was assessed clinically or by using an APRI cutoff value for severe fibrosis of > 0.462. On this regard, liver biopsy may not be the optimal procedure for the diagnosis of CFLD due to the patchy pattern of liver involvement and the variety of liver diseases that can be associated with CF.[100] Therefore for the diagnosis of CFLD, physical examination, serum blood tests, and ultrasound evaluation are recommended by the best practice guidance, and CFLD should be considered if at least two of these criteria are positive.[101] It must be highlighted that some CFLD patients may have large regenerative nodules that may lead to an underestimation of liver stiffness.

By using a pSWE technique in a study that enrolled 72 patients with CF and 60 healthy controls, it has been found that a threshold of 1.27 m/s (4.84 kPa) was able to detect children with CFLD with 56.5% sensitivity and 90.5% specificity.[102]

Studies have shown that the delta change of liver stiffness over time is a very useful parameter for identifying patients with CF that develop CFLD.[103] A study showed a more rapid progression of liver stiffness by VCTE (0.94 kPa/yr vs. 0.23 kPa/yr, $P < 0.02$) in patients who developed CFLD.[104] It is worth mentioning that the update to the SRU consensus has proposed that each subject becomes their own control, using the percentage of the liver stiffness change over time to evaluate the efficacy of the treatment or the progression of disease independently of the etiology of the underlying liver disease.[3]

CONFOUNDERS

As ultrasound SWE is a surrogate marker for liver fibrosis, it is worth noting that other tissue processes can affect liver stiffness and thus elastography measurements. The confounders are similar to those observed in adults, even though fewer studies have been published.

An association between liver fibrosis and laboratory inflammation was found using VCTE in children and young adults with F0–F2 histologic liver fibrosis (interestingly, there was no such association in patients with more advanced liver fibrosis).[105] A positive relationship between LSMs and histologic inflammation has also been shown using pSWE in children.[88]

Liver congestion due to increased hepatic afterload, such as following Fontan palliation of single ventricle congenital heart disease, is another potential confounder of liver stiffness measurements. A marked liver stiffening immediately following the Fontan operation due to rerouting of inferior vena cava blood flow away from the heart to the pulmonary arteries (thus, bypassing the heart) has been reported (Fig. 7.15)[106]. In a cohort of 18 children, liver stiffness increased from a mean of 1.18 m/s (4.18 kPa) prior to surgery to a mean of 2.28 m/s (15.60 kPa) 1–3 days after Fontan completion surgery. This marked liver stiffening persisted both at the time of hospital discharge as well as in the outpatient setting as individuals returned for follow-up care. In adolescent and adult Fontan patients with substantially increased LSMs, it becomes impossible to determine how much stiffening is due to congestion versus fibrosis (Fig. 7.16).

PEDIATRIC APPLICATIONS: CONCLUSIONS

Ultrasound SWE is feasible in the pediatric population. A variety of techniques (e.g., VCTE, pSWE, 2D-SWE) are available, with normal liver stiffness values slightly differing by technique and ultrasound system. While exact liver stiffness cutoff values can be challenging to use in clinical practice for the purpose of precise liver staging, SWE techniques can be used to separate normal patients from abnormal patients as well as serially monitor individuals over time for disease progression or regression in the treatment setting. Ultrasound elastographic methods have multiple advantages over MRE in children, including increased availability, lower cost, and overall ease of use.

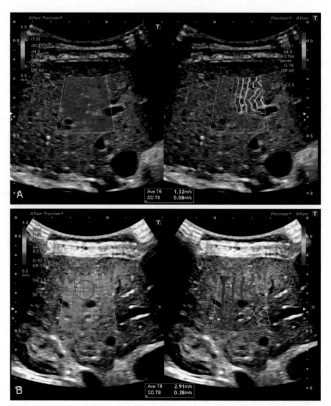

Fig. 7.15 A 3-year-old child with single ventricle congenital heart disease immediately before and after the Fontan operation. (A) Preoperative two-dimensional shear wave elastography (2D-SWE) image shows a normal liver stiffness (1.32 m/s, 5.23 kPa). (B) Postoperative 2D-SWE image shows marked liver stiffening (2.91 m/s, 25.4 kPa) due to elevated central venous pressure and increased hepatic afterload. The degree of liver stiffening is typical of that seen in the setting of cirrhosis. The propagation images on the *right* of figure parts A and B have expected appearances, with the postoperative image having fewer parallel lines that are farther apart, indicative of increased shear wave speed.

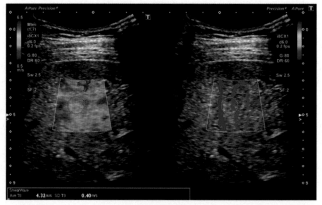

Fig. 7.16 An 18-year-old boy with single ventricle congenital heart disease palliated with the Fontan operation. Two-dimensional shear wave elastography shows marked liver heterogeneity and stiffening with a liver stiffness measurement of 4.32 m/s (55.99 kPa). The wave image on the *right* confirms rapid shear wave propagation. It is uncertain how much of the increased liver stiffness is due to fibrosis versus venous and lymphatic congestion from elevated central venous pressure and increased hepatic afterload.

KEY POINTS

1. With the availability of SWE techniques, the number of liver biopsies performed for staging liver fibrosis in several clinical settings has drastically decreased. Indeed, liver biopsy is now seldom required outside the research setting.
2. The spectrum of advanced fibrosis (METAVIR F3 stage) and cirrhosis (METAVIR F4 stage) is a continuum in asymptomatic patients, and distinguishing between the two is often not possible on clinical grounds. Therefore the term *compensated advanced chronic liver disease* (cACLD), which includes F3 and F4 stages, has been proposed by the Baveno conference.
3. From a clinical point of view, it is more important to rule in or rule out significant disease (cACLD) than it is to provide an exact stage of liver fibrosis by using a histological scoring system.
4. For the staging of liver fibrosis in patients with chronic viral hepatitis and NAFLD, the "rule of 5" has been proposed for VCTE and the "rule of 4" for the ARFI techniques (pSWE and 2D-SWE).
5. Liver stiffness cutoffs obtained in untreated patients with viral hepatitis cannot rule out the presence of advanced fibrosis and guide screening strategies in patients that achieve SVR.
6. Elastography has been proposed as a tool to predict the risk of death or complications in patients with advanced chronic liver disease.
7. In patients with chronic viral hepatitis, the risk of developing liver-related events cannot be completely eliminated even in those who achieve complete virological response; this risk is mainly related to the degree of liver fibrosis before starting the treatment.
8. In ALD patients, cACLD is the main predictor of long-term survival, therefore it is of utmost importance to diagnose patients with advanced fibrosis before decompensation occurs to promote abstinence and improve survival.
9. In children, SWE can be used to separate normal patients from abnormal patients as well as serially monitor individuals over time for disease progression or regression in the treatment setting.

References

1. Marcellin P, Kutala BK. Liver diseases: a major, neglected global public health problem requiring urgent actions and large-scale screening. *Liver Int.* 2018;38(suppl 1):2-6.
2. Scaglione S, Kliethermes S, Cao G, et al. The epidemiology of cirrhosis in the United States: a population-based study. *J Clin Gastroenterol.* 2015;49:690-696.
3. Barr RG, Wilson SR, Rubens D, Garcia-Tsao G, Ferraioli G. Update to the society of radiologists in ultrasound liver elastography consensus statement. *Radiology.* 2020;296:263-274.
4. Wong GL. Non-invasive assessments for liver fibrosis: the crystal ball we long for. *J Gastroenterol Hepatol.* 2018;33:1009-1015.
5. de Franchis R, Baveno VI Faculty. Expanding consensus in portal hypertension: report of the Baveno VI Consensus Workshop: stratifying risk and individualizing care for portal hypertension. *J Hepatol.* 2015;63:743-752.
6. Dietrich CF, Bamber J, Berzigotti A, et al. EFSUMB guidelines and recommendations on the clinical use of liver ultrasound elastography, update 2017 (Long Version). *Ultraschall Med.* 2017;38:e16-e47.
7. Ferraioli G, Wong VW, Castera L, et al. Liver ultrasound elastography: an update to the world federation for ultrasound in medicine and biology guidelines and recommendations. *Ultrasound Med Biol.* 2018;44:2419-2440.
8. Ferraioli G, De Silvestri A, Lissandrin R, et al. Evaluation of inter-system variability in liver stiffness measurements. *Ultraschall Med.* 2019;40:64-75.
9. Mózes FE, Lee JA, Selvaraj EA, et al. Diagnostic accuracy of non-invasive tests for advanced fibrosis in patients with NAFLD: an individual patient data meta-analysis. *Gut.* 2021:gutjnl-2021-324243.
10. Singh S, Facciorusso A, Loomba R, Falck-Ytter YT. Magnitude and kinetics of decrease in liver stiffness after antiviral therapy in patients with chronic hepatitis C: a systematic review and meta-analysis. *Clin Gastroenterol Hepatol.* 2018;16:27-38.
11. Tachi Y, Hirai T, Kojima Y, et al. Liver stiffness measurement using acoustic radiation force impulse elastography in hepatitis C virus-infected patients with a sustained virological response. *Aliment Pharmacol Ther.* 2016;44:346-355.

12. Mauro E, Crespo G, Montironi C, et al. Portal pressure and liver stiffness measurements in the prediction of fibrosis regression after sustained virological response in recurrent hepatitis C. *Hepatology.* 2018;67:1683-1694.

13. Garcia-Tsao G. Regression of HCV cirrhosis: time will tell. *Hepatology.* 2018;67:1651-1653.

14. Kim JH, Kim MN, Han KH, Kim SU. Clinical application of transient elastography in patients with chronic viral hepatitis receiving antiviral treatment. *Liver Int.* 2015;35:1103-1115.

15. Liang X, Xie Q, Tan D, et al. Interpretation of liver stiffness measurement-based approach for the monitoring of hepatitis B patients with antiviral therapy: a 2-year prospective study. *J Viral Hepat.* 2018;25:296-305.

16. Ji D, Chen Y, Shang Q, et al. Unreliable estimation of fibrosis regression during treatment by liver stiffness measurement in patients with chronic hepatitis B. *Am J Gastroenterol.* 2021;116(8):1676-1685.

17. Dillon A, Galvin Z, Sultan AA, Harman D, Guha IN, Stewart S. Transient elastography can stratify patients with Child-Pugh A cirrhosis according to risk of early decompensation. *Eur J Gastroenterol Hepatol.* 2018;30:1434-1440.

18. Singh S, Fujii LL, Murad MH, et al. Liver stiffness is associated with risk of decompensation, liver cancer, and death in patients with chronic liver diseases: a systematic review and meta-analysis. *Clin Gastroenterol Hepatol.* 2013;11:1573-1584.

19. Wang J, Li J, Zhou Q, et al. Liver stiffness measurement predicted liver-related events and all-cause mortality: a systematic review and nonlinear dose-response meta-analysis. *Hepatol Commun.* 2018;2:467-476.

20. Pons M, Simón-Talero M, Millán L, et al. Basal values and changes of liver stiffness predict the risk of disease progression in compensated advanced chronic liver disease. *Dig Liver Dis.* 2016;48:1214-1219.

21. Vutien P, Kim NJ, Moon AM, et al. FibroScan liver stiffness after anti-viral treatment for hepatitis C is independently associated with adverse outcomes. *Aliment Pharmacol Ther.* 2020;52:1717-1727.

22. Trebicka J, Gu W, de Ledinghen V, et al. Two-dimensional shear wave elastography predicts survival in advanced chronic liver disease. *Gut.* 2022;71(2):402-414.

23. Ferraioli G. Beyond the AJR: "Two-dimensional shear wave elastography predicts survival in advanced chronic liver disease". *AJR Am J Roentgenol.* 2021;217:1012.

24. Wong GL, Chan HL, Wong CK, et al. Liver stiffness-based optimization of hepatocellular carcinoma risk score in patients with chronic hepatitis B. *J Hepatol.* 2014;60:339-345.

25. Lee HW, Yoo EJ, Kim BK, et al. Prediction of development of liver-related events by transient elastography in hepatitis B patients with complete virological response on antiviral therapy. *Am J Gastroenterol.* 2014;109:1241-1249.

26. Yang HI, Yuen MF, Chan HL, et al. Risk estimation for hepatocellular carcinoma in chronic hepatitis B (REACH-B): development and validation of a predictive score. *Lancet Oncol.* 2011;12:568-574.

27. Papatheodoridis GV, Sypsa V, Dalekos GN, et al. Hepatocellular carcinoma prediction beyond year 5 of oral therapy in a large cohort of Caucasian patients with chronic hepatitis B. *J Hepatol.* 2020;72:1088-1096.

28. Chon HY, Lee JS, Lee HW, et al. Predictive performance of CAGE-B and SAGE-B models in Asian treatment-naïve patients who started entecavir for chronic hepatitis B. *Clin Gastroenterol Hepatol.* 2022;20(4):e794-e807.

29. Calvaruso V, Cabibbo G, Cacciola I, et al. Incidence of hepatocellular carcinoma in patients with HCV-associated cirrhosis treated with direct-acting antiviral agents. *Gastroenterology.* 2018;155:411-421.

30. Carrat F, Fontaine H, Dorival C, et al. Clinical outcomes in patients with chronic hepatitis C after direct-acting antiviral treatment: a prospective cohort study. *Lancet.* 2019;393:1453-1464.

31. Ioannou GN, Beste LA, Green PK, et al. Increased risk for hepatocellular carcinoma persists up to 10 years after HCV eradication in patients with baseline cirrhosis or high FIB-4 scores. *Gastroenterology.* 2019;157:1264-1278.

32. Pons M, Rodríguez-Tajes S, Esteban JI, et al. Non-invasive prediction of liver-related events in patients with HCV-associated compensated advanced chronic liver disease after oral antivirals. *J Hepatol.* 2020;72:472-480.

33. Ravaioli F, Conti F, Brillanti S, et al. Hepatocellular carcinoma risk assessment by the measurement of liver stiffness variations in HCV cirrhotics treated with direct acting antivirals. *Dig Liver Dis.* 2018;50:573-579.

34. Moreno C, Mueller S, Szabo G. Non-invasive diagnosis and biomarkers in alcohol-related liver disease. *J Hepatol.* 2019;70:273-283.

35. European Association for the Study of the Liver. Clinical Practice Guideline Panel; Chair: EASL Governing Board representative; Panel members. EASL Clinical Practice Guidelines on non-invasive tests for evaluation of liver disease severity and prognosis - 2021 update. *J Hepatol.* 2021;75(3):659-689.
36. Hagström H, Thiele M, Roelstraete B, Söderling J, Ludvigsson JF. Mortality in biopsy-proven alcohol-related liver disease: a population-based nationwide cohort study of 3453 patients. *Gut.* 2021;70: 170-179.
37. Hazeldine S, Hydes T, Sheron N. Alcoholic liver disease - the extent of the problem and what you can do about it. *Clin Med (London, England).* 2015;15:179-185.
38. European Association for the Study of the Liver. EASL Clinical Practice Guidelines: management of alcohol-related liver disease. *J Hepatol.* 2018;69(1):154-181.
39. Liangpunsakul S, Crabb DW. Early detection of alcoholic liver disease: are we a step closer? *Gastroenterology.* 2016;150:29-31.
40. Mann RE, Smart RG, Govoni R. The epidemiology of alcoholic liver disease. *Alcohol Res Health.* 2003;27:209-219.
41. Pose E, Ginès P. Transient elastography for alcoholic liver disease: a step forward. *Lancet Gastroenterol Hepatol.* 2018;3:589-591.
42. Lackner C, Spindelboeck W, Haybaeck J. Histological parameters and alcohol abstinence determine long-term prognosis in patients with alcoholic liver disease. *J Hepatol.* 2017;66:610-618.
43. Thiele M, Detlefsen S, Sevelsted Moller L, et al. Transient and 2-dimensional shear-wave elastography provide comparable assessment of alcoholic liver fibrosis and cirrhosis. *Gastroenterology.* 2016;150: 123-133.
44. Nguyen-Khac E, Thiele M, Voican C, et al. Non-invasive diagnosis of liver fibrosis in patients with alcohol-related liver disease by transient elastography: an individual patient data meta-analysis. *Lancet Gastroenterol Hepatol.* 2018;3:614-625.
45. Cho Y, Choi YI, Oh S, et al. Point shear wave elastography predicts fibrosis severity and steatohepatitis in alcohol-related liver disease. *Hepatol Int.* 2020;14:270-280.
46. Zhang D, Li P, Chen M, et al. Non-invasive assessment of liver fibrosis in patients with alcoholic liver disease using acoustic radiation force impulse elastography. *Abdominal Imaging.* 2015;40:723-729.
47. Trabut JB, Thepot V, Nalpas B, et al. Rapid decline of liver stiffness following alcohol withdrawal in heavy drinkers. *Alcohol Clin Exp Res.* 2012;36:1407-1411.
48. Gelsi E, Dainese R, Truchi R, et al. Effect of detoxification on liver stiffness assessed by FibroScan in alcoholic patients. *Alcohol Clin Exp Res.* 2011;35:566-570.
49. Gianni E, Forte P, Galli V, Razzolini G, Bardazzi G, Annese V. Prospective evaluation of liver stiffness using transient elastography in alcoholic patients following abstinence. *Alcohol Alcohol.* 2017;52: 42-47.
50. Mueller S, Millonig G, Sarovska L, et al. Increased liver stiffness in alcoholic liver disease: differentiating fibrosis from steatohepatitis. *World J Gastroenterol.* 2010;16:966-972.
51. Legros L, Bardou-Jacquet E, Turlin B, et al. Transient elastography accurately screens for compensated advanced chronic liver disease in patients with ongoing or recent alcohol withdrawal. *Clin Gastroenterol Hepatol.* 2021;S1542-3565(21)00155-5.
52. Dyson J, Jones D. Diagnosis and management of patients with primary biliary cirrhosis. *Clin Liver Dis (Hoboken).* 2014;3:52-55.
53. Corpechot C, Carrat F, Poujol-Robert A, et al. Noninvasive elastography-based assessment of liver fibrosis progression and prognosis in primary biliary cirrhosis. *Hepatology.* 2012;56:198-208.
54. Corpechot C, Gaouar F, El Naggar A, et al. Baseline values and changes in liver stiffness measured by transient elastography are associated with severity of fibrosis and outcomes of patients with primary sclerosing cholangitis. *Gastroenterology.* 2014;146:970-979.
55. Gines P, Graupera I, Lammert F, et al. Screening for liver fibrosis in the general population: a call for action. *Lancet Gastroenterol Hepatol.* 2016;1:256-260.
56. Roulot D, Costes JL, Buyck JF, et al. Transient elastography as a screening tool for liver fibrosis and cirrhosis in a community-based population aged over 45 years. *Gut.* 2011;60:977-984.
57. Wong VW, Chu WC, Wong GL, et al. Prevalence of non-alcoholic fatty liver disease and advanced fibrosis in Hong Kong Chinese: a population study using proton-magnetic resonance spectroscopy and transient elastography. *Gut.* 2012;61:409-415.

58. Castera L. Diagnosis of non-alcoholic fatty liver disease/non-alcoholic steatohepatitis: non-invasive tests are enough. *Liver Int.* 2018;38(suppl 1):67-70.

59. Koehler EM, Plompen EP, Schouten JN, et al. Presence of diabetes mellitus and steatosis is associated with liver stiffness in a general population: the Rotterdam study. *Hepatology.* 2016;63:138–147.

60. Kwok R, Choi KC, Wong GL, et al. Screening diabetic patients for non-alcoholic fatty liver disease with controlled attenuation parameter and liver stiffness measurements: a prospective cohort study. *Gut.* 2016;65:1359–1368.

61. Harman DJ, Ryder SD, James MW, et al. Direct targeting of risk factors significantly increases the detection of liver cirrhosis in primary care: a cross-sectional diagnostic study utilising transient elastography. *BMJ Open.* 2015;5:e007516.

62. Ferraioli G, Filice C, Castera L, et al. WFUMB guidelines and recommendations for clinical use of ultrasound elastography: Part 3: liver. *Ultrasound Med Biol.* 2015;41:1161-1179.

63. Barr RG, Ferraioli G, Palmeri ML, et al. Elastography assessment of liver fibrosis: Society of Radiologists in Ultrasound consensus conference statement. *Radiology.* 2015;276:845-861.

64. Goyal NP, Schwimmer JB. The progression and natural history of pediatric nonalcoholic fatty liver disease. *Clin Liver Dis.* 2016;20:325-338.

65. Regev A, Berho M, Jeffers LJ, et al. Sampling error and intraobserver variation in liver biopsy in patients with chronic HCV infection. *Am J Gastroenterol.* 2002;97:2614-2618.

66. Northern NA, Dillman JR, Trout AT. Frequency of technical success of two-dimensional ultrasound shear wave elastography in a large pediatric and young adult cohort: a clinical effectiveness study. *Pediatr Radiol.* 2019;49:1025-1031.

67. Jung C, Groth M, Petersen KU, et al. Hepatic shear wave elastography in children under free-breathing and breath-hold conditions. *Eur Radiol.* 2017;27:5337-5343.

68. Yoon HM, Cho YA, Kim JR, et al. Real-time two-dimensional shear-wave elastography for liver stiffness in children: interobserver variation and effect of breathing technique. *Eur J Radiol.* 2017;97:53-58.

69. Dillman JR, Chen S, Davenport MS, et al. Superficial ultrasound shear wave speed measurements in soft and hard elasticity phantoms: repeatability and reproducibility using two ultrasound systems. *Pediatr Radiol.* 2015;45:376-385.

70. Galina P, Alexopoulou E, Zellos A, et al. Performance of two-dimensional ultrasound shear wave elastography: reference values of normal liver stiffness in children. *Pediatr Radiol.* 2019;49:91-98.

71. Fontanilla T, Cañas T, Macia A, et al. Normal values of liver shear wave velocity in healthy children assessed by acoustic radiation force impulse imaging using a convex probe and a linear probe. *Ultrasound Med Biol.* 2014;40:470-477.

72. Trout AT, Dillman JR, Xanthakos S, et al. Prospective assessment of correlation between US acoustic radiation force impulse and MR elastography in a pediatric population: dispersion of US shear-wave speed measurement matters. *Radiology.* 2016;281:544-552.

73. Mandelia C, Kabbany MN, Worley S, Conjeevaram Selvakumar PK. Performance characteristics, intra- and inter-operator agreement of transient elastography in pediatric nonalcoholic fatty liver disease. *J Pediatr Gastroenterol Nutr.* 2021;72:430-435.

74. Li DK, Khan MR, Wang Z, et al. Normal liver stiffness and influencing factors in healthy children: an individual participant data meta-analysis. *Liver Int.* 2020;40:2602-2611.

75. Hanquinet S, Courvoisier D, Kanavaki A, Dhouib A, Anooshiravani M. Acoustic radiation force impulse imaging-normal values of liver stiffness in healthy children. *Pediatr Radiol.* 2013;43:539-544.

76. Matos H, Trindade A, Noruegas MJ. Acoustic radiation force impulse imaging in paediatric patients: normal liver values. *J Pediatr Gastroenterol Nutr.* 2014;59:684-688.

77. Mjelle AB, Mulabecirovic A, Havre RF, et al. Normal liver stiffness values in children: a comparison of three different elastography methods. *J Pediatr Gastroenterol Nutr.* 2019;68:706-712.

78. Trout AT, Xanthakos SA, Bennett PS, Dillman JR. Liver shear wave speed and other quantitative ultrasound measures of liver parenchyma: prospective evaluation in healthy children and adults. *AJR Am J Roentgenol.* 2020;214:557-565.

79. Franchi-Abella S, Corno L, Gonzales E, et al. Feasibility and diagnostic accuracy of supersonic shear-wave elastography for the assessment of liver stiffness and liver fibrosis in children: a pilot study of 96 patients. *Radiology.* 2016;278:554-562.

80. Engelmann G, Gebhardt C, Wenning D, et al. Feasibility study and control values of transient elastography in healthy children. *Eur J Pediatr.* 2012;171:353-360.

81. Lee MJ, Kim MJ, Han KH, Yoon CS. Age-related changes in liver, kidney, and spleen stiffness in healthy children measured with acoustic radiation force impulse imaging. *Eur J Radiol.* 2013;82:e290-e294.

82. Hanquinet S, Rougemont AL, Courvoisier D, et al. Acoustic radiation force impulse (ARFI) elastography for the noninvasive diagnosis of liver fibrosis in children. *Pediatr Radiol.* 2013;43:545-551.

83. Kim DW, Park C, Yoon HM, et al. Technical performance of shear wave elastography for measuring liver stiffness in pediatric and adolescent patients: a systematic review and meta-analysis. *Eur Radiol.* 2019;29:2560-2572.

84. Kim JR, Suh CH, Yoon HM, Lee JS, Cho YA, Jung AY. The diagnostic performance of shear-wave elastography for liver fibrosis in children and adolescents: a systematic review and diagnostic meta-analysis. *Eur Radiol.* 2018;28:1175-1186.

85. Trout AT, Sheridan RM, Serai SD, et al. Diagnostic performance of MR elastography for liver fibrosis in children and young adults with a spectrum of liver diseases. *Radiology.* 2018;287:824-832.

86. de Lédinghen V, Le Bail B, Rebouissoux L, et al. Liver stiffness measurement in children using FibroScan: feasibility study and comparison with FibroTest, aspartate transaminase to platelets ratio index, and liver biopsy. *J Pediatr Gastroenterol Nutr.* 2007;45:443-450.

87. Fitzpatrick E, Quaglia A, Vimalesvaran S, Basso MS, Dhawan A. Transient elastography is a useful noninvasive tool for the evaluation of fibrosis in paediatric chronic liver disease. *J Pediatr Gastroenterol Nutr.* 2013;56:72-76.

88. Dillman JR, Heider A, Bilhartz JL, et al. Ultrasound shear wave speed measurements correlate with liver fibrosis in children. *Pediatr Radiol.* 2015;45:1480-1488.

89. Alhashmi GH, Gupta A, Trout AT, Dillman JR. Two-dimensional ultrasound shear wave elastography for identifying and staging liver fibrosis in pediatric patients with known or suspected liver disease: a clinical effectiveness study. *Pediatr Radiol.* 2020;50:1255-1262.

90. Farmakis SG, Buchanan PM, Guzman MA, Hardy AK, Jain AK, Teckman JH. Shear wave elastography correlates with liver fibrosis scores in pediatric patients with liver disease. *Pediatr Radiol.* 2019;49: 1742-1753.

91. Garcovich M, Veraldi S, Di Stasio E, et al. Liver stiffness in pediatric patients with fatty liver disease: diagnostic accuracy and reproducibility of shear-wave elastography. *Radiology.* 2017;283:820-827.

92. Dardanelli EP, Orozco ME, Lostra J, et al. Bidimensional shear-wave elastography for assessing liver fibrosis in children: a proposal of reference values that correlate with the histopathological Knodell-Ishak score. *Pediatr Radiol.* 2020;50:817-826.

93. Tutar O, Beşer ÖF, Adaletli I, et al. Shear wave elastography in the evaluation of liver fibrosis in children. *J Pediatr Gastroenterol Nutr.* 2014;58:750-755.

94. Hwang JY, Yoon HM, Kim JR, et al. Diagnostic performance of transient elastography for liver fibrosis in children: a systematic review and meta-analysis. *AJR Am J Roentgenol.* 2018;211:W257-W266.

95. Dana J, Girard M, Debray D. Hepatic manifestations of cystic fibrosis. *Curr Opin Gastroenterol.* 2020;36:192-198.

96. Boëlle PY, Debray D, Guillot L, Clement A, Corvol H, French CF, Modifier Gene Study Investigators. Cystic fibrosis liver disease: outcomes and risk factors in a large cohort of French patients. *Hepatology.* 2019;69:1648-1656.

97. Lewindon PJ, Puertolas-Lopez MV, Ramm LE, et al. Accuracy of transient elastography data combined with APRI in detection and staging of liver disease in pediatric patients with cystic fibrosis. *Clin Gastroenterol Hepatol.* 2019;17:2561-2569.

98. Lam S, Nettel-Aguirre A, Van Biervliet S, et al. Transient elastography in the evaluation of cystic fibrosis-associated liver disease: systematic review and meta-analysis. *J Can Assoc Gastroenterol.* 2019; 2:71-80.

99. Calvopina DA, Noble C, Weis A, et al. Supersonic shear-wave elastography and APRI for the detection and staging of liver disease in pediatric cystic fibrosis. *J Cyst Fibros.* 2020;19:449-454.

100. Koh C, Sakiani S, Surana P, et al. Adult-onset cystic fibrosis liver disease: diagnosis and characterization of an underappreciated entity. *Hepatology.* 2017;66:591-601.

101. Debray D, Kelly D, Houwen R, et al. Best practice guidance for the diagnosis and management of cystic fibrosis-associated liver disease. *J Cyst Fibros.* 2011;10(suppl 2):S29-S36.

102. Cañas T, Maciá A, Muñoz-Codoceo RA, et al. Hepatic and splenic acoustic radiation force impulse shear wave velocity elastography in children with liver disease associated with cystic fibrosis. *Biomed Res Int.* 2015;2015:517369.

103. Ferraioli G, Barr RG, Dillman JR. Elastography for pediatric chronic liver disease: a review and expert opinion. *J Ultrasound Med.* 2021;40:909-928.

104. Gominon AL, Frison E, Hiriart JB, et al. Assessment of liver disease progression in cystic fibrosis using transient elastography. *J Pediatr Gastroenterol Nutr.* 2018;66:455-460.

105. Raizner A, Shillingford N, Mitchell PD, et al. Hepatic inflammation may influence liver stiffness measurements by transient elastography in children and young adults. *J Pediatr Gastroenterol Nutr.* 2017;64:512-517.

106. DiPaola FW, Schumacher KR, Goldberg CS, Friedland-Little J, Parameswaran A, Dillman JR. Effect of Fontan operation on liver stiffness in children with single ventricle physiology. *Eur Radiol.* 2017;27:2434-2442.

CHAPTER 8

The Role of Ultrasound in Portal Hypertension

Davide Roccarina ■ Richard G. Barr

Introduction

Portal hypertension (PH) is a clinical syndrome characterized by an increase of the pressure gradient between the portal vein (PV) and the inferior vena cava (IVC) above 5 mmHg and develops when there is a resistance in the portal–venous system exacerbated by an increased splanchnic and portal–collateral blood flow.

There are different types of PH, depending on the site of the increased resistance. Most often the resistance occurs within the liver (intrahepatic PH), as in liver cirrhosis; however, it can also be prehepatic, as is the case of portal vein thrombosis (PVT), or posthepatic, as in Budd-Chiari syndrome (BCS), congestive heart failure, constrictive pericarditis, and tricuspidal valve diseases.[1]

Liver cirrhosis represents the most common cause of PH in Western countries, whereas in other parts of the world, schistosomiasis and PVT remain the main cause.[2]

In liver cirrhosis, two different components take part to the increased resistance as structural and dynamic changes, according to the Ohm's electricity law described by the equation *Pressure (P) = Resistance (R) × Flow (F)*. Structural changes are caused by distortion of the liver microcirculation by fibrosis, regenerative nodules, angiogenesis, and vascular occlusion. Dynamic changes happen when there is contraction of activated hepatic stellate cells and myofibroblasts that surround hepatic sinusoids and are in the fibrous septa and vascular smooth muscle cells of the hepatic vasculature. The dynamic changes are due to the increased production of local vasoconstrictors (e.g., endothelins, angiotensin-II, norepinephrine, thromboxane A2) and the reduced release of endothelial vasodilators (e.g., nitric oxide). Moreover, there are also dynamic changes that occur in the splanchnic circulation as vascular endothelial growth factor, nitric oxide, and other splanchnic vasodilators that cause splanchnic arteriolar vasodilation and angiogenesis are released; this leads to collaterals formation, plasma volume expansion, and increased cardiac output. All these factors contribute to the rise of the portal pressure by increasing the blood flow toward the liver and play a key role in the development of hypotension, hyperdynamic syndrome, and ascites.[3]

The gold standard for PH assessment in cirrhosis is the measurement of hepatic venous pressure gradient (HVPG), which is obtained by evaluating the difference between wedged hepatic venous pressure (WHVP) and free hepatic venous pressure (FHVP) by a balloon-tipped catheter guided under fluoroscopic control through the right atrium and IVC into the main right hepatic vein (HV). FHVP is obtained by maintaining the tip of the catheter free in the HV, near its opening into the IVC, whereas WHVP is measured after the occlusion of the HV by inflating the balloon at the tip of the catheter. Values of HVPG ≤5 mmHg are normal, whereas an HVPG between 5 and 10 mmHg defines the presence of PH in the absence of clinical manifestations. An HVPG ≥10 mmHg is representative of clinically significant PH (CSPH), which is what matters in the clinical practice because it is associated with the risk of clinical decompensation and onset of complications such as ascites, gastroesophageal varices (GEV) bleeding, hepatic encephalopathy, and hepatorenal syndrome, which represent the main cause of death or liver transplantation. An HVPG $\geq$12 mmHg is strongly related with high risk of gastrointestinal bleeding, a life-threatening condition.[1] Once cirrhosis is diagnosed and CSPH is confirmed, the clinical management of the patient comprises endoscopy screening for GEV, which allows clinicians to identify the presence of varices and to describe their size and the potential presence of red marks that are indicators of high risk of rupture. However, although HVPG represents the reference standard technique to assess the presence of PH, it is invasive, expensive, implies risks, and is not widely available.

B-mode and Doppler ultrasound (US), integrated in the last years by liver and spleen elastography, represent the first-line imaging in the diagnosis of PH and should be performed every time this condition is suspected because it is noninvasive, repeatable, inexpensive, and able not only to highlight the presence of chronic liver disease (CLD), as it is the case of cirrhotic PH, but also to find other features that reveal the mechanism that leads to PH in cases of noncirrhotic PH. However, the interpretation of US findings of PH needs to be always integrated with clinical and laboratory data.

Which Equipment Do We Need and How Do We Perform Ultrasound to Assess the Presence of Portal Hypertension?

Every time we suspect the presence of PH, the liver, spleen, and portal–venous system should be properly examined. US is performed using convex transducers (mean frequencies 3.5–5 MHz). Higher frequency transducers (linear transducers, mean frequencies 7.5–10 MHz) might be needed for children or very lean adult patients or to properly assess the liver surface. The US system needs to have color/power Doppler modes to assess the patency of vessels and to detect hemodynamic parameters of portal and splanchnic arterial and venous circulation. Patients need to fast for at least 6 hours before the examination and are examined in a supine position after 5–10 minutes of rest (food ingestion, posture, and exercise cause hemodynamic changes). Quantitative Doppler measurements should be taken in a suspended normal respiration because deep inspiration/expiration might cause hemodynamic changes.[4,5] Age,[6] fever, smoking, and vasoactive drugs or diuretics can modify the hemodynamic parameters of the portal and splanchnic circulation, and they need to be taken into account and properly reported when Doppler measurements are collected.

LIMITATIONS OF ULTRASOUND EXAMINATION

The limitations of US for PH assessment are the same as for general abdominal US. The main limitation is bowel gas interposition as it does not allow visualization and examination of the abdominal organs and vessels. US imaging can also be impaired by the presence of massive ascites. Moreover, quantitative Doppler measurements are affected by the interobserver and interequipment variability. For this reason, even though the application of standardized protocols has been proved to reduce such variability, it is preferable the examination be performed by the same operator and using the same US equipment in case of patients in follow-up.[7-10]

Ultrasound Features of Portal Hypertension in Advanced Chronic Liver Disease: Intrahepatic Portal Hypertension

B-MODE ULTRASOUND

Patients with advanced chronic liver disease (ACLD) or known liver cirrhosis may already have signs of CSPH evaluated by HVPG even when in the compensated ACLD (cACLD) stage.

Therefore signs of liver cirrhosis should be always investigated. A normal-looking liver has the left lobe usually smaller than the right lobe, a regular surface, homogeneous echotexture, a sharp margin, and a normal-sized caudate lobe (Fig. 8.1).

Liver cirrhosis is usually characterized by changes in liver volume distribution (right lobe hypotrophy, left lobe hypertrophy, caudate lobe hypertrophy), surface nodularity, rounded margins, heterogeneity, brightness, and coarsening of the hepatic architecture. Several studies have shown an overall B-mode US sensitivity of 65%–95% for ACLD diagnosis, with a positive predictive value of 98%. The most accurate single sign of liver cirrhosis is a nodular surface, which is more sensitive on the posterior surface of the liver than on the anterior surface (86% vs. 53%, respectively). Moreover, the sensitivity improves when the liver surface is assessed using a high-frequency linear transducer[11-13] (Fig. 8.2).

Caudate lobe hypertrophy and caudate/right lobe (C/RL) ratio are also used in the assessment of liver cirrhosis in which there is hypotrophy/atrophy of the right lobe with hypertrophy of the caudate lobe. To calculate the C/RL ratio we use an axial slice image immediately below the bifurcation of the main PV. Then we draw three lines:

- line 1: a parasagittal line drawn through the right lateral border of the PV;
- line 2: a parasagittal line drawn through the left lateral border of the caudate lobe; and
- line 3: line orthogonal to lines 1 and 2 midway between the PV and the IVC extended to the right liver edge.

The right lobe is measured along line 3, from right liver edge to line 1. The caudate lobe is measured along line 3, between line 1 and line 2. A C/RL ratio <0.60 is considered normal, whereas a value of >0.65 or >0.73 is 96% and 99% likely to be representative of cirrhosis, respectively.[14]

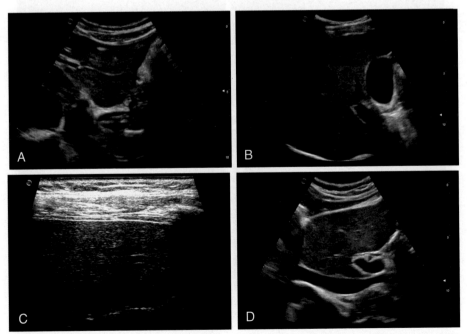

Fig. 8.1   Normal looking liver. (A) Sharp margin. (B) Smooth surface and homogeneous echotexture. (C) Smooth surface assessed with high-frequency transducer. (D) Normal-sized caudate lobe.

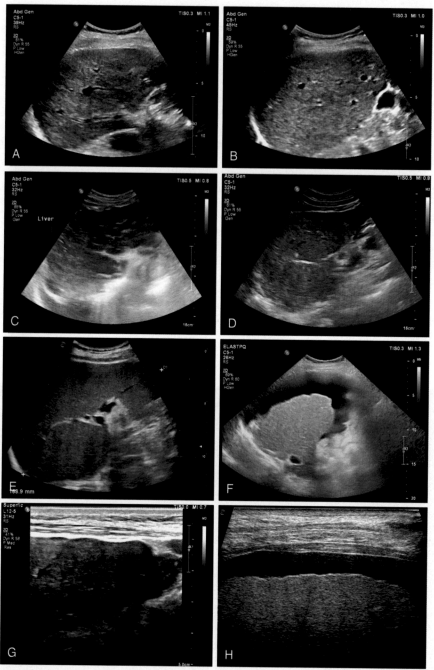

Fig. 8.2 Liver with ultrasound features of advanced chronic disease/cirrhosis. (A) Heterogeneous parenchyma echotexture. (B) Coarse echotexture and posterior nodular surface. (C) Grossly heterogeneous parenchyma echotexture, nodular surface. (D) Echocoarse pattern, anterior and posterior nodular surface, caudate hypertrophy. (E) Heterogeneous echotexture, hepatomegaly, and caudate hypertrophy. (F) Shrunken right lobe with nodular surface and perihepatic ascites. (G) Nodular surface and rounded margin assessed with high-frequency transducer. (H) Nodular surface and perihepatic ascites assessed with high-frequency transducer.

An alternative placement of line 1 has been proposed by Awaya et al. as being more sensitive and specific. Rather than line 1 intersecting the right lateral border of the main PV, they describe drawing line 1 through the right lateral aspect of the right PV bifurcation.[15]

However, it is the combination of different signs that increases the accuracy of US for the diagnosis of cirrhosis (Table 8.1).

Once cirrhosis has been diagnosed, US provides important information on the presence and severity of PH. Even though the majority of studies have been performed using the presence of GEV instead of HVPG values and the correlation between HVPG and US parameters is only slight/moderate, US signs have a very high positive predictive value for the noninvasive diagnosis

TABLE 8.1 ■ B-Mode and Color-Doppler Features of Intrahepatic Portal Hypertension

Ultrasound	Finding	Normal	Clinically Significant Portal Hypertension (HVPG ≥ 10 mmHg)*
Liver surface		Regular	• Irregular/nodular
Liver echotexture		Homogeneous	• Heterogeneous • Coarse
Caudate lobe hypertrophy		No	• Yes
C/RL		<0.65	• >0.65 • >0.73
Spleen	Bipolar length Area	≤12 cm ≤45 cm²	• >12 cm • >45 cm²
PV	Diameter	≤13 mm	>13 mm
	Velocity	≥14–16 cm/s (TAMV) ≥20–24 cm/s (TAPV)	≤14–16 cm/s ≤20–24 cm/s
	Flow direction	Hepatopetal	• Hepatofugal • Alternate
	Congestive index	<0.075	≥0.08
SMV	Diameter	<11 mm	≥11 mm
	Respiratory variation of diameter	≥40%	≤40%
	Flow direction	Hepatopetal	• Hepatofugal • Alternate
SV	Diameter	<11 mm	≥11 mm
	Respiratory variation of diameter	≥40%	≤40%
	Flow direction	Hepatopetal	• Hepatofugal • Alternate
Portosystemic collaterals		Absent	Paraumbilical vein recanalization, left gastric vein, short gastric veins, perigastric, perisplenic, splenorenal shunt, paravertebral, pericholecystic, others

Continued on following page

TABLE 8.1 ■ B-Mode and Color-Doppler Features of Portal Hypertension (Continued)

Ultrasound	Finding	Normal	Clinically Significant Portal Hypertension (HVPG ≥ 10 mmHg)*
HA	RI	≤0.70	>0.70
	PI	≤1.20	>1.20
SA	RI	≤0.63	>0.63
	PI	≤1	>1
RA	RI	≤0.65	>0.65
SMA	RI	≥0.84	<0.84
	PI	≥2.70	<2.70
HVs	Phasicity	Triphasic	Biphasic Flat

*All findings reported in this column have varying degrees of sensitivity and specificity and they may not be present even in cases of severe portal hypertension. HVPG, hepatic venous pressure gradient.
C/RL, Caudate/right lobe; HA, hepatic artery; HVs, hepatic veins; PI, pulsatility index; PV, portal vein; RA, renal artery; RI, resistive index; SA, splenic artery; SMA, superior mesenteric artery; SMV, superior mesenteric vein; SV, splenic vein; TAMV, time averaged medium velocity; TAPV, time averaged pick velocity.

of CSPH. Therefore the diagnosis of CSPH can be confidently established when a US sign or a combination of US signs are detected. However, it is important to bear in mind that the absence of US signs of PH cannot definitely rule out the presence of CSPH.[16]

One of the most common signs of PH is splenomegaly, which is defined by a bipolar diameter (craniocaudal length) >12 cm (13 cm in very tall persons) or an area >45 cm^2 measured by a left intercostal approach and using the splenic hilum as landmark to have a reproducible value (Fig. 8.3).

Splenomegaly is detected in 60%–80% of patients with cirrhosis of different etiologies who have developed PH. There is a good correlation between spleen diameter and HVPG values, and spleen size is significantly associated with CSPH.[17]

Splenomegaly is frequently found in patients with a more severe disease as in patients with decompensated liver cirrhosis[18] and esophageal varices (EVs).[19,20] Moreover, spleen diameter also correlates with the presence and size of EVs in patients with compensated cirrhosis.[21,22] However, in 20% of patients the spleen size can be normal despite the presence of CSPH, especially in alcoholic cirrhosis,[23,24] and splenomegaly might be present in many other conditions especially in hematological and infectious diseases. Sometimes, millimetric hyperechoic spots without acoustic shadowing may be found scattered throughout the splenic parenchyma in severe PH (Fig. 8.4). These splenic siderotic and fibrosiderotic nodules, also known as Gamna-Gandy bodies of the spleen, are small focal deposits of iron and calcium within fibrous tissue and elastic fibers followed by fibroblast reaction, and they are the result of microhemorrhage.[25]

Other sonographic findings commonly associated with PH include enlarged diameter of the PV >13 mm, measured at the crossing point of PV by the hepatic artery (HA), and lack of respiratory variation in the splenic vein (SV; see Table 8.1). Even though PV dilation has a specificity of 95% for the diagnosis of PH and seems to be consistently associated with the presence of EVs,[26] the sensitivity of this sign is quite poor, ranging from 50%–70% in published studies, meaning that a normal-sized PV does not rule out the presence of PH. Dilation of splenic and mesenteric veins more than 11 mm and the reduction of the respiratory variations of their diameter less than 40% are also very specific signs, and they should be routinely explored (see Table 8.1; Fig. 8.5).[27]

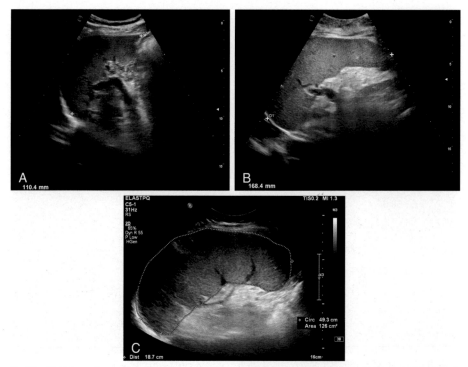

Fig. 8.3 (A) Spleen of normal size. (B) Splenomegaly (bipolar length). (C) Splenomegaly (bipolar length and area).

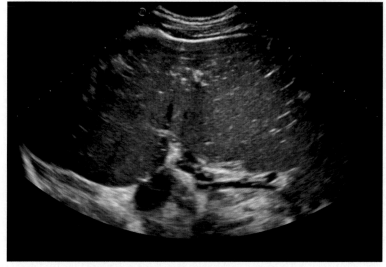

Fig. 8.4 Splenomegaly with Gamna-Gandy bodies.

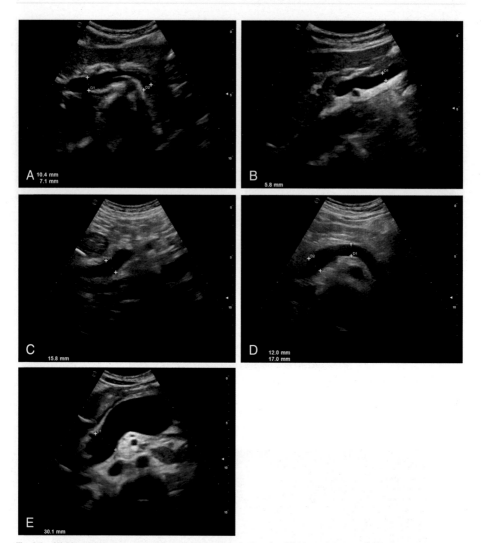

Fig. 8.5 (A) Normal appearance of portal vein and splenic vein. (B) Normal appearance of superior mesenteric vein. (C) Portal vein dilation in liver cirrhosis. (D) Portal vein and splenic vein dilation in liver cirrhosis. (E) Portal vein dilation in idiopathic portal hypertension.

When the resistance to the blood flow through the liver increases, many alternate pathways called portosystemic collaterals, from which the blood from the gut reaches the systemic circulation, might develop. US imaging is a useful tool to detect the presence of the portosystemic collaterals such as a patent paraumbilical vein, dilated left gastric (coronary) vein, short gastric veins, splenic collaterals, and splenorenal shunt. In patients with known PH, portosystemic abdominal collaterals can be observed in approximately 70%–80% of cases, and they are 100% specific signs of PH. The left gastric or coronary vein is the most common portosystemic shunt, occurring in 80% to 90% of patients, and is imaged in the epigastric region posterior to the left lobe of the liver. The recanalized paraumbilical vein is easily sonographically recognized as a tubular structure at the falciform ligament, exits the anterior aspect of the liver and courses under the skin surface to

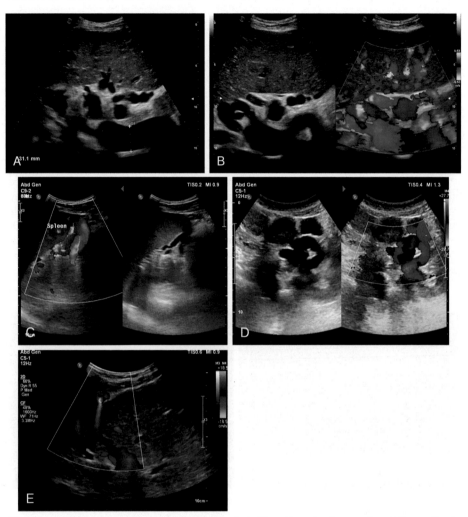

Fig. 8.6 (A) Splenic vein dilation, collaterals at the splenic hilum (B-mode ultrasound), and Gamna-Gandy bodies in the splenic parenchyma. (B) Splenic vein dilation and collaterals at the splenic hilum (B-mode and color-Doppler ultrasound). (C) Collaterals at the inferior pole of the spleen. (D) Epigastric collaterals (collaterals of the gastric vein). (E) Paraumbilical vein recanalization.

the umbilicus where a "caput medusa" can be observed. Short gastric collaterals are located in the left hypochondrium, posterior to the upper splenic pole. Other portosystemic collateral vessels include gastric, retroperitoneal/paravertebral, and gallbladder varices. Gastric varices might be seen around the stomach in the epigastrium posterior to the left lobe of the liver and near the spleen. Retroperitoneal/paravertebral varices are very difficult to visualize with US. Careful scanning may reveal tortuous vessels also between the liver and right kidney. A splenorenal shunt might be detected scanning the splenorenal region and represents a connection between the splenic and left renal vein (see Table 8.1; Fig. 8.6).

Subclinical ascites is an accurate sign of PH in the context of decompensated liver cirrhosis, and US is extremely sensitive to detect it. The perihepatic space is the most usual site of visualization of minimal ascites, and high-frequency transducers improve the sensitivity of its diagnosis (see Table 8.1).

COLOR-DOPPLER AND PULSED-DOPPLER

The PV normally exhibits a monophasic, low-velocity Doppler signal with slight respiratory variation. The normal range of portal flow velocity is large but is usually between 20 and 40 cm/s (time averaged peak velocity). The flow is continuous, hepatopetal (from the gut and spleen toward the liver), and should demonstrate little pulsatility. The flow in the splenic vein (SV) and superior mesenteric vein (SMV) is hepatopetal and exhibits a low-velocity and monophasic pattern. HA blood flow is in the same direction as the PV (hepatopetal) and shows a low-resistance (resistive index [RI] <0.70) waveform with continuous forward flow throughout the cardiac cycle. The HVs drain blood from the liver into the IVC. The normal Doppler waveform obtained from the HVs is triphasic (Fig. 8.7).

Portal blood flow reversal develops when the intrahepatic resistance is greater than the resistance inside the portosystemic collaterals. It is a 100% specific sign of PH, and it can be observed in any tract of the portal system (SV, SMV, portal trunk, and lobar portal branches) and in collaterals (coronary/gastric vein, paraumbilical vein). Hepatofugal portal blood flow is usually associated with a more severe liver disease with compromised liver function and with the presence of large shunts, mainly a splenorenal shunt. Slow flow that alternates in direction between anterograde and retrograde is also a sign of PH (Fig. 8.8).[28]

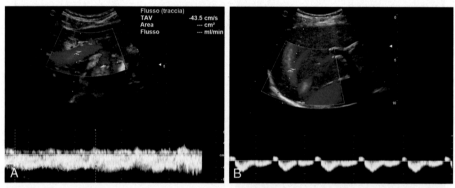

Fig. 8.7 (A) Hepatopetal blood flow with normal flow velocity in the portal vein. (B) Normal triphasic blood flow in the right hepatic vein.

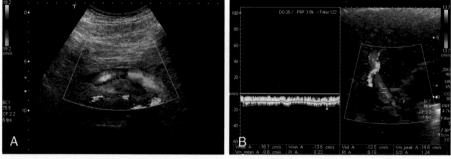

Fig. 8.8 (A) Hepatofugal blood flow in the splenic vein. (B) Hepatofugal blood flow in the right intrahepatic portal branch. (Courtesy Dr. Umberto Arena.)

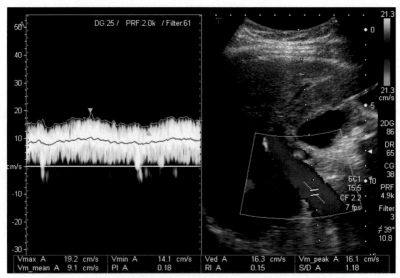

Fig. 8.9 Slow hepatopetal portal blood flow. (Courtesy Dr. Umberto Arena.)

Prominent pulsatility of the PV is also abnormal and may be indicative of PH but also of other conditions such as right heart failure, tricuspid regurgitation, and HV/PV fistula.

PV blood flow velocity can be assessed with good reproducibility if some technical rules aimed to reduce the intraobserver and interobserver variability are carefully followed.[8] The landmark where the portal blood flow velocity should be measured is the crossing point of the PV by the HA. The PV blood flow velocity reduces as the resistance and then the PH increase. A time averaged peak velocity <16 cm/s is strongly suggestive of CSPH, whereas a value <24 cm/s is indicative of cirrhosis.[29,30] In some cases the blood flow inside the PV can slow so much as to become stagnant, increasing the risk of developing PVT (see Table 8.1; Fig. 8.9).

Among other Doppler US parameters, the congestion index, which is the ratio of the cross-sectional area of the PV derived from its diameter and the PV blood flow velocity, ≥0.075 seems to be well-related to CSPH and the presence of EVs (see Table 8.1).[31]

Flattening of physiological phasicity of the HVs' Doppler flow pattern represents another sign that seems to correlate with PH even though data are controversial and further validations are required. This is mainly due to the collagen deposition and nodular regeneration, which narrow and compress the HVs. This causes HVs to lose their triphasic pattern, which progressively becomes biphasic and then flattens (see Table 8.1; Fig. 8.10).[32,33]

As a consequence of the reduced PV blood flow, arterial vascularization that leads to hepatic parenchymal arterialization takes place. For this reason, there is usually an increased size of the HA (HA hypertrophy) followed by an increase in arterial peak systolic velocity (PSV; >60 cm/s) and diminished HA end-diastolic velocity (EDV), resulting in increased HA RI (RI >0.70) and pulsatility index ([PI] >1.20) unless a shunt between the HA and HV (arterial–venous shunt) or between the HA and PV (arterial–portal shunt) has been formed, with a drop in the peripheral resistance of the arterial blood flow and a HA waveform changing from high to low resistance (see Table 8.1).[34]

The splenic congestion due to PH generates a hypertrophy and hyperplasia of some tissue elements of the spleen, which causes an increased arterial blood flow through the splenic artery (SA) that shows both a high PSV and EDV and results in an increased RI (>0.63) and PI (>1); in some studies, these results showed the highest accuracy in diagnosing CSPH (see Table 8.1).[35,36]

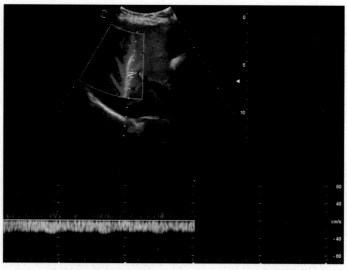

Fig. 8.10 Monophasic blood flow in the right hepatic vein.

As a consequence of the hyperdynamic circulation, secondary splanchnic vasodilation may occur and a reduction in the superior mesenteric artery RI (<0.84) and PI (<2.70) is frequently found during fasting (see Table 8.1).[37,38]

Systemic vasodilation results in diminished renal perfusion, and this leads to intrarenal vasoconstriction and an increased intrarenal RI (>0.70), which is the final stage of the systemic hemodynamic derangement that occurs in patients with cirrhosis and PH. An increase of the intraparenchymal renal artery RI greater than 0.70 seems associated with severe PH (HVPG ≥16 mmHg), and, from a clinical point of view, this sign has been associated with the presence of a life-threatening condition, hepatorenal syndrome (see Table 8.1).[39]

Although all these Doppler parameters have been shown to correlate with PH and were largely used in the past, they represent additional findings and should be used as an integration rather than as independent factors for PH diagnosis.

Prehepatic Portal Hypertension: Portal Vein Thrombosis

PVT might be the consequence of blood flow stagnation due to severe liver cirrhosis–related PH or can be secondary to other conditions and in this case represents the most common cause of noncirrhotic PH. Primary or secondary hypercoagulable states as well as myeloproliferative diseases can result in thrombosis of the PV directly or indirectly through thrombosis in the SV or SMV. Pancreatitis and other inflammatory processes most commonly cause thrombosis that begins in the SV or SMV and extend to the PV. PV compression by lymphadenopathy or a tumor mass, or tumor infiltration, usually by an infiltrating hepatocellular carcinoma or metastases, can also result in thrombosis (the latter named neoplastic PVT).

Echogenic material partially or completely occupying the lumen of the vessel can be visible using B-mode US. Usually, a recent thrombosis appears hypoechoic, whereas hyperecogenicity, wall vessel calcifications, and vessel dilation are features of longstanding thrombosis. Moreover, the wall of the vessel is intact and clearly visible, and no color-Doppler signals are detected unless the thrombosis is partial. When the thrombus is consequent to a tumor invasion, the vessel wall is disrupted or sometimes not even recognizable due to the tumor infiltration. Moreover, color-Doppler US can sometimes aid in the differentiation of benign thrombosis from tumor infiltration by demonstrating tiny vessels with low-resistance arterial signals within the tumor-filled vein as effectively as contrast-enhanced US even though Doppler is less sensitive (Fig. 8.11).

Due to the hepatic arterial buffer response, increased flow through the HA with a decrease in resistance is associated with PVT. The HA may appear enlarged with prominent color-Doppler signals. On the contrary, partial thrombosis is not associated with HA blood flow changes.

Cavernous transformation of the PV has been shown to occur within 6–20 days following acute thrombosis. It is readily recognized with color-Doppler US as multiple, tortuous, tiny vessels at the porta hepatis with an absence of a normal PV. Flow is hepatopetal and venous (Fig. 8.12). Sometimes, it can be associated with biliary tract dilation due to an *ab extrinseco* compression/obstruction of the common biliary duct at the hepatic hilum by the collaterals (portal biliopathy).[16]

In PH that is related to PVT, the spleen is always very enlarged, and abdominal collaterals as in cases of cirrhotic PH can be observed. If PVT is not a complication of cirrhosis, the liver is usually normal-looking or might have some slight features of chronic disease in the case of long-standing PVT without a cirrhotic appearance.

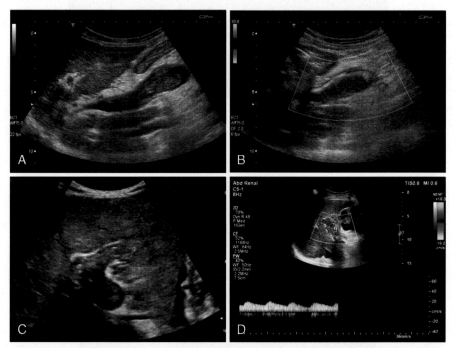

Fig. 8.11 (A) Nonobstructive benign portal vein thrombosis at B-mode ultrasound. (B) Nonobstructive benign portal vein thrombosis at color-Doppler ultrasound that does not show vascular signals inside the thrombus. (C) Neoplastic thrombosis of the left intrahepatic portal branch at B-mode ultrasound. (D) Neoplastic thrombosis of the right intrahepatic portal branch at color-Doppler ultrasound that shows arterial vascular signals with low resistance inside the thrombus.

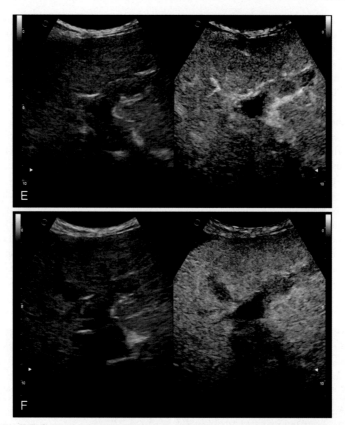

Fig. 8.11, cont'd (E-F) Contrast-enhanced ultrasound of neoplastic thrombosis of the left intrahepatic portal branch: hyperenhancement of the thrombus during the arterial phase of the dynamic study (E) and washout of the thrombus compared with the liver parenchyma during the portal and late phase of the dynamic study (F). (A and B, Courtesy Dr. Umberto Arena.)

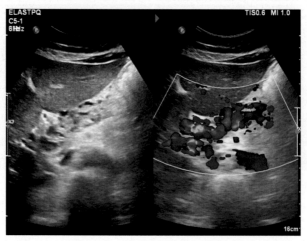

Fig. 8.12 Cavernoma transformation.

Posthepatic Portal Hypertension

BUDD-CHIARI SYNDROME

Since US permits the evaluation of IVC and HVs, it allows clinicians to diagnose posthepatic causes of PH such as HV thrombosis as in cases of BCS. The most common US findings in acute BCS are lack of color-Doppler signal in one or more HVs, thrombus filling the vein, vein stenosis, or vein obstruction due to a tumor compressing or invading the vessel. BCS might be also due to a thrombosis of the IVC just above the HV's ostium, but this represents a rather rare condition. The liver has a normal appearance, and no other features of PH are detectable.

The most common US findings in subacute and chronic BCS are the presence of a fibrous tract replacing the obstructed HV and the presence of intrahepatic collaterals and caudate lobe hypertrophy due to the presence in this lobe of short veins (caudate lobe veins) that drain directly into the IVC without connecting with the HVs. In chronic BCS the caudate lobe can be so enlarged to cause a compression of the retrohepatic IVC.[40,41] The liver is usually enlarged due to vascular congestion, and the echotexture is commonly heterogeneous. Moreover, all other signs of PH such as collaterals, dilated PV, an enlarged spleen, and a slow/inverted PV flow can be found (Fig. 8.13).

HEART DISEASES

Right heart failure, tricuspid valve diseases, and constrictive pericarditis can also induce PH due to the increased right cardiac filling pressure, and the most common US features are the consequences of high central venous pressure values such as dilated HVs (>10 mm) and IVC (>21 mm) as well as the typical changes in the HV's waveform detected by color-Doppler US.[42] Moreover, all other signs of PH such as collaterals, dilated PV, an enlarged spleen, and a

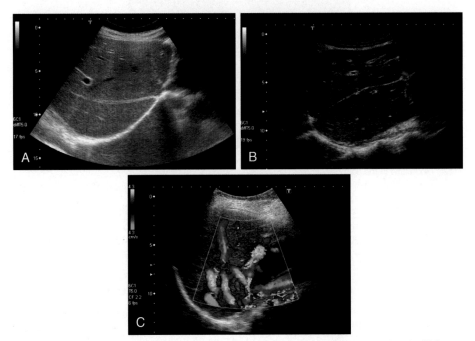

Fig. 8.13 Chronic Budd-Chiari syndrome. (A) Fibrous tract replacing the obstructed hepatic vein. (B) Severe caudate hypertrophy. (C) Intrahepatic collaterals. (Courtesy Dr. Umberto Arena.)

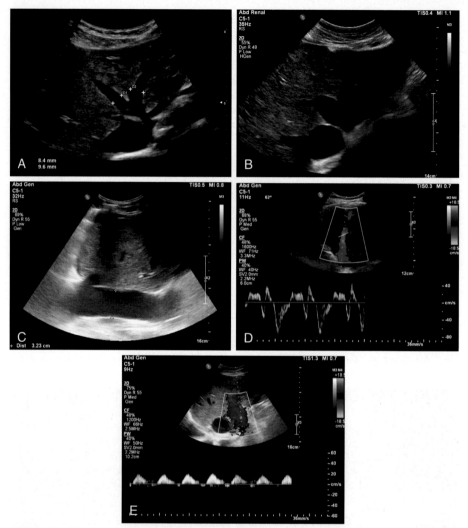

Fig. 8.14 (A) Normal size hepatic veins. (B) Enlarged hepatic veins. (C) Enlarged inferior vena cava. (D) Tetraphasic blood flow in the right hepatic vein. (E) phasic flow in the portal vein.

slow/inverted (or more commonly a phasic/oscillating) PV flow can be found. The liver is usually enlarged due to the congestion. In case of a longstanding hepatic congestion, features of cirrhosis such as heterogeneous echotexture and irregular/nodular surface or even signs of decompensation such as ascites might be seen (cardiac cirrhosis) (Fig. 8.14).

Other Causes of Noncirrhotic Portal Hypertension

Intrahepatic and extrahepatic arterioportal fistulae and SA–SV fistulae due to congenital malformation (in idiopathic PH), fistulae secondary to trauma or invasive procedures, and (only rarely) liver cirrhosis–related fistulae generate a marked increase in portal–venous inflow and can be causes of PH. In B-mode US the fistulae might appear as anechoic rounded structures connecting a branch of the HA to a portal branch. Using color-Doppler US, they might be seen as a web of

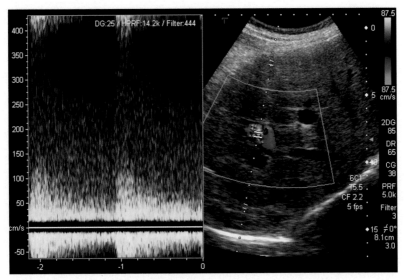

Fig. 8.15 Intrahepatic arterioportal fistula. (Courtesy Dr. Umberto Arena.)

vascular channels with the aliasing phenomenon at low pulse repetition frequency values due to high flow velocity and then turbulent flow at the site of the arteriovenous connection. The portal flow can acquire a pulsatile spectrum, and, in the case of a large fistula, a hepatofugal flow might be observed in one or both intrahepatic portal branches or even in the portal trunk. A difference ≥25% in resistive Doppler indexes between the right and left HA branches suggests the presence of an intrahepatic fistula in the side where the indexes are lower. The same findings can be observed in the case of a splenic arteriovenous fistula. The absence of liver surface nodularity should raise the suspicion of other causes of arteriovenous fistula and then of noncirrhotic PH (Fig. 8.15).[43-45]

Chronic hepatic schistosomiasis represents a common cause of presinusoidal intrahepatic PH in Africa and Latin America, and it is characterized by the US finding of wall thickening of the PV and its branches, which is associated with increased echogenicity due to an increased amount of fibrous tissue (bull's eye sign).[46]

In PH due to suspected hereditary hemorrhagic telangiectasia, there is an increased diameter of the common HA (>7mm), an increased HA blood flow velocity, and the presence of intrahepatic hypervascularization and subcapsular vascular spots with a high-velocity arterial blood flow and low RI represented by very small hepatic arteriovenous malformations[47-49] (Fig. 8.16).

In the case of sinusoidal obstruction syndrome, US findings are not specific, and the suspicion arises when there is hepatomegaly, ascites, gallbladder wall thickening and decreased or reversed portal–venous flow in patients with recent bone marrow transplantation or exposure to systemic chemotherapy for solid neoplasia.[50] More details about sinusoidal obstruction syndrome are given in Chapter 9.

The Role of Elastography in Portal Hypertension

CIRRHOTIC PORTAL HYPERTENSION

In cases of cirrhosis-related CSPH, patients are at high risk of developing complications such as decompensation, spontaneous bacterial peritonitis, hepatorenal syndrome, and GEV, which might rupture and cause a life-threatening bleed. For this reason, gastroscopy is routinely used to

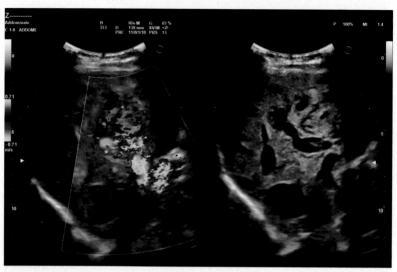

Fig. 8.16   Intrahepatic arteriovenous malformations in patient with hereditary hemorrhagic telangiectasia.

screen for varices once the diagnosis of cirrhosis is confirmed. In cases in which varices are detected, gastroscopy offers different therapeutic opportunities.[51,52] Although gastroscopy is an important procedure for its diagnostic and therapeutic applications, HVPG still represents the gold standard test for PH diagnosis. It gives information not only on the site of the underlying increased resistance but also on the prognosis in the case of cirrhosis-related PH; a value above 10 mmHg is independently associated with a high risk of complications and death. However, HVPG is an invasive and expensive procedure performed in theater, needing a general anesthesia and is not available in all clinical settings.[53-58] The need for noninvasive techniques for diagnosing CSPH has driven successful research efforts. All elastographic techniques are repeatable, largely available, and provide information on the presence of PH with a liver stiffness measurement (LSM) that is related to the amount of hepatic fibrosis.[59-61] Therefore liver elastography provides information on PH by detecting the static component of portal pressure and shows an excellent correlation within certain values of HVPG. However, it is necessary to bear in mind that other confounding factors might contribute to an increase in the hepatic stiffness independently from the fibrosis stage, such as cholestasis, hepatitis, congestion due to heart failure, etc. When PH becomes more severe, dynamic components such as intrahepatic vasoconstriction and splanchnic vasodilation contribute to the portal pressure value, and the correlation between HVPG and LSM is partly lost.[62] The liver receives blood through the PV directly from the spleen via the SV, which continues into the portal trunk. This results in the increased portal pressure being transmitted to the spleen, and generates an increased intrasplenic pressure. Therefore the spleen stiffness measurement (SSM), which is still a matter of research and not currently implemented in routine clinical practice, might represent a more reliable marker in the case of more severe PH. Another area of noninvasive assessment of PH under investigation is subharmonic pressure estimates using contrast-enhanced US, a technique named *subharmonic-aided pressure estimation (SHAPE)*. Subharmonic imaging transmits at double the microbubble resonance frequency and receives at half that frequency. The nonlinear response of microbubbles depends strongly on the incidence acoustic pressure and undergoes three stages: occurrence, growth, and saturation. In the growth stage, the subharmonic microbubble signals have the highest sensitivity to pressure changes and an inverse linear relationship with the ambient hypostatic pressure. Early investigations suggest that SHAPE allows for identification of patients with PH and those at elevated risk of variceal bleeding among at-risk populations.[63]

In all studies aimed at validating liver elastography for PH diagnosis, upper endoscopy and HVPG have been used as reference standard. Currently, liver elastography is so widely used in clinical practice that guidelines have been issued on how to correctly perform the technique and on its clinical application (see Chapter 10).

Liver Stiffness Measurement

Vibration Controlled Transient Elastography

Vibration controlled transient elastography (VCTE) was the first method introduced to assess liver fibrosis. Since then, many studies have been published regarding the correlation between stiffness values measured by VCTE and HVPG, and 12 of these (8 prospective and 4 retrospective) have been included in a metaanalysis.[64] The total sample size was of 1491 patients. Ten studies provided information about both the correlation between VCTE and HVPG and the accuracy of VCTE to detect CSPH. The summary correlation coefficient was 0.78, suggesting a quite good correlation. However, the two techniques do not seem to correlate as well in the case of severe PH, probably due to the greater contribution of dynamic components in the portal pressure. VCTE showed a good diagnostic performance in detecting CSPH with a summary sensitivity and specificity of 87% and 85%, respectively. Encouraging results were also reported by another metaanalysis published in the same year that included eight studies with a total sample size of 1356 patients.[65] However, the LSM cutoff values were wide in both metaanalyses, ranging from 8.74 to 25 kPa, which may be due to the inclusion of patients without CSPH and patients with different etiologies of liver disease, such as alcoholic liver disease (ALD) and nonalcoholic fatty liver disease in which inflammation is well established to overestimate the LSM. A seminal study performed in 2014 showed that an LSM ≥ 25 kPa had an excellent accuracy to rule in CSPH, whereas a cutoff value ≥ 13.6 kPa was able to identify patients with high risk of CSPH with a good diagnostic performance only in the presence of a low platelet count ($<150,000/mm^3$) and US features of cirrhosis.[66] These results were further confirmed 2 years later in the "Anticipate" study in which simple parameters such as LSM, platelet count, and spleen longitudinal size combined in a score called LSPS (liver stiffness-spleen size-to-platelet ratio score) were able to identify up to 80% of patients with CSPH.[67]

Many studies have been published regarding the accuracy of LSM measured by VCTE in predicting the presence of EVs and EVs at high-risk of bleeding. Fifteen of these studies, with a total sample size of 2697 patients, were included in a metaanalysis published in 2017. The summary sensitivity, specificity, and area under the receiver operating characteristic (AUROC) curve were 84%, 62%, and 0.82 and 78%, 76%, and 0.82 for the detection of EVs and large EVs, respectively. The cutoff ranged from 12 to 29.7 kPa and from 19 to 48 kPa for EVs and large EVs, respectively. Also in this case, the wide range of cutoffs can be explained by the different etiologies of liver disease included in the studies, with cutoffs lower for viral etiologies and higher for ALD.[68]

Several milestone studies[66,67,69-71] demonstrated that LSM measured by VCTE had an excellent accuracy to detect EVs at high risk of bleeding when combined with parameters such as platelet count and spleen longitudinal diameter in very simple scores using LSPS.

On the basis of these results, the Baveno VI consensus proposed to combine LSM by VCTE and platelet count for a noninvasive approach to rule out patients with cACLD and Child-Pugh A cirrhosis who can safely avoid screening endoscopy. In particular, patients with an LSM <20 KPa and a platelet count $>150,000/mm^3$ have a very low risk of having varices needing treatment (VNT) and can safely avoid screening endoscopy. These patients can be followed up by yearly repetition of VCTE and platelet count. If the LSM increases or the platelet count declines, these patients should undergo screening endoscopy.[72] Multiple studies since 2015 have confirmed that by applying these criteria, VNT are missed in less than 5% of patients. However, the number of spared endoscopies was still low (20%) with a total of 38% of unneeded gastroscopies performed.[73] For this reason, the Baveno VI criteria have been expanded with new criteria (expanded Baveno VI) in the "Anticipate" study with a derivation cohort and two additional validation cohorts from London (309 patients) and Barcelona (117 patients).[74] According to these new criteria, patients with a platelet count >110,000/mm³ and LSM <25 kPa have a low risk of having VNT. With the application of the expanded Baveno VI criteria, the number of missed VNT was still reasonably low (1.6%), but the number of spared endoscopies was much higher compared with Baveno VI (40% vs. 20%).[74] It is important to bear in mind that these new criteria perform well in patients with cACLD due to chronic hepatitis C virus infection, ALD, and nonalcoholic steatohepatitis.

The performance of Baveno VI and expanded Baveno VI in predicting the absence of VNT has been assessed in a multicenter retrospective study including 227 patients with cholestatic liver disease (primary sclerosing cholangitis and primary biliary cholangitis, respectively). The conclusion was that Baveno VI criteria can be applied in patients with cACLD due to cholestatic liver disease, which would result in saving 30%–40% of endoscopies with an acceptable percentage of missed high-risk EVs. However, expanded criteria in primary biliary cholangitis would lead to false negative results >5%, and this could be due to the presinusoidal component of PH in this cohort of patients.[75]

Acoustic Radiation Force Impulse Techniques

Although there are fewer published studies compared with VCTE, acoustic radiation force impulse (ARFI) techniques are now widely used for assessing PH.[76]

Since ARFI technology is implemented into US systems, one of the major advantages compared with VCTE is the availability to detect features of CLD and PH using B-mode and color-Doppler US modes. Moreover, as the tissue inside the liver is directly displaced in a precise area rather than from skin compression, the technique is less sensitive to the presence of ascites and obesity, which represent technical limitations when VCTE is used. However, while VCTE-based elastography is a simple technique that can be performed by anyone after a short training period, ARFI techniques are critically dependent on the experience of the US operator even though the accuracy can be improved by following quality criteria (see Chapters 6 and 7 for more details).[77]

Although there are fewer data compared with VCTE on the usefulness of point shear wave elastography (pSWE), results are encouraging since studies show a good diagnostic accuracy for detecting CSPH with AUROCs ranging from 0.82 to 0.97 and cutoff values from 2.17 to 3.29 m/s. Data are less encouraging regarding the detection of EVs, because the AUROCs range from 0.58 to 0.96 and from 0.58 to 0.95 with cutoff values from 2.55 to 3.41 m/s and from 3.30 to 3.51 m/s for the prediction of any EVs and VNT, respectively.[76,78]

Few data are available for two-dimensional shear wave elastography (2D-SWE).[76] However, rules about how to correctly perform it, quality criteria to improve its diagnostic accuracy, interpretation of results, and clinical application have been established.[79] Although there is strong evidence for the value of 2D-SWE-based LSM for fibrosis assessment, studies on the value of 2D-SWE-based LSM to assess CSPH and for screening of EVs are limited. The few published studies showed a good diagnostic performance of 2D-SWE to detect CSPH, with AUROC ranging from 0.79 to 0.95 and specificity and sensitivity around 85%. However, the cutoffs ranged from 15.2 to 24.6 kPa. Regarding the accuracy of any EVs or VNT prediction, AUROCs range from 0.58 to 0.89 and cutoffs range from 13.9 to 19.7 kPa.[76]

Moreover, LSM measured with ARFI techniques seems to have a better diagnostic performance for CSPH when used alone than when integrated with spleen size and platelet count.[80,81]

This may be due to the nonlinear relationship between spleen size and PH since splenomegaly is not only due to passive congestion development, but also to lymphoid hyperplasia, angiogenesis, and fibrogenesis and does not represent a consistent finding in patients with PH. For these reasons, its clinical utility is controversial and scores combining spleen parameters noninvasively assessed as spleen size and area have not been widely developed and pursued.

The cutoff range of ARFI techniques is wide, and this might depend not only on different etiologies and grade of severity of the underlying liver disease included in the studies but also on the different US systems used. However, according to the consensus by the Society of Radiologists in Ultrasound, in patients affected by hepatitis C virus and nonalcoholic steatohepatitis-related cACLD, an LSM greater than 17 kPa (2.4 m/s) is highly suggestive of CSPH although further tests might be required.[79] For other causes of liver disease such as ALD, primary biliary cholangitis, primary sclerosing cholangitis, Wilson disease, autoimmune hepatitis, and drug-induced liver disease, data are still scarce and a conclusion cannot be made.

Spleen Stiffness Measurement

As already discussed, the correlation between liver stiffness and HVPG values becomes poor for high HVPG values. This is due to the major role played by dynamic extrahepatic factors over liver fibrosis in severe PH. All these changes lead to splenic congestion, hyperplasia, and fibrosis. In this scenario, SSM seems to better perform compared with LSM in assessing the risk of CSPH as well as detecting the presence of EVs. Unfortunately, data on this matter are still scarce as of early 2022. The acquisition technique is the same as that for the liver, except that the measurements are between the left ribs with the patient in supine or slightly lateral position and the left arm extended up to the head. Measurements should be taken at 15 mm from the splenic surface with the region of interest placed perpendicularly to the splenic capsule (Fig. 8.17). Using pSWE techniques, the median value of 10 valid measurements with an interquartile range/median (IQR/M) ≤30% (for values in kPa) is necessary for a reliable result. For 2D-SWE, five valid measurements are enough if the IQR/M ≤30% (for values in kPa) is applied.[79] In healthy subjects, the spleen is stiffer than the liver. SSM should be measured only in patients with cACLD (METAVIR F ≥3 and F = 4; VCTE liver stiffness ≥15 kPa; ARFI liver stiffness ≥13 kPa) since a significant increase of portal pressure is not expected in patients with lower stages of liver fibrosis unless there is an idiopathic PH.

Several studies using VCTE have shown the superiority of SSM compared with LSM for assessing the risk of CSPH and the presence of EVs. However, the range of cutoffs is wide, ranging from 47.6 to 56.3 kPa for CSPH, and from 40.8 to 65 kPa for detecting any EVs. For large varices cutoffs are narrow, ranging from 54 to 54.5 kPa but only few studies have been published. The

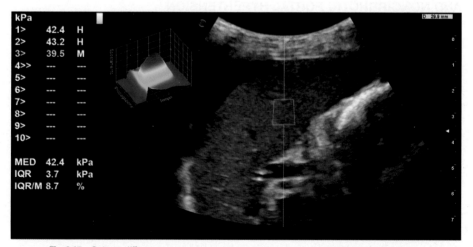

Fig. 8.17 Spleen stiffness measurement with a point shear wave elastography technique.

diagnostic performance is reasonably good; the specificity and sensitivity are greater than 70% in most of the cases. The wideness of the cutoff range is mainly due to different etiologies and the grade of severity of the underlying liver disease included in the studies.[73] The rate of unsuccessful measurements is significantly high, mainly in patients with normal or low spleen size since the measurement is taken in a blind manner unless a conventional US system is available. Moreover, in all these studies the VCTE system used was the standard 50-Hz frequency FibroScan used to assess the liver stiffness, with a ceiling stiffness threshold of 75 kPa. However, a new 100-Hz setting installed in an US system provided a better correlation with HVPG and a higher accuracy for EV and VNT detection than the standard 50 Hz. Furthermore, the combination of Baveno VI criteria and an SSM cutoff of 38.3 kPa measured with the 100-Hz system significantly increased the spared endoscopy rate compared with Baveno VI criteria alone or combined with SSM measured by the standard 50 Hz.[82] Although these data seem interesting, the level of evidence is still too low to recommend SSM taken with VCTE in the work-up of patients with liver cirrhosis.

Regarding ARFI techniques, the overall rate of successful measurements ranges from 66% to 80%, and predictors of failure are a high body mass index and smaller spleen. Normal values of SSM with ARFI-based techniques range from 20.5 to 24.4 kPa (2.6 to 2.85 m/s).[83-85]

Using a pSWE technique, a study showed a high incidence of bleeding from EVs when the SSM was ≥39 kPa (3.64 m/s).[86] Using a 2D-SWE technique, a study reported that an SSM of 26.6 kPa was able to rule out CSPH.[87]

In a multicenter study, LSM and SSM were combined to create an algorithm to rule out and rule in CSPH in patients who underwent HVPG. According to the results of this study, an LSM ≤16 kPa (2.3 m/s) together with an SSM ≥21.7 kPa (2.7 m/s) are able to rule out CSPH with a specificity >92%. On the other hand, CSPH can be confidently (specificity >92%) ruled in in case of LSM of 29.5 kPa (3.2 m/s) or more and SSM greater than 35.6 kPa (3.5 m/s). If a higher LSM (>38 kPa [3.6 m/s]) is considered, an SSM value of 27.9 kPa (3.2 m/s) or more suffices to rule in CSPH with sensitivity and specificity of 89% and 91%, respectively.[88] However, these results have not been further confirmed and validated in a larger cohort of patients since the false positive rate was too high (specificity 52%).[89]

Even though the literature data seem to be promising, as of early 2022 the level of evidence is still too low to recommend SSM taken with ARFI techniques in the work-up of patients with liver cirrhosis.

PORTAL HYPERTENSION OF UNKNOWN CAUSE AND NONCIRRHOTIC PORTAL HYPERTENSION

Although liver biopsy remains crucial in the work-up of patients with PH without evident cause and features of cACLD, liver and spleen assessment by elastography can help the clinician in the initial assessment of PH. In the case of idiopathic PH, LSM is usually only moderately increased; however, in this population, SSM is elevated, reaching values similar to or even higher than those of cirrhotic PH. Since cirrhotic PH and idiopathic PH can show the same features on imaging, the ratio between LSM and SSM can improve the ability of the clinicians to suspect idiopathic PH.

In extrahepatic PVT, LSM is usually normal or only slightly increased, whereas SSM is elevated mostly in patients who already had an episode of bleeding. In this case the ratio between LSM and SSM can help make a differential diagnosis and stratify the severity of PH in patients in whom HVPG is not helpful by definition (prehepatic PH). No data are available regarding BCS.[76]

FACTORS THAT MIGHT INFLUENCE LIVER AND SPLEEN STIFFNESS

Food, physical exercise, and other medications such as vasoactive drugs and diuretics can make hemodynamic changes that might influence LSM and SSM values, and for this reason, they need to be clearly stated in the final report.

Few papers have been published on the influence of nonselective beta-blocker treatment on LSM and SSM. A study showed that the correlation of HVPG with LSM in patients with an initial HVPG >12 mmHg improved after starting the treatment due to the restoration of the linear correlation between HVPG and LSM.[90] These results were confirmed in another cohort composed of patients receiving nonselective beta-blockers; the diagnostic performance of LSM and SSM assessed by VCTE in predicting varices was better than in untreated patients.[91]

Few studies have been published about the influence of transjugular intrahepatic portosystemic shunt (TIPS) placement on LSM and SSM measured by ARFI techniques. In one study, only SSM seemed to change after TIPS insertion, and the authors concluded that it could be used as a marker in monitoring the TIPS function.[92] In another study, TIPS insertion significantly modified both LSM and SSM, even though SSM decreased significantly more than LSM and therefore seemed to be superior in detecting the reduction of portal pressure induced by TIPS.[93] Although data regarding the accuracy of spleen stiffness in monitoring the TIPS function seem to be promising, they are still inconsistent and spleen stiffness cannot be suggested as a noninvasive tool for such purpose in the clinical practice.

KEY POINTS

1. Although the measurement of HVPG is the gold standard for evaluation of PH, newer noninvasive US techniques are available that can aid in the clinical work-up of patients.
2. It is important to recognize the cause of the PH as the treatments are different depending on the etiology.
3. An HVPG ≥10 mmHg is representative of CSPH and is associated to the risk of clinical decompensation and onset of complications that represent the main cause of death or liver transplantation.
4. An HVPG ≥12 mmHg is strongly related to high risk of gastrointestinal bleeding, a life-threatening condition.
5. In patients with known PH, the presence of portosystemic abdominal collaterals is a 100% specific sign of PH.
6. The absence of B-mode US signs of PH cannot definitely rule out the presence of CSPH.
7. Doppler parameters have been shown to correlate with PH and were largely used in the past; however, they represent additional findings and should be used as an integration rather than independently for PH diagnosis.
8. The use of elastography evaluating liver and spleen stiffness in patients with compensated cirrhosis have been used to estimate portal pressures; however, as of early 2022, the use of splenic stiffness is not recommended until further studies validate the cutoff values.
9. Since ARFI technology is implemented into US systems, one of the major advantages compared with VCTE is the availability to detect features of CLD and PH using B-mode and color-Doppler US modes.

References

1. Bosch J, Groszmann RJ, Shah VH. Evolution in the understanding of the pathophysiological basis of portal hypertension: how changes in paradigm are leading to successful new treatments. *J Hepatol.* 2015;62(suppl 1):S121-S130.
2. Berzigotti A, Seijo S, Reverter E, Bosch J. Assessing portal hypertension in liver diseases. *Expert Rev Gastroenterol Hepatol.* 2013;7:141-155.
3. Garcia-Pagan JC, Gracia-Sancho J, Bosch J. Functional aspects on the pathophysiology of portal hypertension in cirrhosis. *J Hepatol.* 2012;57:458-461.
4. Gaiani S, Bolondi L, Li Bassi S, Santi V, Zironi G, Barbara L. Effect of meal on portal hemodynamics in healthy humans and in patients with chronic liver disease. *Hepatology.* 1989;9:815-819.
5. Ohnishi K, Saito M, Nakayama T, et al. Portal venous hemodynamics in chronic liver disease: effects of posture change and exercise. *Radiology.* 1985;155:757-761.

6. Berzigotti A, Castaldini N, Rossi V, et al. Age dependency of regional impedance indices regardless of clinical stage in patients with cirrhosis of the liver. *Ultraschall Med.* 2009;30:277-285.
7. Sabba C, Weltin GG, Cicchetti DV, et al. Observer variability in echo-Doppler measurements of portal flow in cirrhotic patients and normal volunteers. *Gastroenterology.* 1990;98:1603-1611.
8. Sabba C, Merkel C, Zoli M, et al. Interobserver and interequipment variability of echo-Doppler examination of the portal vein: effect of a cooperative training program. *Hepatology.* 1995;21:428-433.
9. Sacerdoti D, Gaiani S, Buonamico P, et al. Interobserver and interequipment variability of hepatic, splenic, and renal arterial Doppler resistance indices in normal subjects and patients with cirrhosis. *J Hepatol.* 1997;27:986-992.
10. Zoli M, Merkel C, Sabba C, et al. Interobserver and inter-equipment variability of echo-Doppler sonographic evaluation of the superior mesenteric artery. *J Ultrasound Med.* 1996;15:99-106.
11. Colli A, Fraquelli M, Andreoletti M, Marino B, Zuccoli E, Conte D. Severe liver fibrosis or cirrhosis: accuracy of US for detection—analysis of 300 cases. *Radiology.* 2003;227:89-94.
12. Vigano M, Visentin S, Aghemo A, Rumi MG, Ronchi G. US features of liver surface nodularity as a predictor of severe fibrosis in chronic hepatitis C. *Radiology.* 2005;234:641.
13. Soresi M, Giannitrapani L, Cervello M, Licata A, Montalto G. Noninvasive tools for the diagnosis of liver cirrhosis. *World J Gastroenterol.* 2014;20:18131-18150.
14. Harbin WP, Robert NJ, Ferrucci Jr JT. Diagnosis of cirrhosis based on regional changes in hepatic morphology: a radiological and pathological analysis. *Radiology.* 1980;135:273-283.
15. Awaya H, Mitchell DG, Kamishima T, Holland G, Ito K, Matsumoto T. Cirrhosis: modified caudate-right lobe ratio. *Radiology.* 2002;224:769-774.
16. Berzigotti A, Piscaglia F. Ultrasound in portal hypertension—part 1. *Ultraschall Med.* 2011;32:548-568.
17. Berzigotti A, Gilabert R, Abraldes JG, et al. Noninvasive prediction of clinically significant portal hypertension and esophageal varices in patients with compensated liver cirrhosis. *Am J Gastroenterol.* 2008;103:1159-1167.
18. Piscaglia F, Donati G, Cecilioni L, et al. Influence of the spleen on portal haemodynamics: a non-invasive study with Doppler ultrasound in chronic liver disease and haematological disorders. *Scand J Gastroenterol.* 2002;37:1220-1227.
19. Chalasani N, Imperiale TF, Ismail A, et al. Predictors of large esophageal varices in patients with cirrhosis. *Am J Gastroenterol.* 1999;94:3285-3291.
20. Thomopoulos KC, Labropoulou-Karatza C, Mimidis KP, Katsakoulis EC, Iconomou G, Nikolopoulou VN. Non-invasive predictors of the presence of large oesophageal varices in patients with cirrhosis. *Dig Liver Dis.* 2003;35:473-478.
21. Schepis F, Camma C, Niceforo D, et al. Which patients with cirrhosis should undergo endoscopic screening for esophageal varices detection? *Hepatology.* 2001;33:333-338.
22. Medhat A, Iber FL, Dunne M, Baum R. Ultrasonographic findings with bleeding and nonbleeding esophageal varices. *Am J Gastroenterol.* 1988;83:58-63.
23. Berzigotti A, Zappoli P, Magalotti D, Tiani C, Rossi V, Zoli M. Spleen enlargement on follow-up evaluation: a noninvasive predictor of complications of portal hypertension in cirrhosis. *Clin Gastroenterol Hepatol.* 2008;6:1129-1134.
24. Kashani A, Salehi B, Anghesom D, Kawayeh AM, Rouse GA, Runyon BA. Spleen size in cirrhosis of different etiologies. *J Ultrasound Med.* 2015;34:233-238.
25. Minami M, Itai Y, Ohtomo K, et al. Siderotic nodules in the spleen: MR imaging of portal hypertension. *Radiology.* 1989;172:681-684.
26. Cottone M, D'Amico G, Maringhini A, et al. Predictive value of ultrasonography in the screening of non-ascitic cirrhotic patients with large varices. *J Ultrasound Med.* 1986;5:189-192.
27. Bolondi L, Gandolfi L, Arienti V, et al. Ultrasonography in the diagnosis of portal hypertension: diminished response of portal vessels to respiration. *Radiology.* 1982;142:167-172.
28. von Herbay A, Frieling T, Haussinger D. Color Doppler sonographic evaluation of spontaneous porto-systemic shunts and inversion of portal venous flow in patients with cirrhosis. *J Clin Ultrasound.* 2000;28:332-339.
29. Bolondi L, Gaiani S, Barbara L. Accuracy and reproducibility of portal flow measurement by Doppler US. *J Hepatol.* 1991;13:269-273.
30. Zoli M, Marchesini G, Cordiani MR, et al. Echo-Doppler measurement of splanchnic blood flow in control and cirrhotic subjects. *J Clin Ultrasound.* 1986;14:429-435.

31. Moriyasu F, Nishida O, Ban N, et al. "Congestion index" of the portal vein. *AJR Am J Roentgenol.* 1986;146:735-739.
32. Bolondi L, Li Bassi S, Gaiani S, et al. Liver cirrhosis: changes of Doppler waveform of hepatic veins. *Radiology.* 1991;178:513-516.
33. Kim MY, Baik SK, Park DH, et al. Damping index of Doppler hepatic vein waveform to assess the severity of portal hypertension and response to propranolol in liver cirrhosis: a prospective nonrandomized study. *Liver Int.* 2007;27:1103-1110.
34. McNaughton DA, Abu-Yousef MM. Doppler US of the liver made simple. *Radiographics.* 2011;31:161-188.
35. Bolognesi M, Sacerdoti D, Merkel C, et al. Splenic Doppler impedance indices: influence of different portal hemodynamic conditions. *Hepatology.* 1996;23:1035-1040.
36. Piscaglia F, Donati G, Serra C, et al. Value of splanchnic Doppler ultrasound in the diagnosis of portal hypertension. *Ultrasound Med Biol.* 2001;27:893-899.
37. Piscaglia F, Gaiani S, Gramantieri L, Zironi G, Siringo S, Bolondi L. Superior mesenteric artery impedance in chronic liver diseases: relationship with disease severity and portal circulation. *Am J Gastroenterol.* 1998;93:1925-1930.
38. Taourel P, Blanc P, Dauzat M, et al. Doppler study of mesenteric, hepatic, and portal circulation in alcoholic cirrhosis: relationship between quantitative Doppler measurements and the severity of portal hypertension and hepatic failure. *Hepatology.* 1998;28:932-936.
39. Berzigotti A, Casadei A, Magalotti D, et al. Renovascular impedance correlates with portal pressure in patients with liver cirrhosis. *Radiology.* 2006;240:581-586.
40. Bargallo X, Gilabert R, Nicolau C, Garcia-Pagan JC, Bosch J, Bru C. Sonography of the caudate vein: value in diagnosing Budd-Chiari syndrome. *AJR Am J Roentgenol.* 2003;181:1641-1645.
41. Valla DC. Hepatic vein thrombosis (Budd-Chiari syndrome). *Semin Liver Dis.* 2002;22:5-14.
42. Scheinfeld MH, Bilali A, Koenigsberg M. Understanding the spectral Doppler waveform of the hepatic veins in health and disease. *Radiographics.* 2009;29:2081-2098.
43. Billing JS, Jamieson NV. Hepatic arterioportal fistula: a curable cause of portal hypertension in infancy. *HPB Surg.* 1997;10:311-314.
44. Lafortune M, Breton G, Charlebois S. Arterioportal fistula demonstrated by pulsed Doppler ultrasonography. *J Ultrasound Med.* 1986;5:105-106.
45. Bolognesi M, Sacerdoti D, Bombonato G, Chiesura-Corona M, Merkel C, Gatta A. Arterioportal fistulas in patients with liver cirrhosis: usefulness of color Doppler US for screening. *Radiology.* 2000;216:738-743.
46. Nompleggi DJ, Farraye FA, Singer A, Edelman RR, Chopra S. Hepatic schistosomiasis: report of two cases and literature review. *American J Gastroenterol.* 1991;86:1658-1664.
47. Caselitz M, Bahr MJ, Bleck JS, et al. Sonographic criteria for the diagnosis of hepatic involvement in hereditary hemorrhagic telangiectasia (HHT). *Hepatology.* 2003;37:1139-1146.
48. Ocran K, Rickes S, Heukamp I, Wermke W. Sonographic findings in hepatic involvement of hereditary haemorrhagic telangiectasia. *Ultraschall Med.* 2004;25:191-194.
49. Faughnan ME, Palda VA, Garcia-Tsao G, et al. International guidelines for the diagnosis and management of hereditary haemorrhagic telangiectasia. *J Med Genet.* 2011;48:73-87.
50. Hashiguchi M, Okamura T, Yoshimoto K, et al. Demonstration of reversed flow in segmental branches of the portal vein with hand-held color Doppler ultrasonography after hematopoietic stem cell transplantation. *Bone Marrow Transplant.* 2005;36:1071-1075.
51. Beppu K, Inokuchi K, Koyanagi N, et al. Prediction of variceal hemorrhage by esophageal endoscopy. *Gastrointest Endosc.* 1981;27:213-218.
52. North Italian Endoscopic Club for the Study and Treatment of Esophageal Varices. Prediction of the first variceal hemorrhage in patients with cirrhosis of the liver and esophageal varices. A prospective multicenter study. *N Engl J Med.* 1988;319:983-989.
53. Merkel C, Bolognesi M, Bellon S, et al. Prognostic usefulness of hepatic vein catheterization in patients with cirrhosis and esophageal varices. *Gastroenterology.* 1992;102:973-979.
54. Moitinho E, Escorsell A, Bandi JC, et al. Prognostic value of early measurements of portal pressure in acute variceal bleeding. *Gastroenterology.* 1999;117:626-631.
55. Ripoll C, Banares R, Rincon D, et al. Influence of hepatic venous pressure gradient on the prediction of survival of patients with cirrhosis in the MELD Era. *Hepatology.* 2005;42:793-801.
56. Tsochatzis EA, Bosch J, Burroughs AK. New therapeutic paradigm for patients with cirrhosis. *Hepatology.* 2012;56:1983-1992.

57. Ripoll C, Groszmann R, Garcia-Tsao G, et al. Hepatic venous pressure gradient predicts clinical decompensation in patients with compensated cirrhosis. *Gastroenterology*. 2007;133:481-488.
58. Ripoll C, Groszmann RJ, Garcia-Tsao G, et al. Hepatic venous pressure gradient predicts development of hepatocellular carcinoma independently of severity of cirrhosis. *J Hepatol*. 2009;50:923-928.
59. Castera L, Pinzani M, Bosch J. Noninvasive evaluation of portal hypertension using transient elastography. *J Hepatol*. 2012;56:696-703.
60. Tsochatzis EA, Gurusamy KS, Ntaoula S, Cholongitas E, Davidson BR, Burroughs AK. Elastography for the diagnosis of severity of fibrosis in chronic liver disease: a meta-analysis of diagnostic accuracy. *J Hepatol*. 2011;54:650-659.
61. Crossan C, Tsochatzis EA, Longworth L, et al. Cost-effectiveness of non-invasive methods for assessment and monitoring of liver fibrosis and cirrhosis in patients with chronic liver disease: systematic review and economic evaluation. *Health Technol Assess*. 2015;19:1-409, v-vi.
62. Vizzutti F, Arena U, Rega L, Pinzani M. Non invasive diagnosis of portal hypertension in cirrhotic patients. *Gastroenterol Clin Biol*. 2008;32:80-87.
63. Gupta I, Eisenbrey JR, Machado P, et al. Diagnosing portal hypertension with noninvasive subharmonic pressure estimates from a US contrast agent. *Radiology*. 2021;298:104-111.
64. You MW, Kim KW, Pyo J, et al. A meta-analysis for the diagnostic performance of transient elastography for clinically significant portal hypertension. *Ultrasound Med Biol*. 2017;43:59-68.
65. Kim G, Kim MY, Baik SK. Transient elastography versus hepatic venous pressure gradient for diagnosing portal hypertension: a systematic review and meta-analysis. *Clin Mol Hepatol*. 2017;23:34-41.
66. Augustin S, Millan L, Gonzalez A, et al. Detection of early portal hypertension with routine data and liver stiffness in patients with asymptomatic liver disease: a prospective study. *J Hepatol*. 2014;60:561-569.
67. Abraldes JG, Bureau C, Stefanescu H, et al. Noninvasive tools and risk of clinically significant portal hypertension and varices in compensated cirrhosis: The "Anticipate" study. *Hepatology*. 2016;64:2173-2184.
68. Pu K, Shi JH, Wang X, et al. Diagnostic accuracy of transient elastography (FibroScan) in detection of esophageal varices in patients with cirrhosis: a meta-analysis. *World J Gastroenterol*. 2017;23:345-356.
69. Kim BK, Han KH, Park JY, et al. A liver stiffness measurement-based, noninvasive prediction model for high-risk esophageal varices in B-viral liver cirrhosis. *Am J Gastroenterol*. 2010;105:1382-1390.
70. Berzigotti A, Seijo S, Arena U, et al. Elastography, spleen size, and platelet count identify portal hypertension in patients with compensated cirrhosis. *Gastroenterology*. 2013;144:102-111.
71. Ding NS, Nguyen T, Iser DM, et al. Liver stiffness plus platelet count can be used to exclude high-risk oesophageal varices. *Liver Int*. 2016;36:240-245.
72. de Franchis R, Baveno VI Faculty. Expanding consensus in portal hypertension: Report of the Baveno VI Consensus Workshop: stratifying risk and individualizing care for portal hypertension. *J Hepatol*. 2015;63:743-752.
73. Roccarina D, Rosselli M, Genesca J, Tsochatzis EA. Elastography methods for the non-invasive assessment of portal hypertension. *Expert Rev Gastroenterol Hepatol*. 2018;12:155-164.
74. Augustin S, Pons M, Maurice JB, et al. Expanding the Baveno VI criteria for the screening of varices in patients with compensated advanced chronic liver disease. *Hepatology*. 2017;66:1980-1988.
75. Moctezuma-Velazquez C, Saffioti F, Tasayco-Huaman S, et al. Non-invasive prediction of high-risk varices in patients with primary biliary cholangitis and primary sclerosing cholangitis. *Am J Gastroenterol*. 2019;114:446-452.
76. Berzigotti A. Non-invasive evaluation of portal hypertension using ultrasound elastography. *J Hepatol*. 2017;67:399-411.
77. Ferraioli G, De Silvestri A, Reiberger T, et al. Adherence to quality criteria improves concordance between transient elastography and ElastPQ for liver stiffness assessment-a multicenter retrospective study. *Dig Liver Dis*. 2018;50:1056-1061.
78. Paternostro R, Reiberger T, Bucsics T. Elastography-based screening for esophageal varices in patients with advanced chronic liver disease. *World J Gastroenterol*. 2019;25:308-329.
79. Barr RG, Wilson SR, Rubens D, Garcia-Tsao G, Ferraioli G. Update to the society of radiologists in ultrasound liver elastography consensus statement. *Radiology*. 2020;296:263-274.
80. Elkrief L, Rautou PE, Ronot M, et al. Prospective comparison of spleen and liver stiffness by using shear-wave and transient elastography for detection of portal hypertension in cirrhosis. *Radiology*. 2015;275:589-598.
81. Kim TY, Jeong WK, Sohn JH, Kim J, Kim MY, Kim Y. Evaluation of portal hypertension by real-time shear wave elastography in cirrhotic patients. *Liver Int*. 2015;35:2416-2424.

82. Stefanescu H, Marasco G, Cales P, et al. A novel spleen-dedicated stiffness measurement by FibroScan improves the screening of high-risk oesophageal varices. *Liver Int*. 2020;40:175-185.
83. Cho YS, Lim S, Kim Y, Sohn JH, Jeong JY. Spleen stiffness measurement using 2-dimensional shear wave elastography: the predictors of measurability and the normal spleen stiffness value. *J Ultrasound Med*. 2019;38:423-431.
84. Procopet B, Berzigotti A, Abraldes JG, et al. Real-time shear-wave elastography: applicability, reliability and accuracy for clinically significant portal hypertension. *J Hepatol*. 2015;62:1068-1075.
85. Ferraioli G, Tinelli C, Lissandrin R, et al. Ultrasound point shear wave elastography assessment of liver and spleen stiffness: effect of training on repeatability of measurements. *Eur Radiol*. 2014;24:1283-1289.
86. Takuma Y, Nouso K, Morimoto Y, et al. Portal hypertension in patients with liver cirrhosis: diagnostic accuracy of spleen stiffness. *Radiology*. 2016;279:609-619.
87. Jansen C, Bogs C, Verlinden W, et al. Algorithm to rule out clinically significant portal hypertension combining shear-wave elastography of liver and spleen: a prospective multicentre study. *Gut*. 2016;65: 1057-1058.
88. Jansen C, Bogs C, Verlinden W, et al. Shear-wave elastography of the liver and spleen identifies clinically significant portal hypertension: a prospective multicentre study. *Liver Int*. 2017;37:396-405.
89. Elkrief L, Ronot M, Andrade F, et al. Non-invasive evaluation of portal hypertension using shear-wave elastography: analysis of two algorithms combining liver and spleen stiffness in 191 patients with cirrhosis. *Aliment Pharmacol Ther*. 2018;47:621-630.
90. Reiberger T, Ferlitsch A, Payer BA, et al. Non-selective beta-blockers improve the correlation of liver stiffness and portal pressure in advanced cirrhosis. *J Gastroenterol*. 2012;47:561-568.
91. Wong GL, Kwok R, Chan HL, et al. Measuring spleen stiffness to predict varices in chronic hepatitis B cirrhotic patients with or without receiving non-selective beta-blockers. *J Dig Dis*. 2016;17:538-546.
92. Gao J, Ran HT, Ye XP, Zheng YY, Zhang DZ, Wang ZG. The stiffness of the liver and spleen on ARFI imaging pre and post TIPS placement: a preliminary observation. *Clin Imaging*. 2012;36:135-141.
93. De Santis A, Nardelli S, Bassanelli C, et al. Modification of splenic stiffness on acoustic radiation force impulse parallels the variation of portal pressure induced by transjugular intrahepatic portosystemic shunt. *J Gastroenterol Hepatol*. 2018;33:704-709.

CHAPTER 9

Liver Stiffness Beyond the Staging of Liver Fibrosis

Giovanna Ferraioli ■ Richard G. Barr

Introduction

Shear wave elastography (SWE) assesses stiffness, not fibrosis. In addition to fibrosis, there are some factors or clinical conditions that may lead to an increase of liver stiffness (LS). They are known as confounding factors for fibrosis staging: liver inflammation, mostly gauged using transaminase values, which are indirect biomarkers; acute hepatitis; obstructive cholestasis; liver congestion; and infiltrative liver diseases.[1-3]

The first report of an increase in LS in a patient with hepatic vascular congestion due to cardiac insufficiency dates back to 2008.[4] The authors describe the case of a patient infected with hepatitis C virus after two heart transplants for severe ischemic cardiopathy followed by primary nonfunction of the graft. The patient had heart failure and showed a very stiff liver measuring 44.3 kPa at vibration controlled transient elastography (VCTE), with signs of cardiac hepatopathy but without liver cirrhosis at histology. One year after a third heart transplantation, a liver biopsy showed that there was a significant improvement of the cardiac hepatopathy, and the VCTE value was 3.8 kPa (i.e., within the normal range). The authors highlighted that vascular hepatic congestion can considerably increase LS up to values that are definitely diagnostic for liver cirrhosis. They also underscored that this increase is entirely reversible upon correction of cardiovascular dysfunction.

Since that report, several studies have investigated the role of the LS in patients with congestive heart disease and without a primary liver disease.[5-18]

Heart Diseases

Any disease affecting the right heart may lead to an increase of the pressure in the right atrium, the inferior vena cava (IVC), and the hepatic veins. Hepatic veins do not have valves, thus an increase of pressure in the IVC directly affects the sinusoidal bed, causing centrilobular congestion and sinusoidal dilation. The liver is covered by a minimally distensible but nonelastic capsule; therefore hepatic congestion may lead to an increase of stiffness.

CONGESTIVE HEART DISEASE

Heart failure is a major health problem with a considerable risk of morbidity and mortality. In patients with congestive heart disease, right-heart catheterization is the gold standard to measure central venous pressure (CVP). However, the procedure is invasive, not readily available, and not useful for following up patients. An indirect noninvasive parameter of the right atrial pressure (RAP), recommended by the guidelines of the American Society of Echocardiography, is the IVC diameter and its changes with breathing (Fig. 9.1).[5] The guidelines recommend IVC diameter be measured

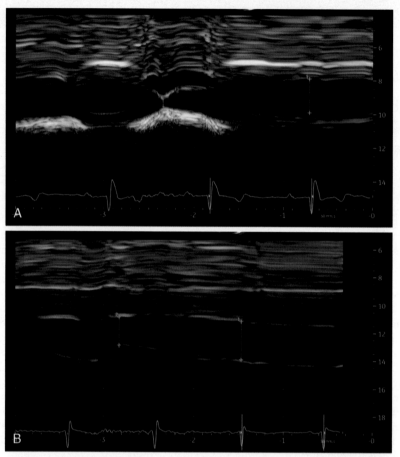

Fig. 9.1   (A) M-mode image of the inferior vena cava (IVC) with respiration in an 81-year-old female with chest pain. The IVC changes from 2.0 to 0.4 cm during respiration. With a diameter ≤2.1 cm that collapses >50% with a breath, this suggests the patient has a normal right atrial pressure (3 mmHg; range, 0–5 mmHg). (B) M-mode image of the IVC in a 68-year-old male with a pericardial effusion. The IVC has an abnormal response to respiration changing from 2.8 to 2.0 cm. With an IVC diameter >2.1 cm that collapses <50% with a breath this suggests the patient has a high right atrial pressure (15 mmHg; range, 10–20 mmHg).

just proximal to the entrance of hepatic veins. IVC diameter ≤2.1 cm that collapses >50% with a breath suggests normal RAP (3 mmHg; range, 0–5 mmHg), whereas IVC diameter >2.1 cm that collapses <50% with a breath suggests high RAP (15 mmHg; range, 10–20 mmHg). If IVC diameter and collapse do not fit this paradigm, an intermediate value (8 mmHg; range, 5–10 mmHg) may be inferred or other indices of RAP should be integrated to downgrade to normal or upgrade to high RAP values. It is also underscored that in young athletes the IVC may be dilated in the presence of normal pressure and that the IVC is commonly dilated and may not collapse in patients on ventilators, so it should not be used in such cases for RAP estimate.[5]

In patients with right-sided heart failure, the LS measurement could be a useful parameter for assessing RAPs and can be repeated over short periods of time.

Millonig and coworkers[6] published the pivotal study in 2010 reporting that the LS is directly influenced by CVP. They showed that the clamping of the IVC in landrace pigs created a visible swelling of the liver and an increase in LS from 3.9 to 27.8 kPa. The reopening of the vein led to a rapid decrease in LS down to 5.1 kPa within 5 minutes ($P < 0.05$). The reversible elevation of LS by increased venous pressure was highly reproducible in all five animals, suggesting that LS is directly controlled by the intravenous pressure in the absence of fibrosis or other causes of LS. For a direct correlation between hydrostatic pressure and LS, the authors also used the model of an isolated pig liver by clamping the portal vein, hepatic artery, and IVC distal and proximal to the liver. The IVC was then cannulated and the intravenous hydrostatic pressure was increased by infusion of isotonic saline solution. LS linearly increased with increasing intravenous pressures, and at a 36-cm water column, the maximum measurable LS with VCTE. (i.e., 75 kPa) was reached. The increase in LS was completely reversible and almost reached initial levels (5.5 kPa) within 5 minutes after resetting hydrostatic pressure back to a 0-cm water column.

Moreover, in a group of 10 patients with decompensated congestive heart disease that clinically recovered over a mean hospitalization interval of 7.2 days, they found a significant decrease of the LS from a median initial LS of 40.7 to 15.3 kPa. Thus treatment of cardiac insufficiency by diuretic therapy, concomitant weight loss, and clinical resolution of edema resulted in a decrease of initially elevated LS.[6]

The decrease of the LS in patients with congestive heart disease who had a clinical improvement after treatment was confirmed in another small series of patients.[7]

A study reported that LS could be an indirect marker of the RAP in patients with right-sided heart failure that was more accurate than IVC findings.[8] In the study, both LS and IVC parameters were obtained within 3 hours before right-sided cardiac catheterization. There was a high correlation (r) between LS and RAP assessed with right-heart catheterization (r = 0.95), and the regression equation to predict RAP was $-5.8 + (6.7 \times$ natural logarithm of LS value in kilopascals). The authors found that an LS cutoff value of 10.6 kPa (with VCTE) identified RAP >10 mmHg with sensitivity and accuracy higher than the IVC parameters (sensitivity 0.85 vs. 0.56, accuracy 0.90 vs. 0.74, $P < 0.05$ for both).

The authors outline that IVC diameter and respiratory variation offer only semiquantitative assessment of RAP and may lead to erroneous inference, especially in patients with intermediate values, whereas LS gives a quantitative assessment of RAP and remains reliable even in patients on mechanical ventilation and with severe tricuspid regurgitation in which the use of echocardiography is usually limited.

However, it should be noted that 16 of the 105 (15.2%) patients who were screened were excluded. This is not a negligible percentage and may raise concern on the applicability of the technique in this setting. On the other hand, it should be highlighted that congestive heart disease may lead to organic liver disease, and this latter may be a confounder when the LS is used to noninvasively assess the CVP. For that reason it is of utmost importance to exclude cases with suspected organic liver disease in research studies.

Despite the improvements in the management of heart failure, there is still a high rate of hospital readmission due to heart failure. The same group of the previous study has assessed the prognostic value of the LS by VCTE in a series of hospitalized patients with heart failure.[9] Of the 226 patients who were screened, 55 (24.3%) were excluded (37 for organic liver disease and 18 for invalid LS measurement). The LS was assessed before discharge in the remaining 171 patients and was stratified into three groups on the basis of the LS value: Group1: ≤4.7 kPa, corresponding to a RAP of 4.6 mmHg on the basis of the regression equation found in their previous study[8]; Group2: 4.7 to ≤6.9 kPa, estimated RAP 6.9 mmHg; Group3: >6.9 kPa, estimated RAP ≥7.0 mmHg. The authors found that the patients in Group3 were in the advanced New York Heart Association functional class and that they had a significantly higher risk of death or readmission to the hospital for heart failure than those in the other two groups. The LS value was able to predict cardiac events with a hazard ratio of 1.13 per 1-kPa increase in LS. LS showed a good predictive value for worse outcomes in patients regardless of severity of diastolic dysfunction. IVC diameter was also associated with the incidence of cardiac events; however, this parameter did not show significant predictive ability in the model that included both LS and IVC.

An LS value of 10.1 kPa had 0.73 sensitivity and 0.90 specificity for predicting worse short-term cardiac events. Notably, LS showed an incremental prognostic value when combined with previously established variables for predicting worse outcomes, including B-type natriuretic peptide. The results of this study indicate that the value of LS at discharge in patients with heart failure can be used as a reliable indicator of subclinical residual liver congestion, which reflects the severity of heart failure and adverse cardiac events, even in patients with optimized treatment and without visible edema or elevated liver function tests.

The prognostic value of the LS in patients with decompensated heart failure has been investigated in a few studies. Of note, the applicability of the technique in these studies is affected by the presence of other factors that could likely increase the LS, and invalid LS measurement or patients lost to follow-up should also be taken into account. In a study that excluded some 30% of patients for the previously mentioned reasons, 105 patients with acute decompensated heart failure were divided into two groups using an arbitrary LS value of 8.8 kPa by VCTE.[10] In a median follow-up period of about 5 months, cardiac events (i.e., death or readmission to hospital) occurred in 54% of patients with LS ≥8.8 kPa and 25% of patients with LS <8.8 kPa ($P =$ 0.001). After adjusting for age, sex, and indices related to organ congestion, an LS ≥8.8 kPa was still significantly associated with cardiac events.

Another study assessed LS with VCTE both on admission to the hospital and the day of discharge in a series of 149 patients with acute decompensated heart failure.[11] Overall there was a significant decrease of the LS during the hospitalization. An LS value higher than 13 kPa on admission and an LS value higher than 5 kPa at discharge was associated with an increased risk of 1-year all-cause death or readmission to the hospital. The authors highlight that LS increase is a nonspecific sign, therefore it would be difficult to use as the method for the differential diagnosis of liver dysfunction. However, in the clinical setting of an already established diagnosis of heart failure, after excluding other confounding factors, this limitation is not so relevant, and LS increase and its associations with negative prognosis in acute decompensated heart failure may be interpreted through two interrelated mechanisms of congestive hepatopathy: parenchymal congestion and congestion-induced fibrosis, both related to unfavorable outcomes.

Using a point shear wave elastography (pSWE) technique in patients with heart failure, it was reported that the changes in LS in patients with heart failure significantly correlated with changes in CVP in multivariate analysis and that an LS cutoff value of 7 kPa could predict a CVP >10 mmHg with 89.6% sensitivity and 87.5% specificity.[12,13] Another group reported that a high LS value on admission was an independent determinant of worse clinical outcomes in patients with acute decompensated heart failure.[14]

All the published studies confirm that LS can be a marker of congestive heart failure; however, it is not yet clear what cutoff value should be used to define the risk of adverse cardiac events. In fact, this value ranges from >5 to 8.8 kPa. Of note, the "rule of 5" proposed by the Baveno VI consensus on portal hypertension has proposed that LS value with VCTE up to 5 kPa may exclude liver fibrosis.[15]

It should also be emphasized that there is an interaction between the liver and the heart: heart failure and liver disease often coexist, because of systemic disorders and factors/diseases that affect both organs (alcohol abuse, drugs, inflammation, autoimmunity, infections).[16] Moreover, there is a complex interaction between the heart and the liver: heart failure may lead to irreversible liver disease; conversely, liver disease may cause cardiac dysfunction and failure in the absence of other cardiovascular abnormalities. Therefore, in some cases, the increase in LS may be due to both liver congestion due to heart disease and liver disease, even when other causes of primary liver disease are excluded.[16] Extensive fibrosis can be seen in chronic or severe cases of congestive hepatopathy. On this regard, it is worth mentioning that liver biopsy data were not available in the majority of the studies reported previously.

A study in a small series of patients with end-stage chronic heart failure who underwent left ventricular assist device implantation reported that the LS values were affected both by the central venous congestion and by the histologic changes of the liver.[17] On the other hand, in patients with severe heart failure who required a left ventricular assist device, it has been observed that the incidence of major adverse events was lower when the LS was ≤12.5 kPa.[18]

CONGENITAL HEART DISEASES AND VALVULAR HEART DISEASES

The usefulness of LS as a noninvasive tool for the evaluation of CVP in patients with congenital heart disease and valvular disease has been assessed in several studies.

One study that included both children and adults with congenital heart disease undergoing cardiac catheterization reported that LS significantly correlated with CVP (r = 0.75).[19] When the two subgroups were analyzed separately, the correlation was significantly higher in the adults (r = 0.68 in children vs. r = 0.84 in adults, $P < 0.0001$). Overall, the area under the receiver operating characteristic (AUROC) curve of the LS for identifying a CVP >10 mmHg was 0.97, and the optimal cutoff value of LS for detection of CVP >10 mmHg was 8.8 kPa with 92% sensitivity and 96% specificity. Considering the children separately (n = 60) from adults (n = 36), the AUROC curve of LS for identification of CVP >10 mmHg was 0.99 with an optimal LS cutoff value of 6.8 kPa (100% sensitivity, 90.5% specificity) in children and 0.95 with an 8.8 kPa cutoff value (100% sensitivity, 89% specificity) in adults.

The LS with a two-dimensional shear wave elastography (2D-SWE) technique was measured in 79 patients aged <20 years old with congenital heart disease and without liver disease who underwent cardiac catheterization.[20] Of them, 34 (43.0%) had Fontan physiology. As observed in adult patients with heart failure, CVP was the only factor that independently and significantly correlated with LS (r = 0.78). This correlation was also present in the subgroups of patients with biventricular disease and those who underwent the Fontan procedure.

In a series of 131 patients with various degrees of tricuspid valve regurgitation secondary to left-sided heart valve disease, it was found that the individuals with severe regurgitation had higher LS than those with moderate regurgitation.[21] Moreover, the LS values were associated with the parameters that noninvasively assess the severity of tricuspid regurgitation, such as the area of the regurgitant orifice, the RAP, and the IVC diameter.

The change over time of the LS value was assessed in a series of 32 consecutive patients undergoing surgery for valve replacement or repair.[22] All patients had tricuspid valve regurgitation secondary to left-sided heart valve disease. It was reported that LS decreased significantly at 3 months after corrective surgery, from 8.4 to 6.0 kPa ($P = 0.03$).

Therefore LS could be proposed as a tool to evaluate, noninvasively, the effects of medical therapy, transcatheter interventions, or mechanical devices on CVP.

FONTAN CIRCULATION

The Fontan operation was proposed for the surgical repair of tricuspid atresia, and it still is the palliative standard procedure for patients with univentricular physiology.[23] The Fontan procedure leads to physiological pulmonary blood flow restoration obtained by diverting the inferior and superior vena cava blood to the pulmonary arteries through cava-pulmonary anastomoses. Doing so, the right atrium is "ventriclized" and oxygenated blood only returns to the left heart. In a Fontan circulation there is no pump to propel blood into the pulmonary arteries, because the systemic veins are directly connected to the pulmonary arteries, and there is a critical bottle-neck with obligatory upstream congestion and downstream decreased flow that account for most of the clinical and physiological disorders in a Fontan circuit.[24] The elevated pressure is trans-mitted to the liver directly through the IVC and the hepatic veins.

The advances in the surgical techniques and in the management of patients with single ven-tricle physiology, congenital heart disease, and Fontan circulation have led to a longer survival of Fontan-palliated patients who now reach adulthood in the majority of cases.

However, the altered hemodynamics lead to disfunction of several organs, especially the liver. In fact, cardiac cirrhosis is quite common in Fontan-palliated patients during their adulthood. The pathologic changes in the liver are sinusoidal dilatation and fibrosis, likely due to high ve-nous pressures, hypoxia, and diminished cardiac output.

Using a 2D-SWE technique in patients with Fontan circulation, a study demonstrated that the LS values correlated with the stage of histopathologic fibrosis and that the LS values were significantly higher (15.6 kPa vs. 5.5 kPa, $P < 0.0001$) than in healthy controls.[25] Forty-one patients with Fontan physiology and 65 controls were enrolled, and a small number of Fontan patients underwent transjugular liver biopsy. LS on average was 13.4 kPa in patients with METAVIR fibrosis stage F <2 (n = 4) and 19.8 kPa in patients with F ≥2 (n = 6). These LS values are significantly higher than that observed in other causes of chronic liver disease likely due to the combination of fibrosis and congestion. It was also found that portal vein blood flow assessed with Doppler flowmetry was decreased, whereas the celiac and mesenteric arterial resistive indices were higher and that the LS correlated both with ventricular end-diastolic pressure and pulmonary artery wedge pressure as well as the degree of liver fibrosis. All these findings clearly indicate there is interplay between the hepatic afterload and the histological changes.

Hepatic complications are correlated with the duration of the Fontan circulation. Using VCTE, a study in 39 patients with Fontan circulation reported a significant correlation between the stage of fibrosis and the interval of time since the Fontan surgery, with a sharp increase in the number of patients with significant liver fibrosis at 5 years after the operation.[26] Moreover, there was a relationship between the LS and the inspiration/expiration diameter ratio of the IVC (i.e., a sign of liver congestion).

A study performed with a pSWE technique in 64 Fontan patients demonstrated that patients with a fenestration had significant lower mean LS than patients without (1.75 vs. 2.03 m/s, $P = 0.003$).[27]

A study in a small series of Fontan patients (n = 10) with liver biopsy results available re-ported that the VCTE cutoffs obtained in patients with mixed causes of chronic liver disease would have overestimated fibrosis by at least one stage in 70% of subjects and by at least two stages in 50% of subjects.[28] There was no agreement with liver biopsy results when using the 2D-SWE cutoffs obtained in patients with chronic hepatitis C in a small cohort that included 14 Fontan patients who underwent liver biopsy.[29]

The Fontan procedure leads to a significant increase in LS caused by hepatic congestion.[30,31] This increase persists chronically, therefore the evaluation of liver fibrosis in this setting is chal-lenging because it is not possible to separate the two factors (i.e., congestion and fibrosis) and it could lead to an overestimation of fibrosis.[32]

Using pSWE in 18 children undergoing the Fontan operation (stage 3), an immediate marked increase in LS from 1.18 to 2.28 m/s, on average, simply due to increased hepatic systemic venous afterload and increased CVP was observed; this increase in LS persisted to the time of hospital discharge and beyond.[30] In a small series (9 children; age range, 3.5–5.6 years), it was observed that LS increased from 6.2 ± 1.5 kPa in the preoperative period to 11.2 ± 4 kPa at a mean follow-up of 4 months.[31]

For the follow-up and longitudinal monitoring of Fontan patients, the assessment of the delta changes in LS over time as suggested by the update to the Society of Radiologists in Ultrasound consensus statement can be applied and provides valuable information.[33] This approach helps overcome the lack of reliable cutoff values and our current inability to distinguish if the increased stiffness is caused by congestion or fibrosis.[32] An increase of LS over time is indicative of worsening fibrosis and/or congestion and may indicate additional clinical investigation is needed.

Liver Diseases Beyond the Staging of Fibrosis

LS assessment is a reliable and noninvasive method for the staging of liver fibrosis in several clinical scenarios, and it is an accepted biomarker of portal hypertension.[15,34,35] The potential role of LS in evaluating liver disease beyond the stage of liver fibrosis has been investigated in hepatic sinusoidal obstruction syndrome (SOS), Budd-Chiari syndrome, and biliary atresia (BA).

HEPATIC SINUSOIDAL OBSTRUCTION SYNDROME

Hepatic SOS, previously named *hepatic venoocclusive disease,* is caused by toxic damage to the hepatic sinusoidal endothelial cells that leads to loss of sinusoidal wall integrity, endothelium detachment, and embolization toward the centrolobular zone of the hepatic acinus.[36,37] These events hamper the liver blood outflow, with sinusoidal obstruction resulting in congestion and ultimately development of postsinusoidal portal hypertension.[37]

SOS may be a result of cytoreductive therapy prior to hematopoietic stem cell transplantation following oxaliplatin-containing adjuvant or neoadjuvant chemotherapy for colorectal liver metastases, after the ingestion of alkaloid toxins, and in other particular settings such as the autosomal recessive condition of venoocclusive disease with immunodeficiency or after high-dose radiation therapy.[36]

SOS is a life-threatening disease in its severe forms.[37] The diagnosis is based on clinical criteria including weight gain, hepatomegaly, right-upper quadrant pain, ascites, and jaundice.[37] The use of defibrotide for the treatment of severe forms has reduced the high mortality rate. The mortality is lower when the treatment is started earlier, therefore an earlier diagnosis is of utmost importance. On this regard, studies suggest that elastography could play an important role.

In 2011 Fontanilla and coworkers[38] reported an increase of LS assessed by a pSWE technique (2.75 m/s and 2.58 m/s) in two adult patients diagnosed with SOS. They observed that LS decreased to normal values after successful treatment.

The potential role of LS assessment in this setting has been investigated in rat models of acute and severe SOS or chronic, mild, and reversible SOS.[39] In both SOS models, LS values were significantly higher than in the matched control rats. In the chronic and reversible SOS models there was a significant decrease of LS after a treatment-free period of 2 weeks.

The role of LS in predicting SOS syndrome has been investigated in a series of 25 pediatric patients who received hematopoietic stem cell transplant and in those whom LS by pSWE technique was assessed at three scheduled time points.[40] Five of them developed SOS. In respect to the patients who did not develop SOS, they had a significant increase of LS at day +5 and at day +14 after transplant. LS increase occurred on average 9 and 11 days before clinical and conventional ultrasound (US) diagnosis of SOS. Therefore an LS increase seems to be an early marker of SOS development, allowing an early diagnosis and the possibility to timely start an effective treatment.

Similar findings were observed in a series of 78 adult patients who underwent hematopoietic stem cell transplantation.[41] The median baseline LS value assessed by VCTE was 4.2 kPa. Four patients (5.1%) presented with SOS, and in all of them LS showed a significant increase in respect to baseline values 2–12 days before the clinical manifestation of SOS. The three patients who were successfully treated with defibrotide showed a decrease of LS, which reached pretransplantation value within 2–4 weeks after the diagnosis of SOS, whereas in the patient with severe SOS who died 20 days after the diagnosis of SOS, there was not any decrease of LS.

An algorithm has been proposed for the diagnostic work-up of patients undergoing hematopoietic stem cell transplantation.[37] A baseline assessment with US and SWE is recommended within 1 month before the procedure. As per the guidelines,[42] after the transplantation the patient must be screened daily to rule out the onset of SOS. US and SWE should be performed weekly to detect any morphological, Doppler, and LS changes. In the absence of clinical signs but with a sudden increase in stiffness compared with the baseline value, a close clinical follow-up is required and could be combined with US or radiological (magnetic resonance imaging [MRI]/computed tomography [CT]) studies. This follow-up is needed because there is a high likelihood that SOS will develop in the following days. If there is an agreement between the clinical evaluation and the radiological findings, the diagnosis of SOS can be confirmed; otherwise, an invasive approach is necessary to confirm or rule out SOS.

BUDD-CHIARI SYNDROME

Budd-Chiari syndrome is due to hepatic venous outflow obstruction in the absence of cardiac or pericardial disease that leads to hepatic congestion and portal hypertension. The outflow obstruction can be partial or complete and may occur in small or large hepatic veins, the suprahepatic segment of the IVC, or the right atrium. The clinical manifestations are highly variable, ranging from fulminant or acute liver failure to subacute, chronic, or asymptomatic forms. Important clinical features include abdominal pain, ascites, hepatosplenomegaly, and prominent venous collaterals secondary to the obstruction of the IVC. Budd-Chiari syndrome can be primary or secondary, depending on the cause of the hepatic venous outflow obstruction.[43] It is classified as secondary when the hepatic flow is obstructed by compression or invasion of a lesion outside the hepatic venous outflow. Primary cases are, in the majority of cases in the Western world, caused by an underlying hypercoagulable or prothrombotic state resulting from several congenital conditions (such as protein C deficiency, protein S deficiency, antithrombin deficiency, factor V Leiden mutation) or myeloproliferative disorders, paroxysmal nocturnal hemoglobinuria, hyperhomocysteinemia, Behçet's disease, oral contraceptive intake, antiphospholipid antibody, malignancy, and few other conditions. Anatomical anomalies of the IVC, such as membranous obstruction, are less frequent and more common in Asian populations.[43]

Noninvasive imaging such Doppler ultrasonography, CT, or MRI play a crucial role in the diagnosis of Budd-Chiari syndrome, demonstrating the hepatic venous outflow.

Rather than a diagnostic tool, SWE can potentially be used in the follow-up of patients. Few studies have been published so far.

The role of LS in monitoring short- and long-term outcome after angioplasty was assessed in a series of 25 patients with Budd-Chiari syndrome.[44] There was a significant decrease of LS values within 24 hours after intervention from 62.8 to 26.3 kPa. In the patients for whom liver histology results were available, the changes in LS did not show any significant difference between cases with mild fibrosis and significant fibrosis. There was also a significant difference between LS values obtained at 24 hours and those at 3 months after treatment (26.3 kPa vs. 20.9 kPa; $P = 0.003$). It is suggested that LS measurement can be used as a surveillance tool to longitudinally assess the outcome of the vascular intervention, irrespective of preintervention fibrosis stage.

Likewise, a significant decrease of LS 2 days after the treatment from 35.2 to 20.1 kPa was observed in a series of 32 patients with Budd-Chiari syndrome successfully treated with angioplasty.[45] The patients were followed up with for 6 months. With respect to baseline values, there was a significant decrease at 3 months; thereafter, LS values remained stable even though the liver was still in the cirrhotic stage.

In a case report, LS with the pulsed Doppler waveform of the hepatic veins was used to follow-up at 3-month intervals with a patient who presented with restenosis of the IVC after balloon dilation. A sharp increase of LS (from 14.3 to 20.5 kPa) and a monophasic pattern of the hepatic vein flow at pulsed Doppler were markers of restenosis confirmed by x-ray venography.[46]

BILIARY ATRESIA

BA is a progressive fibroinflammatory process that causes obliteration of the extra- and intrahepatic biliary tree and that clinically presents during the first few weeks of life with persistent jaundice and elevated conjugated bilirubin. It is the most common cause of chronic cholestasis in infants, and it leads to secondary biliary cirrhosis in the first months of life and to death in early childhood if untreated. Kasai hepatic portoenterostomy (HPE) is the standard treatment for BA, and early HPE (before 46 days of life) results in a higher rate of survival with native liver and better long-term clinical outcomes, and thus a high index of suspicion is needed for investigation of infants with persistent jaundice.[47,48]

The diagnosis of BA is often based on some combination of B-mode US imaging, hepatobiliary scintigraphy, liver biopsy, and intraoperative cholangiography.[49] Early diagnosis is of utmost importance to reestablish bile flow from the liver into the small bowel and provide the best patient outcomes.[50] Conventional B-mode US is recommended for BA diagnosis. It has a good diagnostic performance; however, the B-mode findings do not rule out nonsyndromic BA.[48]

In BA the liver may become very stiff, and there is evidence in the literature that SWE can be used to help differentiate BA from other nonsurgical causes of neonatal jaundice.[51]

In a study on 48 cholestatic neonates, 15 of whom had BA, an LS cutoff value of >7.7 kPa by VCTE had 80% sensitivity and 97% specificity for diagnosing BA.[52]

A study in 41 patients, 13 of whom were diagnosed with BA, reported that LS by pSWE was significantly higher in patients with BA (1.95 vs. 1.21 m/s), and a cutoff value >1.53 m/s had 76.9% sensitivity and 78.6% specificity.[53] In the same study, a cutoff value of LS by 2D-SWE >1.84 m/s had 92.3% sensitivity and 78.6% specificity.

The utility of LS measurement by 2D-SWE and several commonly used biomarkers in differentiating BA from other causes of cholestasis (non-BA) patients within 45 days and in predicting the postoperative prognosis has been investigated in a series of 156 patients, consisting of BA (n = 83) and non-BA (n = 73) cases.[54] 2D-SWE and serum gamma-glutamyl transferase showed better discriminative utility. The optimal cutoff values for 2D-SWE and gamma-glutamyl transferase were >7.10 kPa and >195.4 U/L, with the AUROC curves of 0.82 and 0.87, respectively. Subgroup analysis showed an increased discriminative performance of 2D-SWE with age.

The survival rate with a native liver after a successful HPE is >50% at 10 years and 30%–40% at 20 years, whereas orthotopic liver transplantation has a 10-year survival rate of 86%.[55] Literature data suggest that liver and spleen SWE could be a valuable tool to monitor liver disease and portal hypertension after the Kasai operation. In a study on 31 patients with BA who had undergone a Kasai portoenterostomy, the optimal LS cutoff by VCTE for predicting esophageal varices was >10.6 kPa (87% sensitivity, 87.5% specificity, and 0.92 AUROC curve).[55]

In a series of 69 patients who underwent HPE and performed VCTE before and 3 months after HPE, LS value was the most powerful independent factor of the development of liver-related events. The cutoff value of 19.9 kPa had 85.3% sensitivity, 95.2% specificity, and 0.94 AUROC curve.[56]

KEY POINTS

1. SWE techniques have largely been used for the assessment of LS related to liver fibrosis, and their use in the clinical practice is now accepted by guidelines.
2. SWE measures the stiffness, not just fibrosis, thus its use can be extended to the evaluation of other conditions as well. Several studies have shown that, beyond liver fibrosis assessment, LS is a useful parameter for the evaluation of liver congestion that occurs in the case of right-sided heart failure, some congenital and valvular diseases, hepatic SOS, or Budd-Chiari syndrome.
3. The literature shows that SWE can be used to help differentiate BA from other nonsurgical causes of neonatal jaundice.
4. In these scenarios, LS assessment may also play a role in monitoring changes over time, therefore it could be a marker of clinical outcome rather than a diagnostic tool.

References

1. Ferraioli G, Wong VW, Castera L, et al. Liver ultrasound elastography: an update to the World Federation for Ultrasound in Medicine and Biology guidelines and recommendations. *Ultrasound Med Biol.* 2018;44:2419-2440.
2. Dietrich CF, Bamber J, Berzigotti A, et al. EFSUMB guidelines and recommendations on the clinical use of liver ultrasound elastography, update 2017 (short version). *Ultraschall Med.* 2017;38:377-394.
3. Barr RG, Ferraioli G, Palmeri ML, et al. Elastography assessment of liver fibrosis: Society of Radiologists in Ultrasound consensus conference statement. *Ultrasound Q.* 2016;32:94-107.
4. Lebray P, Varnous S, Charlotte F, Varaut A, Poynard T, Ratziu V. Liver stiffness is an unreliable marker of liver fibrosis in patients with cardiac insufficiency. *Hepatology.* 2008;48:2089.
5. Rudski LG, Lai WW, Afilalo J, et al. Guidelines for the echocardiographic assessment of the right heart in adults: a report from the American Society of Echocardiography endorsed by the European Association of Echocardiography, a registered branch of the European Society of Cardiology, and the Canadian Society of Echocardiography. *J Am Soc Echocardiogr.* 2010;23:685-713.
6. Millonig G, Friedrich S, Adolf S, et al. Liver stiffness is directly influenced by central venous pressure. *J Hepatol.* 2010;52:206-210.
7. Colli A, Pozzoni P, Berzuini A, et al. Decompensated chronic heart failure: increased liver stiffness measured by means of transient elastography. *Radiology.* 2010;257:872-878.
8. Taniguchi T, Sakata Y, Ohtani T, et al. Usefulness of transient elastography for noninvasive and reliable estimation of right-sided filling pressure in heart failure. *Am J Cardiol.* 2014;113:552-558.
9. Taniguchi T, Ohtani T, Kioka H, et al. Liver stiffness reflecting right-sided filling pressure can predict adverse outcomes in patients with heart failure. *JACC Cardiovasc Imaging.* 2019;12:955-964.
10. Saito Y, Kato M, Nagashima K, et al. Prognostic relevance of liver stiffness assessed by transient elastography in patients with acute decompensated heart failure. *Circ J.* 2018;82:1822-1829.
11. Soloveva A, Kobalava Z, Fudim M, et al. Relationship of liver stiffness with congestion in patients presenting with acute decompensated heart failure. *J Card Fail.* 2019;25:176-187.
12. Yoshitani T, Asakawa N, Sakakibara M, et al. Value of virtual touch quantification elastography for assessing liver congestion in patients with heart failure. *Circ J.* 2016;80:1187-1195.
13. Demirtas AO, Koc AS, Sumbul HE, et al. Liver stiffness obtained by ElastPQ ultrasound shear wave elastography independently determines mean right atrial pressure. *Abdom Radiol (NY).* 2019;44:3030-3039.
14. Omote K, Nagai T, Asakawa N, et al. Impact of admission liver stiffness on long-term clinical outcomes in patients with acute decompensated heart failure. *Heart Vessels.* 2019;34:984-991.
15. de Franchis R, Baveno VI Faculty. Expanding consensus in portal hypertension: Report of the Baveno VI Consensus Workshop: stratifying risk and individualizing care for portal hypertension. *J Hepatol.* 2015;63:743-752.
16. Xanthopoulos A, Starling RC, Kitai T, Triposkiadis F. Heart failure and liver disease: cardiohepatic interactions. *JACC Heart Fail.* 2019;7:87-97.
17. Potthoff A, Schettler A, Attia D, et al. Liver stiffness measurements and short-term survival after left ventricular assist device implantation: a pilot study. *J Heart Lung Transplant.* 2015;34:1586-1594.

18. Nishi H, Toda K, Miyagawa S, et al. Novel method of evaluating liver stiffness using transient elastography to evaluate perioperative status in severe heart failure. *Circ J*. 2015;79:391-397.

19. Jalal Z, Iriart X, De Lédinghen V, et al. Liver stiffness measurements for evaluation of central venous pressure in congenital heart diseases. *Heart*. 2015;101:1499-1504.

20. Terashi E, Kodama Y, Kuraoka A, et al. Usefulness of liver stiffness on ultrasound shear-wave elastography for the evaluation of central venous pressure in children with heart diseases. *Circ J*. 2019;83:1338-1341.

21. Chen Y, Seto WK, Ho LM, et al. Relation of tricuspid regurgitation to liver stiffness measured by transient elastography in patients with left-sided cardiac valve disease. *Am J Cardiol*. 2016;117:640-646.

22. Chon YE, Kim SU, Park JY, et al. Dynamics of the liver stiffness value using transient elastography during the perioperative period in patients with valvular heart disease. *PLoS One*. 2014;9:e92795.

23. Fontan F, Baudet E. Surgical repair of tricuspid atresia. *Thorax*. 1971;26:240-248.

24. Gewillig M, Brown SC. The Fontan circulation after 45 years: update in physiology. *Heart*. 2016;102: 1081-1086.

25. Kutty SS, Peng Q, Danford DA, et al. Increased hepatic stiffness as consequence of high hepatic afterload in the Fontan circulation: a vascular Doppler and elastography study. *Hepatology*. 2014;59:251-260.

26. Friedrich-Rust M, Koch C, Rentzsch A, et al. Noninvasive assessment of liver fibrosis in patients with Fontan circulation using transient elastography and biochemical fibrosis markers. *J Thorac Cardiovasc Surg*. 2008;135:560-567.

27. Kim SO, Lee SY, Jang SI, et al. Hepatic stiffness using shear wave elastography and the related factors for a Fontan circulation. *Pediatr Cardiol*. 2018;39:57-65.

28. Wu FM, Opotowsky AR, Raza R, et al. Transient elastography may identify Fontan patients with unfavorable hemodynamics and advanced hepatic fibrosis. *Congenit Heart Dis*. 2014;9:438-447.

29. Schachter JL, Patel M, Horton SR, Devane AM, Ewing A, Abrams GA. FibroSure and elastography poorly predict the severity of liver fibrosis in Fontan-associated liver disease. *Congenit Heart Dis*. 2018;13:764-770.

30. DiPaola FW, Schumacher KR, Goldberg CS, Friedland-Little J, Parameswaran A, Dillman JR. Effect of Fontan operation on liver stiffness in children with single ventricle physiology. *Eur Radiol*. 2017;27: 2434-2442.

31. Deorsola L, Aidala E, Cascarano MT, Valori A, Agnoletti G, Pace Napoleone C. Liver stiffness modifications shortly after total cavopulmonary connection. *Interact Cardiovasc Thorac Surg*. 2016;23:513-518.

32. Ferraioli G, Barr RG. Ultrasound liver elastography beyond liver fibrosis assessment. *World J Gastroenterol*. 2020;26:3413-3420.

33. Barr RG, Wilson SR, Rubens D, Garcia-Tsao G, Ferraioli G. Update to the Society of Radiologists in Ultrasound liver elastography consensus statement. *Radiology*. 2020;296:263-274.

34. Paternostro R, Reiberger T, Bucsics T. Elastography-based screening for esophageal varices in patients with advanced chronic liver disease. *World J Gastroenterol*. 2019;25:308-329.

35. Berzigotti A. Non-invasive evaluation of portal hypertension using ultrasound elastography. *J Hepatol*. 2017;67:399-411.

36. Fan CQ, Crawford JM. Sinusoidal obstruction syndrome (hepatic veno-occlusive disease). *J Clin Exp Hepatol*. 2014;4:332-346.

37. Ravaioli F, Colecchia A, Alemanni LV, et al. Role of imaging techniques in liver veno-occlusive disease diagnosis: recent advances and literature review. *Expert Rev Gastroenterol Hepatol*. 2019;13:463-484.

38. Fontanilla T, Hernando CG, Claros JC, et al. Acoustic radiation force impulse elastography and contrast-enhanced sonography of sinusoidal obstructive syndrome (veno-occlusive disease): preliminary results. *J Ultrasound Med*. 2011;30:1593-1598.

39. Park SH, Lee SS, Sung JY, et al. Noninvasive assessment of hepatic sinusoidal obstructive syndrome using acoustic radiation force impulse elastography imaging: a proof-of-concept study in rat models. *Eur Radiol*. 2018;28:2096-2106.

40. Reddivalla N, Robinson AL, Reid KJ, et al. Using liver elastography to diagnose sinusoidal obstruction syndrome in pediatric patients undergoing hematopoietic stem cell transplant. *Bone Marrow Transplant*. 2020;55:523-530.

41. Colecchia A, Ravaioli F, Sessa M, et al. Liver stiffness measurement allows early diagnosis of veno-occlusive disease/sinusoidal obstruction syndrome in adult patients who undergo hematopoietic stem cell transplantation: results from a monocentric prospective study. *Biol Blood Marrow Transplant*. 2019;25:995-1003.

42. Mohty M, Malard F, Abecassis M, et al. Revised diagnosis and severity criteria for sinusoidal obstruction syndrome/veno-occlusive disease in adult patients: a new classification from the European Society for Blood and Marrow Transplantation. *Bone Marrow Transplant*. 2016;51:906-912.

43. Khan F, Armstrong MJ, Mehrzad H, et al. Review article: a multidisciplinary approach to the diagnosis and management of Budd-Chiari syndrome. *Aliment Pharmacol Ther*. 2019;49:840-863.

44. Mukund A, Pargewar SS, Desai SN, Rajesh S, Sarin SK. Changes in liver congestion in patients with Budd-Chiari syndrome following endovascular interventions: assessment with transient elastography. *J Vasc Interv Radiol*. 2017;28:683-687.

45. Wang HW, Shi HN, Cheng J, Xie F, Luo YK, Tang J. Real-time shear wave elastography (SWE) assessment of short- and long-term treatment outcome in Budd-Chiari syndrome: a pilot study. *PLoS One*. 2018;13:e0197550.

46. Nakatsuka T, Soroida Y, Nakagawa H, et al. Utility of hepatic vein waveform and transient elastography in patients with Budd-Chiari syndrome who require angioplasty: two case reports. *Medicine (Baltimore)*. 2019;98:e17877.

47. Hartley JL, Davenport M, Kelly DA. Biliary atresia. *Lancet*. 2009;374:1704-1713.

48. Yan H, Du L, Zhou J, et al. Diagnostic performance and prognostic value of elastography in patients with biliary atresia and after hepatic portoenterostomy: protocol for a systematic review and meta-analysis. *BMJ Open*. 2021;11:e042129.

49. Wang L, Yang Y, Chen Y, Zhan J. Early differential diagnosis methods of biliary atresia: a meta-analysis. *Pediatr Surg Int*. 2018;34:363-380.

50. Bezerra JA, Wells RG, Mack CL, et al. Biliary atresia: clinical and research challenges for the twenty-first century. *Hepatology*. 2018;68:1163-1173.

51. Ferraioli G, Barr RG, Dillman JR. Elastography for pediatric chronic liver disease: a review and expert opinion. *J Ultrasound Med*. 2021;40:909-928.

52. Wu JF, Lee CS, Lin WH, et al. Transient elastography is useful in diagnosing biliary atresia and predicting prognosis after hepatoportoenterostomy. *Hepatology*. 2018;68:616-624.

53. Dillman JR, DiPaola FW, Smith SJ, et al. Prospective assessment of ultrasound shear wave elastography for discriminating biliary atresia from other causes of neonatal cholestasis. *J Pediatr*. 2019;212:60-65.

54. Liu Y, Peng C, Wang K, et al. The utility of shear wave elastography and serum biomarkers for diagnosing biliary atresia and predicting clinical outcomes. *Eur J Pediatr*. 2022;181(1):73-82.

55. Colecchia A, Di Biase AR, Scaioli E, et al. Non-invasive methods can predict oesophageal varices in patients with biliary atresia after a Kasai procedure. *Dig Liver Dis*. 2011;43:659-663.

56. Hahn SM, Kim S, Park KI, Han SJ, Koh H. Clinical benefit of liver stiffness measurement at 3 months after Kasai hepatoportoenterostomy to predict the liver related events in biliary atresia. *PLoS One*. 2013;8:e80652.

CHAPTER 10

Liver Shear Wave Elastography: Guidelines

Richard G. Barr ▪ Giovanna Ferraioli

Introduction

Guidelines for the use of elastography in diffuse liver disease have been released by societies or federations of societies. The first set of guidelines was released by European Federation of Societies for Ultrasound in Medicine and Biology (EFSUMB) in 2013.[1] In 2015 the World Federation for Ultrasound in Medicine and Biology (WFUMB) and the Society of Radiologists in Ultrasound (SRU) produced guidelines on this topic, and the European Association for the Study of the Liver (EASL), together with the Asociación Latinoamericana para el Estudio del Hígado (ALEH), released clinical practice guidelines for the use of noninvasive tests in the evaluation of liver disease.[2-5] The advances in the technologies and the rapidly increasing evidence in the past few years have prompted all these societies/federations of societies to update their guidelines: EFSUMB did so in 2017, WFUMB in 2018, SRU in 2020, and EASL in 2021.[6-11]

All guidelines have highlighted that a correct acquisition's protocol is necessary to obtain a liver stiffness measurement (LSM) of good quality and that the literature shows that the acoustic radiation force impulse (ARFI) techniques have similar or better accuracy than vibration controlled transient elastography (VCTE) in the assessment of liver fibrosis even though the evidence is still low. Details about the correct acquisition's protocol are given in Chapter 4. Guidelines have also highlighted that ultrasound (US) shear wave elastography (SWE) techniques measure liver stiffness, not fibrosis. Beside liver fibrosis, there are other factors that may lead to an increase in stiffness. These confounding factors are presented in detail in Chapter 4.

It has been underscored that there is a large overlap of stiffness values between benign and malignant liver lesions and that there is insufficient evidence to make a recommendation on the use of SWE for differentiating and/or characterizing them.[2,8]

For the staging of liver fibrosis in patients with chronic viral hepatitis or nonalcoholic fatty liver disease (NAFLD), the "rule of 5" has been proposed for VCTE and "rule of 4" for the ARFI techniques.[8,9] This topic is presented in detail in Chapter 7.

European Federation of Societies for Ultrasound in Medicine and Biology Guidelines[1,6,7]

EFSUMB produced guidelines and recommendations on the clinical applications of US elastography in 2013; the largest section of the document was dedicated to the liver and was mainly based on the use of VCTE because the technique had been available for almost a decade at that time.[1] In 2017 an update of the guidelines, dedicated to the clinical use of the SWE techniques for the assessment of diffuse liver disease, was released.[6,7] Based on literature data, the document evaluated the role of the SWE techniques in different etiologies of liver diseases and in several clinical scenarios.[10] The highest level of evidence was in patients with chronic viral hepatitis, and VCTE was still the most validated technique.

The document contains several recommendations that are listed below. They were graded according to the Oxford Centre for Evidence-Based Medicine in which the level of evidence (LoE) from published studies goes from 1 (the highest level) to 5 (the lowest level). The grade of recommendation (GoR) goes from A (strongest) to D (weakest). The consensus reached through voting of the expert on each recommendation was also reported.

Recommendation 1: The operator must acquire appropriate knowledge and training in US elastography (LoE 5, GoR C; strong consensus).

Recommendation 2: Data acquisition should be undertaken by dedicated and specially trained personnel. For point shear wave elastography (pSWE) and two-dimensional shear wave elastography (2DSWE), experience in B-mode ultrasound is mandatory (LoE 5, GoR C; strong consensus).

Recommendation 3: LSM by SWE should be performed through a right intercostal space in supine position, with the right arm in extension, during breath hold, avoiding deep inspiration prior to the breath hold (LoE 2b, GoR B; strong consensus).

Recommendation 4: LSM by SWE should be performed by experienced operators (LoE 2b, GoR B; strong consensus).

Recommendation 5: LSM by pSWE and 2D-SWE should be performed at least 10 mm below the liver capsule (LoE 1b, GoR A; strong consensus).

Recommendation 6: Patients should fast for a minimum of 2 hours and rest for a minimum of 10 minutes before undergoing LSM with SWE (LoE 2b, GoR B; majority consensus).

Recommendation 7: The major potential confounding factors (liver inflammation indicated by aspartate aminotransferase (AST) and/or alanine aminotransferase (ALT) elevation more than 5 times the normal limits, obstructive cholestasis, liver congestion, acute hepatitis and infiltrative liver diseases) should be excluded before performing LSM with SWE to avoid overestimation of liver fibrosis (LoE 1b, GoR B; broad consensus).

Recommendation 8: SWE within the normal range can rule out significant liver fibrosis when in agreement with the clinical and laboratory background (LoE 2a, GoR B; broad consensus).

Recommendation 9: For VCTE, 10 measurements should be obtained. An interquartile range/ median ≤30% of the 10 measurements is the most important reliability criterion (LoE 1b, GoR A; strong consensus).

Recommendation 10: For VCTE, values obtained with XL probe are usually lower than with the M probe, therefore no recommendation on the cutoffs to be used can be given (LoE 2b, GoR B; broad consensus).

Recommendation 11: Adequate B-mode liver image is a prerequisite for pSWE and 2D-SWE measurements (LoE 5, GoR D; strong consensus).

Recommendation 12: The median value of at least 10 measurements should be used for liver elastography by pSWE (LoE 2b, GoR B; strong consensus).

Recommendation 13: For 2D-SWE, a minimum of three measurements should be obtained; the final result should be expressed as median together with interquartile range (LoE 2b, GoR B; strong consensus).

Recommendation 14: Methods to objectively assess strain are being developed but currently cannot be recommended in clinical practice (LoE 5, GoR D; strong consensus).

Recommendation 15: The results with the lowest variability in comparing different pSWE or 2D-SWE systems were obtained at a depth of 4–5 cm from the transducers (with convex transducers). Accordingly, if this location is technically suitable, it would be recommended (LoE 4, GoR C; broad consensus).

Recommendation 16: VCTE can be used as first-line assessment for the severity of liver fibrosis in patients with chronic viral hepatitis C (HCV). It performs best to rule out cirrhosis (LoE 1b, GoR A; broad consensus).

Recommendation 17: pSWE, as demonstrated with virtual touch quantification (VTQ), can be used as first-line assessment for the severity of liver fibrosis in patients with chronic HCV. It performs best to rule out cirrhosis (LoE 2a, GoR B; broad consensus).

Recommendation 18: 2D-SWE, as demonstrated with the SuperSonic Imagine (SSI) modality, can be used as a first-line assessment for the severity of liver fibrosis in patients with chronic HCV. It performs best to rule out cirrhosis (LoE 1b, GoR A; broad consensus).

Recommendation 19: SWE is not recommended to monitor fibrosis changes during anti-HCV treatment (LoE 3, GoR D; strong consensus).

Recommendation 20: LSM changes after successful anti-HCV treatment should not affect the management strategy (e.g., surveillance for hepatocellular carcinoma [HCC] occurrence in patients at risk) (LoE 3, GoR D; broad consensus).

Recommendation 21: VCTE is useful in patients with chronic hepatitis B virus (HBV) to identify those with cirrhosis. Concomitant assessment of transaminases is required to exclude flare (elevation >5 times upper limit of normal) (LoE 1b, GoR A; broad consensus).

Recommendation 22: VCTE is useful in carriers of inactive HBV to rule out fibrosis (LoE 2, GoR B; strong consensus).

Recommendation 23: pSWE, as demonstrated with VTQ, is useful in patients with chronic HBV to identify those with cirrhosis (LoE 2a, GoR B; strong consensus).

Recommendation 24: 2D-SWE, as demonstrated with SSI, is useful in patients with chronic HBV to identify those with cirrhosis (LoE 3a, GoR C; broad consensus).

Recommendation 25: LSM changes under HBV treatment should not affect the management strategy (e.g., surveillance for HCC occurrence in patients at risk) (LoE 2b, GoR B; strong consensus).

Recommendation 26: VCTE can be used to exclude cirrhosis in patients with NAFLD (LoE 2a, GoR B; broad consensus).

Recommendation 27: VCTE can be used to exclude cirrhosis in patients with alcoholic liver disease, provided that acute alcoholic hepatitis is not present (LoE 2b, GoR B; strong consensus).

Recommendation 28: LSM with VCTE is useful to identify patients with a high likelihood of having clinically significant portal hypertension (hepatic venous pressure gradient [HVPG] ≥10 mmHg) (LoE 2b, GoR B; strong consensus).

Recommendation 29: Liver stiffness using VCTE combined with platelet count is useful to rule out varices requiring treatment. Although preliminary results are encouraging, there is insufficient evidence to recommend pSWE and 2D-SWE in this setting (LoE 2b, GoR B; broad consensus).

World Federation for Ultrasound in Medicine and Biology Guidelines[2,8]

WFUMB released the first set of guidelines for the use of elastographic techniques in 2015. They were composed of three documents: basic principles and terminology, liver elastography, and breast elastography.[2]

The recommendations were based on the international literature and on the expertise of the team designated by WFUMB. The recommendations were not graded because at that time it was felt that there was a great heterogeneity between studies and the available evidence was still low.[10]

An update to the liver guidelines was released in 2018, and this time the recommendations were based on published literature, and the strength of each recommendation was judged according to the Oxford Centre for Evidence-Based Medicine.[8] The recommendations are reported below. There was strong consensus of the expert panel for all the recommendations.

Strain elastography was included in the WFUMB guidelines because this technique was still performed in some Asian countries. However, the limitations of the technique and the fact that it has an accuracy that is not good enough to diagnose any stage of liver fibrosis were also highlighted, and no specific recommendation on its use was given.

Recommendation 1: Cutoffs for staging liver fibrosis are system specific (LoE 1b, GoR A).

Recommendation 2: The impact of hepatic steatosis on liver stiffness is uncertain. Clinicians should exercise caution when interpreting liver stiffness results in patients with severe steatosis and obesity (LoE5, GoR C).

Recommendation 3: SWE is useful to exclude significant fibrosis and diagnose cirrhosis in patients with untreated chronic hepatitis B (LoE1a, GoR A).

Recommendation 4: Liver stiffness usually decreases during antiviral treatment with analogues. Screening for HCC and portal hypertension should continue despite decreased liver stiffness in patients with advanced disease (LoE1b, GoR A).

Recommendation 5: SWE is the preferred method as the first-line assessment for the severity of liver fibrosis in untreated patients with chronic viral hepatitis C. It is useful to rule out advanced disease (LoE1a, GoR A).

Recommendation 6: Liver stiffness decreases significantly after SVR to treatment with interferon-based therapies or direct-acting antiviral agents. However, liver stiffness cannot be used to stage liver fibrosis or rule out cirrhosis, given the loss of accuracy of cutoffs defined in viremic patients. Screening for HCC and portal hypertension should continue despite decrease of liver stiffness in patients with advanced disease (LoE1b, GoR A).

Recommendation 7: SWE can be used for liver stiffness assessment in patients with NAFLD to rule out advanced fibrosis and select patients for further assessment (LoE1a, GoR A).

Recommendation 8: SWE can be used for liver stiffness assessment in patients with ALD to rule out advanced disease. Caution is needed in patients with ongoing alcohol abuse or with acute alcoholic hepatitis (LoE 2a, GoR B).

Recommendation 9: SWE has high diagnostic accuracy for detecting cirrhosis; better at ruling out (high NPV above 90%) than ruling in (LoE 1a, GoR A).

Recommendation 10: LSM of VCTE >20 kPa can be used to identify patients likely bearing clinically significant portal hypertension (HVPG $\geq$10 mmHg) (LoE 2b, GoR B).

Recommendation 11: LSM using VCTE <20–25 kPa combined with platelet count >110,000–150,000/μL is useful to rule out varices needing treatment (LoE 2b, GoR B).

Recommendation 12: LSM holds prognostic value in compensated cirrhosis and the higher the value, the higher the risk of clinical complications (LoE 2b, GoR B).

Recommendation 13: There is insufficient evidence to make a recommendation on the use of SWE for liver stiffness assessment in pediatric patients (LoE 5, GoR D).

Recommendation 14: There is insufficient evidence to make a recommendation on the use of SWE for differentiation between benign and malignant lesions and characterization of focal liver lesions (LoE 5, GoR D).

Recommendation 15: Controlled attenuation parameter is a point of care, standardized and reproducible technique, promising for the detection of liver steatosis. However, for quantifying steatosis, there is a large overlap between adjacent grades, there are no consensual cutoffs, and quality criteria are not well defined (LoE 3, GoR C).

Recommendation 16: Interpretation of liver stiffness measurements needs to be taken in context with the other clinical and laboratory data (LoE 1b, GoR A).

Society of Radiologists in Ultrasound Consensus[3,4,9]

In 2014 the SRU convened a panel of specialists from radiology, hepatology, pathology, and basic science and physics to arrive at a consensus regarding the use of elastography in the assessment of liver fibrosis in chronic liver disease. The results of the panel were published in 2015.[3,4]

The conference statement discussed the burden of chronic liver disease and cirrhosis, predisposing conditions, and the staging of fibrosis. The panel concluded that the histologic reference standard was imperfect with high variability between pathologist. It listed the sources of variability in elastography: (1) origin of underlying disease, (2) patient comorbidities, (3) modality being used, (4) system-specific factors, (5) machine variability, (6) patient physical factors, (7) indication for study, (8) disease prevalence, (9) patient sex, (10) postprandial state, and (11) breath-hold technique. The panel provided a comparison of the elastographic modalities including advantages, expenses, frequency of shear wave generation, limitations, measurement location, region of interest size, value reported, and defining a good measurement.

The panel provided evidence-based best practice for performance of US-based elastography. These included fasting for 4–6 hours, specific positioning of patient, right arm elevated above the head, shallow breath hold, placement of the region of interest, and the acquisition number of measurements.

A review of the pSWE, 2D-SWE, VCTE, and magnetic resonance elastography (MRE) techniques were provided, highlighting the variability of the measurements in noninvasive assessment of liver fibrosis. Due to the large overlap of stiffness values in intermediate levels of fibrosis regardless of which technique was used, a low cutoff value for various systems was provided, below which there was no clinically significant fibrosis and a high cutoff value, above which there was a high probability of compensated advanced chronic liver disease (cACLD). It was recommended that using likelihood ratios was more appropriate than converting the stiffness values in METAVIR scores. A recommendation of what should be included in the report was provided.

In 2020 the SRU published an update to the SRU liver elastography consensus statement.[9] The update again emphasized following the strict protocol recommended in the 2015 document. The experts panel underscored that most patients with HCV are being treated regardless of the degree of fibrosis. Because the overlap of liver stiffness values between METAVIR scores is as large if not larger than the difference between vendors, separate cutoff values for each vendor were not required. It was pointed out that what is most clinically important is diagnosing cACLD. Given the large overlap of stiffness values for mild to moderate fibrosis, the SRU continued to recommend a low cutoff value, below which there is a high probability of no or mild fibrosis and recommended a high cutoff value, above which there is a high probability of cACLD. The recommendations made by the panel are discussed in detail in Chapter 7. Briefly, a vendor neutral "rule of 4" for interpretation of liver stiffness values obtained using ARFI techniques in patients with viral hepatitis and NAFLD was proposed. In patients with chronic HBV or HCV hepatitis successfully treated with antiviral drugs, the cutoffs obtained in treatment-naive patients should not be used because a rapid decline of stiffness values is observed in treated subjects, likely due to the decrease of liver inflammation. Therefore, when liver cirrhosis is evident by B-mode findings, elastography should not be used to rule out the disease because a value in the low range of liver stiffness may only indicate a successful response to antiviral treatment. The panel suggested that the delta change of liver stiffness values over time should be used instead of the absolute values to follow-up patients. Thus every patient becomes their own control. In patients with chronic viral hepatitis who are successfully treated, the baseline liver stiffness value to be used for the follow up should be that obtained after viral eradication or suppression.

For pediatric patients with liver disease or congenital heart disease with Fontan surgery, it was recommended that each subject becomes their own control, using the stiffness delta changes over time to evaluate the efficacy of the treatment or the progression of disease.

The consensus points out that by applying this rule, liver stiffness assessment can be suitable for evaluating all clinical conditions that increase liver stiffness, independent of the disease etiology, including nonfibrotic causes of liver stiffness increase, such as congestive heart failure.

Because there is an approximately 10% variability of the measurements within a vendor and between vendors, the recommendation is that a clinically significant change should be considered when the delta is greater than 10%. The panel recommended using the same equipment for follow-up studies.

Asian-Pacific Association for the Study of the Liver Guidelines[12]

In 2016 the Asian-Pacific Association for the Study of the Liver (APASL) guidelines developed consensus guidelines on the assessment of liver fibrosis that included invasive methods, such as liver biopsy and hepatic venous pressure gradient measurements, and noninvasive methods, such as biomarkers, conventional radiological methods, and elastography techniques. In these guidelines, liver biopsy was considered the gold standard; however, all the limitations of the procedure were highlighted. In the short paragraph dedicated to elastography techniques, it was acknowledged that ARFI-based methods are as accurate as VCTE in staging liver fibrosis.[10]

American Gastroenterological Association Guidelines[13]

The American Gastroenterological Association (AGA) guidelines, published in 2017, were focused on the role of VCTE for the evaluation of liver fibrosis. At that time there was already an abundant literature on this topic, including several metaanalyses; however, all the recommendations were graded as conditional and with low-quality evidence. In the AGA guidelines it is claimed that VCTE is the most commonly used imaging-based technique for fibrosis assessment method in the United States; however, no evidence is provided, thus this statement could be misleading.[10] Moreover, the term elastography is identified with VCTE, and there is no mention of the ARFI techniques or to the literature data showing that these techniques have an accuracy that is at least similar to that reported for VCTE.

European Association for the Study of the Liver Guidelines[5,11]

The first set of EASL guidelines was produced together with the ALEH in 2015.[5] It indicates that, for fibrosis staging, VCTE should be considered the reference standard because it is the most validated. Nonetheless, the EASL–ALEH guidelines acknowledged that the pSWE and 2D-SWE techniques showed the same accuracy of VCTE for the staging of liver fibrosis in published studies, even though the level of available evidence was lower than that of VCTE. This trend has been maintained in the recently released update.[11]

In the update, the noninvasive tests that were analyzed for the evaluation of liver disease severity and prognosis were blood markers, methods assessing physical properties of the liver tissue (e.g., liver stiffness, attenuation, viscosity), and imaging methods assessing the anatomy of the liver and other abdominal organs (e.g., US, MR, and CT).

The panel of experts developed the clinical practice guidelines (CPGs) update according to a format based on P: Patient, Population, or Problem; I: Intervention, Prognostic Factor, or Exposure; C: Comparison or Intervention (if appropriate); and O: Outcome questions. The CPGs were sent to a Delphi Panel for reviewing and voting. The suggested changes were taken into consideration in a revised version, which was then submitted to the EASL Governing Board. The following scenarios were analyzed: general population; alcohol-related liver disease; HCV post-sustained virological response (SVR)/postantiviral therapy; NAFLD/nonalcoholic steatohepatitis (NASH); cholestatic and autoimmune liver disease; cACLD, and portal hypertension. The LoE based on the Oxford Centre for Evidence-Based Medicine and the QUADAS-2 tool for accuracy of diagnostic studies were used to judge the quality of the evidence.

GENERAL POPULATION

It is underscored that, because of the spectrum effect, noninvasive fibrosis tests will likely have lower sensitivity and higher specificity in populations with lower prevalence of the disease.

Noninvasive tests should be preferentially used in patients at risk of advanced fibrosis, such as patients with metabolic risk factors and/or harmful use of alcohol, and not in unselected populations (LoE 2). They should be used to rule out rather than rule in advanced fibrosis (LoE 1). ALT, AST, and platelet count should be part of the routine investigations in primary care in patients with suspected liver disease so that simple non invasive scores can be readily calculated (LoE 2). The automatic calculation and systematic reporting of simple non invasive fibrosis tests such as the fibrosis-4 index for liver fibrosis (FIB-4) in populations at risk of liver fibrosis (individuals with metabolic risk factors and/or harmful use of alcohol) in primary care is recommended to improve risk stratification and linkage to care (LoE 2). In low-prevalence populations, all noninvasive tests can identify advanced fibrosis in patients at risk significantly better than clinical acumen alone (LoE 1).

Individuals at risk for advanced fibrosis should be entered in appropriate risk stratification pathways using noninvasive fibrosis tests (LoE 1). In low-prevalence populations the choice of noninvasive tests and the design of diagnostic pathways should be performed in consultation with a liver specialist (LoE 3).

All these recommendations were graded as strong.

ALCOHOL-RELATED LIVER DISEASE

Accuracy of Noninvasive Methods for Fibrosis Staging Compared to Liver Biopsy

The followings are strong recommendations:
- Liver stiffness values by VCTE <8 kPa can rule out alcohol-related advanced chronic liver disease (ACLD) (LoE 3); values ≥12–15 kPa can diagnose ACLD in high-prevalence populations only after excluding false positive cases (LoE 2).
- In patients with elevated liver stiffness and evidence of hepatic inflammation by blood tests (AST or gamma-glutamyl transferase higher than two times the upper limit of normal), liver stiffness by VCTE should be repeated after at least 1 week of alcohol restraint (LoE 3).

Accuracy of Noninvasive Tests for Predicting Liver-Related Outcomes Compared to Liver Biopsy, HVPG, Child-Pugh Score, or Model for End-Stage Liver Disease

Because of lack of evidence, the panel felt that was not possible to make any recommendations regarding prognostic markers in alcohol-related compensated liver disease.

HCV POST-SVR/POSTANTIVIRAL THERAPY

Accuracy of Noninvasive Tests Compared to Liver Biopsy to Stage Liver Fibrosis in Patients with cACLD Who Achieved SVR After Antiviral Therapy

- The routine use of noninvasive scores and liver stiffness is not recommended because they lack accuracy in detecting fibrosis regression (LoE 3).
- Liver stiffness cutoffs that were obtained in untreated patients with HCV should not be used to stage liver fibrosis after SVR (LoE 4).

These were strong recommendations.

Accuracy of Noninvasive Tests to Predict Clinical Outcomes (Decompensation, HCC) Compared to Liver Biopsy, HVPG, Child-Pugh Score or MELD in Patients with HCV and Patients with cACLD Who Achieved SVR

In patients with cACLD previous to antiviral therapy for HCV, LSM post-SVR could be helpful to refine the stratification of residual risk of liver-related complications and liver stiffness can be repeated yearly (LoE 3). Patients with cACLD prior to treatment should continue to be monitored for HCC and portal hypertension regardless of the results of noninvasive tests post-SVR (LoE 3; strong recommendation).

NAFLD/NASH

Accuracy of Noninvasive Tests for the Diagnosis of Steatosis Compared to Liver Biopsy

The studies performed using serum scores or controlled attenuation parameter were evaluated. The conclusion was that noninvasive scores are not recommended for the diagnosis of steatosis in the clinical practice (LoE 2; strong recommendation), whereas conventional US is recommended as a first-line diagnostic tool despite its well-known limitations (LoE 1; strong recommendation).

Magnetic resonance imaging-estimated proton density fat fraction (MRI-PDFF) is the most accurate noninvasive method for detecting and quantifying steatosis; however, it is not recommended as a first-line tool due to its cost and limited availability (LoE 2; strong recommendation).

Accuracy of Noninvasive Tests to Evaluate NAFLD Severity (Presence of NASH and Staging of Liver Fibrosis) Compared to Liver Biopsy

It is highlighted that liver biopsy is still the reference standard for the diagnosis of NASH, because none of the available noninvasive tests has acceptable accuracy (LoE 2).

In patients with NAFLD, the following tests are recommended to rule out advanced fibrosis in clinical practice (LoE 1, strong recommendation): liver stiffness by VCTE <8 kPa; patented tests: ELF <9.8 or FibroMeter <0.45 or FibroTest < 0.48; nonpatented tests: FIB-4 <1.3 or NAFLD fibrosis score < −1.455. In patients with FIB-4 >1.3, VCTE and/or patented serum tests should be used to rule out or rule in advanced fibrosis (LoE 2; strong recommendation). Even though MRE is the most accurate noninvasive method for staging liver fibrosis, it is only marginally better than other noninvasive tests for the diagnosis of ACLD; therefore it is not recommended as first-line diagnostic test also due to its cost and limited availability (LoE 2; strong recommendation). It can play a role in clinical trials.

Accuracy of Noninvasive Tests to Predict Liver-Related Outcomes in Patients with NAFLD Compared to Liver Biopsy, HVPG, Child-Pugh Score, or MELD

Serum scores and liver stiffness by VCTE should be used to stratify the risk (LoE 3; strong recommendation). Repeated measurements of noninvasive tests can be used to refine stratification of risk of liver-related events in patients with NAFLD/NASH. Even though there is lack of evidence for choosing the optimal interval for the follow-up, the panel deemed it reasonable to repeat the tests every 3 years in patients in early stage of liver fibrosis and every year in patients with ACLD (LoE 3; weak recommendation).

Accuracy of Noninvasive Tests for Patients' Selection and Evaluation of Treatment Response in NAFLD Therapeutic Trials Compared to Liver Biopsy

It was strongly recommended to use liver biopsy for the selection of patients in therapeutic trials and to evaluate NASH resolution and liver fibrosis improvement in this setting. A weak recommendation was given for the use of MRI-PDFF for assessing steatosis changes under treatment because it was felt that the relevant minimal decrease in MRI-PDFF needed to be better defined.

CHOLESTATIC AND AUTOIMMUNE LIVER DISEASE

Accuracy of Noninvasive Tests to Assess Disease Severity in Comparison to Liver Biopsy in Patients with Primary Biliary Cholangitis and Primary Sclerosing Cholangitis

Noninvasive scores and serum markers are not recommended for fibrosis staging in clinical practice (LoE 3; strong recommendation).

In patients with PBC, a cutoff of 10 kPa by VCTE can rule in cACLD (LoE 3; strong recommendation).

In patients with PSC, a value of liver stiffness >9.5 kPa by VCTE can be used to support the diagnosis of advanced fibrosis in compensated patients with normal bilirubin and without high-grade stenosis (LoE 3; weak recommendation).

Accuracy of Noninvasive Tests to Predict Liver-Related Outcomes in Patients with PBC and PSC Compared to Liver Biopsy, HVPG, Child-Pugh Score, or MELD

In patients with PBC, noninvasive discrimination of early and advanced stage disease based on biochemical parameters (normal vs. abnormal albumin and bilirubin) and LSM by VCTE < or >10 kPa is recommended at baseline (LoE 3; strong recommendation). During treatment, risk stratification should be based on the assessment of response to therapy by using continuous (GLOBE and UK-PBC risk scores) and/or qualitative criteria (Paris II, Toronto, Rotterdam, Barcelona, Paris I) and liver stiffness by VCTE (LoE 3; strong recommendation).

In patients with PSC, both the ELF score and liver stiffness by VCTE correlate with outcomes and they should be used for risk stratification both at baseline and during follow-up (LoE 3; strong recommendation). MRI (alone or combined with VCTE values) can be used for prognostic purposes (LoE 3; strong recommendation).

Accuracy of Noninvasive Test to Assess Liver Fibrosis, and to Monitor Disease Course as Compared to Liver Biopsy in Patients with Autoimmune Hepatitis

Liver stiffness by VCTE can be used in treated patients to monitor the disease course together with transaminases and immunoglobulin G and to stage liver fibrosis after at least 6 months of immunosuppressive therapy (LoE 3; weak recommendation).

COMPENSATED ADVANCED CHRONIC LIVER DISEASE AND PORTAL HYPERTENSION

Accuracy of Noninvasive Tests to Diagnose cACLD as Compared to Liver Biopsy

- Patented serum tests or SWE techniques for the diagnosis of cACLD should be used in specialized settings (LoE 2; strong recommendation).
- Patented serum tests (FibroTest, FibroMeter, and ELF) should be used to rule out cACLD if available (LoE 3; strong recommendation).
- A cutoff <8–10 kPa by VCTE rules out cACLD, whereas a cutoff >12–15 kPa rules in the disease. Intermediate values require further testing (LoE 3; strong recommendation).
- pSWE and 2D-SWE should be used to rule out and diagnose cACLD. They have shown AUROCs >0.90 in published metaanalyses (LoE 2; strong recommendation).

- Intersystem variability should be taken into consideration in the interpretation of results obtained with different SWE techniques because values, ranges, and cutoffs are not comparable (LoE 3; strong recommendation).

Accuracy of Noninvasive Tests to Diagnose Clinically Significant Portal Hypertension and to Monitor Portal Hypertension in cACLD in Comparison to HVPG Measurement

- A cutoff of >20–25 kPa by VCTE should be used to diagnose CSPH in patients with cACLD (LoE 1; strong recommendation).
- Platelet count, spleen size, and spleen stiffness should be used as additional noninvasive tests to further improve risk stratification for CSPH (LoE 3; strong recommendation).
- The presence of portosystemic collaterals on US, CT, or MR is a sign of CSPH in patients with cACLD and should be routinely reported (LoE 2; strong recommendation).
- For an exact assessment of the severity of portal hypertension beyond the detection of CSPH and for assessment of the hemodynamic response to treatment, HVPG remains the only validated tool and should not be substituted by noninvasive tests (LoE 1; strong recommendation).

Accuracy of Noninvasive Tests to Diagnose and Exclude High-Risk Gastroesophageal Varices in Comparison to Endoscopy

- In patients with cACLD due to untreated viral hepatitis, HIV–HCV coinfection, alcohol, NAFLD, PBC, and PSC, a liver stiffness by VCTE <20 kPa and platelet count >150,000 /L (Baveno VI criteria) is a validated tool to rule out high-risk varices and avoid endoscopic screening. These criteria should be used whenever VCTE is available (LoE 1a; strong recommendation).
- Spleen stiffness can be used as an additional tool to refine the risk of high-risk varices in cACLD (LoE 2; weak recommendation).
- CT should not be used for primary screening for esophageal and gastric varices; however, in a routine CT, varices should be reported if present (LoE 3; strong recommendation).

Accuracy of Noninvasive Tests to Predict Clinical Decompensation, Hepatocellular Carcinoma, and Mortality in cACLD as Compared to Liver Biopsy, HVPG, Child-Pugh Score, or MELD

- Liver stiffness at diagnosis should be used in addition to liver function tests to stratify the risk of clinical decompensation and mortality (LoE 1; strong recommendation).
- Annual repeated measurements of liver stiffness can be used to refine risk stratification (LoE 5; weak recommendation).
- Liver stiffness can be used in addition to clinical variables and accepted risk scores to stratify the risk of HCC in patients with HBV (LoE 3; weak recommendation).

KEY POINTS

1. All guidelines recommend following a strict protocol for liver stiffness measurements.
2. All guidelines recommend interpreting results in light of the patient's clinical picture including etiology of their chronic liver disease and confounding factors.
3. Understanding artifacts and avoiding them is highlighted in the guidelines.
4. Using quality assessment features is important to ensure the results are accurate, and a statement of the quality of the data set should be included in the report.
5. Confounding factors are pointed out and should be documented and mentioned in the report.

References

1. Cosgrove D, Piscaglia F, Bamber J, et al. EFSUMB guidelines and recommendations on the clinical use of ultrasound elastography, part 2: clinical applications. *Ultraschall Med.* 2013;34:238-253.
2. Ferraioli G, Filice C, Castera L, et al. WFUMB guidelines and recommendations for clinical use of ultrasound elastography: part 3: liver. *Ultrasound Med Biol.* 2015;41:1161-1179.
3. Barr RG, Ferraioli G, Palmeri ML, et al. Elastography assessment of liver fibrosis: Society of Radiologists in Ultrasound consensus conference statement. *Radiology.* 2015;276:845-861.
4. Barr RG, Ferraioli G, Palmeri ML, et al. Elastography assessment of liver fibrosis: Society of Radiologists in Ultrasound Consensus Conference Statement. *Ultrasound Q.* 2016;32:94-107.
5. European Association for Study of Liver, Asociacion Latinoamericana para el Estudio del Higado. EASL-ALEH Clinical Practice Guidelines: non-invasive tests for evaluation of liver disease severity and prognosis. *J Hepatol.* 2015;63:237-264.
6. Dietrich CF, Bamber J, Berzigotti A, et al. EFSUMB guidelines and recommendations on the clinical use of liver ultrasound elastography, update 2017 (long version). *Ultraschall Med.* 2017;38:e16-e47.
7. Dietrich CF, Bamber J, Berzigotti A, et al. EFSUMB guidelines and recommendations on the clinical use of liver ultrasound elastography, update 2017 (short version). *Ultraschall Med.* 2017;38:377-394.
8. Ferraioli G, Wong VW, Castera L, et al. Liver ultrasound elastography: an update to the World Federation for Ultrasound in Medicine and Biology guidelines and recommendations. *Ultrasound Med Biol.* 2018;44:2419-2440.
9. Barr RG, Wilson SR, Rubens D, Garcia-Tsao G, Ferraioli G. Update to the society of radiologists in ultrasound liver elastography consensus statement. *Radiology.* 2020;296:263-274.
10. Ferraioli G. Review of liver elastography guidelines. *J Ultrasound Med.* 2019;38:9-14.
11. European Association for the Study of the Liver. Electronic address: easloffice@easloffice.eu; Clinical Practice Guideline Panel; Chair; EASL Governing Board representative; Panel members. EASL Clinical Practice Guidelines on non-invasive tests for evaluation of liver disease severity and prognosis–2021 update. *J Hepatol.* 2021;75(3):659-689. doi:10.1016/j.jhep.2021.05.025.
12. Shiha G, Ibrahim A, Helmy A, et al. Asian-Pacific Association for the Study of the Liver (APASL) consensus guidelines on invasive and non-invasive assessment of hepatic fibrosis: a 2016 update. *Hepatol Int.* 2017;11:1-30.
13. Lim JK, Flamm SL, Singh S, Falck-Ytter YT, Clinical Guidelines Committee of the American Gastroenterological Association. American Gastroenterological Association Institute Guideline on the role of elastography in the evaluation of liver fibrosis. *Gastroenterology.* 2017;152:1536-1543.

CHAPTER 11

Noninvasive Assessment of Liver Steatosis with Ultrasound Techniques

Giovanna Ferraioli ■ Richard G. Barr

Introduction

Worldwide, obesity has nearly tripled since 1975.[1] The World Health Organization (WHO) reports that, as of 2016, more than 1.9 billion adults 18 years or older were overweight, and, of these, over 650 million were obese. The WHO report underscores that most of the world's population lives in countries where overweight and obesity kills more people than underweight. As for children, the report estimated that over 340 million children and adolescents aged 5–19 years old were overweight or obese in 2016.[1] A modeling study suggests that by 2030, the prevalence of nonalcoholic steatohepatitis (NASH) will increase 63% from the estimation made in 2015, and liver mortality and advanced liver disease are expected to more than double.[2] These increases in the rates of obesity have prompted the WHO to identify obesity as one of the nine global noncommunicable diseases that must be addressed.

Obesity increases the risk of several diseases including nonalcoholic fatty liver disease (NAFLD), which is currently the most prevalent chronic liver disease worldwide. In fact, the prevalence of NAFLD is proportional to the increase in body mass index.[3]

In a large U.S. cohort of asymptomatic middle-aged adults, the prevalence of NAFLD was 38% and the prevalence of NASH was 14%. Factors associated with the presence of NASH were race, obesity, and diabetes.[4]

The rate of individuals affected by type 2 diabetes mellitus, which is another important risk factor for NAFLD and NASH, is also growing worldwide.[5] Of note, it seems that type 2 diabetes mellitus seems to accelerate the course of NAFLD and is a predictor of advanced fibrosis and mortality.[6] Moreover, liver steatosis can negatively affect the disease progression and treatment response in patients with viral hepatitis C and the prognosis of hepatic transplantation recipients.[7]

NAFLD seems the most common cause of abnormal serum aminotransferase levels as well as chronic liver disease in the Western world.[8] It is an umbrella term that includes a disease spectrum ranging from benign steatosis to NASH. The latter may progress to liver cirrhosis with its complications, namely portal hypertension and hepatocellular carcinoma. The prevalence of NAFLD in the general population is about 25% and it increases to over 90% in morbidly obese individuals. The progression to fibrosis is about 40%, and the mean annual rate of progression in NASH is 0.09%.[6] The reason why some patients with NAFLD, even those with a low amount of fat in the liver, will develop NASH is still not clearly understood. The degree of liver steatosis is linked to metabolic syndrome and the cardiovascular risk.[9] On the other hand, it seems that significant steatosis is associated with progression of fibrosis in patients with NAFLD.[10] It also must be highlighted that a recent nationwide study in Sweden has shown in an adult cohort that the hazard ratio for overall mortality was significantly higher in all patients with NAFLD, including those with simple steatosis, than in controls.[11] The results of this study confirm previous findings in small cohorts of patients with NAFLD with paired liver biopsy,[12,13] suggesting that simple steatosis may clearly progress, with around one quarter of patients developing bridging fibrosis over a relatively short time period.[14] Of note, baseline steatosis grade was higher in those with progressive fibrosis.[12] Alarmingly, similar findings were observed in children and young adults with biopsy-confirmed NAFLD: they had significantly higher rates of overall, cancer-, liver- and cardiometabolic-specific mortality compared with matched general population controls.[15] Simple steatosis was associated with a 5.26-fold higher adjusted rate of mortality compared with controls.

Therefore an accurate estimate of the quantity of the fat in the liver is of great importance in the diagnostic work-up of patients with liver steatosis.

A panel of experts has recently proposed to adopt a new term based on a holistic approach to the disease, *metabolic dysfunction–associated fatty liver disease* (MAFLD).[16] The diagnosis of MAFLD is based on the evidence of liver steatosis together with three positive criteria: overweight/obesity, presence of type 2 diabetes mellitus, or evidence of metabolic dysregulation.

In this chapter, we mostly use the term *NAFLD* because of the criteria that were followed to enroll patients in the cited studies.

Reference Standard for Liver Fat Quantification

For decades, liver biopsy has been considered the reference standard for detecting and grading liver steatosis. In the histologic Kleiner classification, the amount of fat in the liver is graded as S0, steatosis in less than 5% of hepatocytes; S1, 5%–33%; S2, 34%–66%; and S3, more than 66%.[17]

Liver biopsy is an invasive procedure with some risks of complications that can be severe in up to 1% of cases.[18,19] On the other hand, the biopsy specimen is obtained from a very small part of liver, and fatty infiltration could be heterogenous. Moreover, a substantial intraobserver and interobserver variability between readings has been reported.[20,21] Considering the obesity epidemic, biopsy is not a practical approach for screening in patients with MAFLD who may have simple steatosis in most cases. Liver steatosis is a dynamic process that may change in short periods of time (weeks), requiring a noninvasive technique that can be repeated at multiple times to accurately assess progression or regression of disease.[7]

Magnetic resonance imaging–derived proton density fat fraction (MRI-PDFF) is a quantitative noninvasive biomarker that objectively estimates the liver fat content and has been accepted as an alternative to the histological assessment of liver steatosis in patients with MAFLD.[22-26] MRI-PDFF is not influenced by confounding factors, including body weight, and is operator-independent. Currently, it is an accepted noninvasive tool to diagnose and quantify liver steatosis and is used in clinical trials as an accurate reference standard method as an alternative to liver biopsy.[27,28] Also, when assessing the performance of new noninvasive tools for the detection and grading of liver steatosis, liver biopsy is not the best reference to compare the results with, given the very small size of the biopsy specimen and the dynamic nature of liver fat content.[29]

The ultrasound (US) attenuation working group of the American Institute of Ultrasound in Medicine (AIUM) and the Radiological Society of North America (RSNA) Quantitative Imaging Biomarkers Alliance (QIBA) Pulse Echo Quantitative Ultrasound (PEQUS) initiative, which was formed to help develop and standardize acquisition protocols and to better understand confounding factors of US-based fat quantification, has recently advised that MRI-PDFF should be used in studies as the reference standard.[30]

Noninvasive Assessment: Ultrasound

B-MODE IMAGING

B-mode US imaging allows to subjectively estimate the degree of fatty infiltration in the liver. The evaluation of liver steatosis is usually based on a series of US findings including liver echogenicity, hepatorenal echo contrast, visualization of intrahepatic vessels, and visualization of the liver parenchyma and the diaphragm. Steatosis is scored as follows: absent (score 0) when there is a normal liver echotexture; mild (score 1) steatosis, in the case of a slight and diffuse increase in fine parenchymal echoes with normal visualization of diaphragm and portal vein borders; moderate (score 2) steatosis, in the case of a moderate and diffuse increase in fine echoes with slightly impaired visualization of portal vein borders and diaphragm; severe (score 3) steatosis, in the case of marked increase of fine echoes with poor or no visualization of portal vein borders, diaphragm, and posterior portion of the right liver lobe.[31,32] Chapter 2 provides a more detailed discussion of the use of B-mode imaging in fat quantification.

The performance of B-mode US imaging for the detection of mild steatosis (fat content ≥5%) is low, with reported sensitivity of 53.3%–63.6%.[33-35] A metaanalysis reported that, for the detection of moderate to severe fatty liver (>20%–30% steatosis), B-mode US had a performance similar to computed tomography or MRI.[36] There is also a substantial interobserver variability. However, it must be underscored that, despite these limitations, B-mode US has been recommended as the preferred first-line diagnostic procedure for imaging of NAFLD in adults by the clinical practice guidelines of the European Association for the Study of the Liver released together with the European Association for the Study of Diabetes and the European Association for the Study of Obesity.[37]

To improve the accuracy of B-mode US imaging, other scoring systems have been proposed and are reported below.

SEMIQUANTITAVE ASSESSMENT

Hamaguchi Score

The Hamaguchi score combines four US findings: hepatorenal echo contrast, bright liver, deep attenuation, and vessel blurring, and a number is assigned to each of them.[38]

Hepatorenal echo contrast is based on the ultrasonographic contrast between the hepatic and right renal parenchyma evaluated in an intercostal scan in the mid-axillary line; bright liver is based on abnormally intense high level echoes arising from the liver parenchyma and is graded as none, mild, or severe in accordance with intensity brightness; deep attenuation is based on the US attenuation in the deep portion of the liver and impaired visualization of the diaphragm; vessel blurring is based on impaired visualization of the borders of the intrahepatic vessels and narrowing of their lumen (Fig. 11.1).

Bright liver and hepatorenal echo contrast are evaluated together, and the score ranges from 0 to 3. If they are both negative, the final score is 0. Deep attenuation goes from 0 to 2, and vessel blurring can be positive (score 1) or negative (score 0).

In a small series of patients undergoing liver biopsy, Hamaguchi et al. found that a score ≥2 had 91.7% sensitivity and 100% specificity for diagnosing NAFLD with an area under the receiver operating characteristic curve (AUROC) of 0.98. A score ≥1 had high specificity (95.1%) to detect visceral obesity. However, this score has not been validated in large series of patients.

Ultrasonographic Fatty Liver Indicator Score

The ultrasonographic fatty liver indicator (US-FLI) score is based on the following features: intensity of liver/kidney contrast, posterior attenuation of the US beam, vessel blurring, difficult visualization of the gallbladder wall, difficult visualization of the diaphragm, and areas of focal

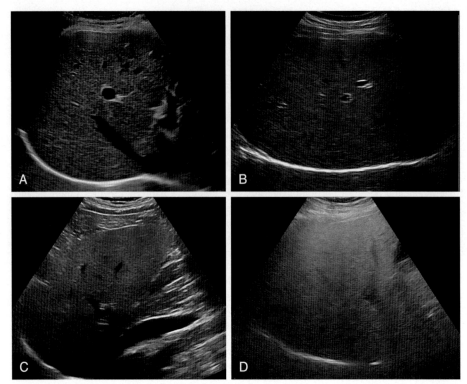

Fig. 11.1 With increasing steatosis (fatty deposition), the echogenicity of the liver increases and visualization of the vascular structures changes. (A) Normal. (B) Grade 1. (C) Grade 2. (D) Grade 3. Note the difference in visualization of the vessels at the various grades of liver steatosis.

sparing.[39] Focal fat sparing is considered to be present when a focal geographic hypoechoic area is observed next to the gallbladder wall, portal vein, or the falciform ligament (Fig. 11.2).

"Conditio sine qua non" is the presence of the contrast between the liver and the kidney, which is scored 2 if mild/moderate and 3 if severe. The presence of each other finding is scored 1.

The score ranges from 2 to 8 and NAFLD is diagnosed by a score at least >2.

In a small series of nonconsecutive patients, using liver histology as the reference, it has been reported that the US-FLI score was an independent predictor of NASH and a US-FLI <4 had a high negative predictive value (94%) in ruling out the diagnosis of severe NASH, but its specificity was low (45.7%). The AUROCs were 0.76 for the diagnosis of NASH and 0.80 for the diagnosis of severe NASH. As for the Hamaguchi score, the US-FLI score still lacks validation.

Hepatorenal Index

The hepatorenal index (HRI) is calculated on the basis of the ratio between the echogenicity of the liver and that of the right kidney cortex (see also Chapter 2).[40]

In the past, free software programs available online were used to analyze the pixels of the images.

To obtain the HRI, two regions of interest (ROIs) are positioned in the liver and the renal cortex. Both must be at the same depth in the hepatic parenchyma and the renal cortex, avoiding vascular and biliary structures or masses. Artifacts, especially from ribs or lung, must be avoided.

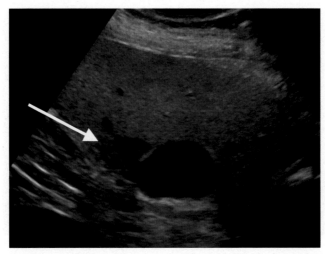

Fig. 11.2 Example of fatty sparing in a patient with moderate steatosis. The *arrow* points to a more hypoechoic area adjacent to the gallbladder. This is a common location for fatty sparing as well as focal fatty infiltration. The area can be mistaken as a mass lesion; however, there is no mass effect, and vessels are not displaced. If there is concern, a contrast-enhanced ultrasound examination can confirm that no mass lesion is present.

Literature data show significant variability with optimal cutoff for the detection of steatosis ranging from 1.24 to 2.2.[30] Moreover, this method is limited by using postprocessing data, which is influenced by the time gain compensation setting as well as other settings.

Currently, most vendors have implemented this feature and the index is directly calculated using preprocessed data and displayed on the monitor of the US equipment (Fig. 11.3). Generally, the intensity data from raw data per pixel are used to calculate the average intensity of pixels. Therefore the influence of gain, dynamic range, time gain compensation, or other scanner parameters is eliminated. However, HRI is affected by operator's experience, depth of measurement, and variability between vendors in calculating this measurement.[30] Moreover, it lacks validation in large series of patients; thus the applicability of the findings to the general population is unclear.

QUANTITATIVE ULTRASOUND IMAGING TECHNIQUES FOR FAT QUANTIFICATION

Currently, the commercially available tools for quantification of liver fat include measuring the attenuation coefficient (AC), the backscatter coefficient (BSC), and the speed of sound. Presently most of them are based on the estimate of the attenuation of the backscattered echo signals originating along the direction of the transmitted US beam. The attenuation is due to absorption and conversion of sound energy into heat, reflecting some sound energy back to transducer, and scattering of the sound energy in several directions.

Attenuation and scattering are important properties of tissue that contribute to diagnostic information in medical US. In conventional gray-scale imaging, these tissue characteristics are acquired from differences in image brightness. However, the brightness displayed on the monitor of the US systems depends on operator settings and system-dependent factors so that attenuation and scattering can only be assessed in a qualitative manner.[41] The algorithms for the quantitative estimate of the attenuation make use of the raw data of the backscattered echo signals, therefore they are not influenced by the system settings.

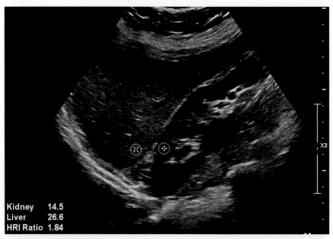

Fig. 11.3 Hepatorenal index *(HRI)* gives a semiquantitative estimate of liver fat content. A region of interest is placed in the renal cortex and the adjacent liver parenchyma at the same depth. The system calculates the ratio of the echogenicity of the liver compared to the renal cortex. This method is best when the raw data are used. Each vendor has a different method of calculating the echogenicity, and therefore cutoff values may vary depending on vendor. In this case the HRI ratio is 1.84, suggesting moderate fatty infiltration of the liver.

Liver steatosis causes an increase of the attenuation of the US beam as it traverses the liver parenchyma. The factors affecting the accuracy of attenuation estimate include backscattering variation, speed of sound variation, focus location, imaging artifacts, imaging resolution, and signal-to-noise ratio. The depth of ROI can be limited by the signal-to-noise ratio level.

Quantitative ultrasound (QUS) methods display the properties of tissue in a numerical way: by using proprietary algorithms, the attenuation can be objectively quantified, and an AC is calculated and usually displayed in decibels per meter (FibroScan) or decibels per centimeter per megahertz (US systems).

Ultrasound Attenuation for Liver Fat Quantification: Some Basic Information

Attenuation measurements are usually performed using backscattered echo signals originating along the direction of the transmitted US beam. The algorithms are generally based on the frequency domain approach in which the signals are divided in windows and for each window the frequency content is calculated. Thereafter, the change of US amplitude for all frequency components in the range of the transducer's bandwidth is calculated over the depth. In fact, attenuation measurement can vary depending on the frequency bandwidth. Measurements performed with a narrow band frequency assume that the intercept is zero. Measurements over a broadband frequency range (i.e., that of the US transducer for clinical use) need to calculate attenuation at discrete frequencies and present the average value.[30]

The attenuation estimate in the frequency domain approach can be obtained through the spectral difference methods or the spectral shift methods. The spectral difference methods assess the decrease of the echo signal power spectra along the path of the transmitted US beam. Spectral shift methods use the presence of a downshift of the power spectra toward lower frequencies as the US beam propagates in the medium. This shift in the power spectra obtained from two different depths is related to the attenuation characteristics of the medium.

The attenuation estimation techniques using a spectral shift are more precise than spectral difference methods but are more prone to local spectral noises and have a difficulty of accounting for the imaging system-dependent factors.

A hybrid method, which combines the advantages of the two methods and overcomes their specific limitations, has been introduced.

How to Perform the Examination

In many US systems the attenuation estimate can be obtained together with liver stiffness estimate. Therefore it is advised that the protocol for accurate liver stiffness values is maintained. The examination should be performed in a supine or slight (<30 degrees) lateral decubitus position in a neutral breath-hold when liver stiffness values are obtained at the same time. As of early 2022, no studies have evaluated different patient positions if only liver fat is quantified. Theoretically, the phase of respiration should not affect the measurement of the AC, but a breath-hold should be used during the measurement. Large blood vessels, artifacts, and masses should be avoided.

As in liver stiffness measurements, reverberation artifact may occur up to 2 cm below the liver capsule; therefore this area should be avoided. When a color map of the attenuation is available, areas that are markedly different from the majority of the color in the ROI should be avoided (Fig. 11.4). A depth dependence of the measurement is likely, although recent studies have obtained clinically acceptable values using vendor guidelines.[42] When there is significant attenuation of the US beam, deep areas may have a marked change in the color map due to the weak signal; these areas should also be avoided. The quality of the measurement is strictly linked to the quality of the B-mode image; that is generally better with the transducer at 90 degrees with respect to the liver capsule.

Currently, it is advisable to perform measurements in a homogeneous area of the liver, avoiding focal fatty deposition or fatty sparing. Presently, the ROI size cannot be changed in most systems, and the ROI is usually large to average over a large portion of the liver as more samples provide a better estimate.

For liver stiffness measurements at least a 4-hour fast is recommended, but the literature suggests that fasting may not be required for liver fat assessment.[30]

It is expert opinion that at least five measurements be performed, and the median value used. The interquartile range/median (IQR/M) and/or the vendor's recommendations should be reported as a quality measure.[30] Presently there are no published studies on this matter. We suggest that the IQR/M be maintained up to 10%–15%.

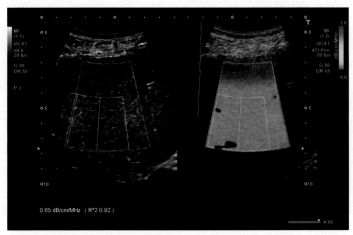

Fig. 11.4 Attenuation imaging *(ATI; Canon Medical Systems)* reverberation artifact. There is a 1-cm-thick orange area in the proximal part of the region of interest. This area must not be included in the measurement box; otherwise, it will lead to an overestimation of liver fat amount.

Commercially Available Algorithms

Controlled Attenuation Parameter (Echosens, France)

Controlled attenuation parameter (CAP) is the algorithm available on the FibroScan system for the quantification of liver steatosis. The AC is given in decibels per meter and ranges from 100 to 400 dB/m; it is calculated together with the liver stiffness value (Fig. 11.5).

The technique is available on the M and XL probe of the FibroScan system, and the choice between the two probes is based on the skin-to-liver capsule distance. Based on this parameter, the system software automatically recommends the choice of the probe. The M probe is used for a skin-to-liver capsule distance up to 25 mm, and the XL probe is used when this distance is greater than 25 mm. A correct choice of the probe is mandatory because the use of the M probe in patients with a skin-to-liver capsule distance greater than 25 mm may lead to an overestimation of liver steatosis. The US attenuation is computed at the US frequency of 3.5 MHz independently from the probe used. The rate of failure, which was initially reported at 7.7% of cases when only the M probe was used, is reported to be around 3% when both probes are available.[43-45]

CAP and vibration controlled transient elastography (VCTE) liver stiffness values are obtained at the same time; therefore, the protocol for measurement is that recommended for liver stiffness measurement with VCTE.

The interobserver reproducibility of the measurements seems high, even though the agreement between observers decreases for CAP values in the normal range (<240 dB/m).[46] This is

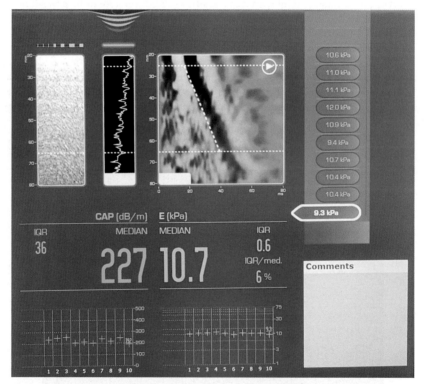

Fig. 11.5 Liver fat quantification with controlled attenuation parameter *(CAP)* in a patient with compensated advanced liver disease due to chronic hepatitis C. The attenuation coefficient is obtained together with liver stiffness measurement and is given in decibels per meter. *IQR,* Interquartile range.

likely due to the uneven distribution of other tissue scatterers that prevail over fat content in determining the attenuation of the US beam.

Generally, the quality criteria that were set for liver stiffness measurements (i.e., median value of 10 acquisitions with an IQR/M up to 30%) are used. Therefore every CAP measurement that is obtained together with a reliable liver stiffness measurement is accepted as reliable. Specific quality criteria for CAP measurements are not yet clearly defined, and the results are conflicting in the literature. A study suggested that the accuracy is significantly decreased when the IQR of the 10 consecutive CAP acquisitions was higher than 40 dB/m; another study reported that the IQR value should be less than 30 dB/m.[45,47] However, these results were not confirmed in a multicenter study and a metaanalysis.[44,48]

CAP is not affected by liver fibrosis. Using CAP, a study found that steatosis was a confounding factor in fibrosis staging with VCTE.[49] However, this finding was not confirmed in another study.[44]

The cutoff for the detection of liver steatosis (≥5%) reported in the literature ranges from 219 dB/m in a cohort of patients with chronic hepatitis C to 294 dB/m in a metaanalysis of patients with NAFLD.[48,50] Therefore uncertainty remains about the cutoff value to be used in the real-world clinical practice for steatosis detection (S >0).[29] It has been suggested that the cutoffs are etiology-specific. However, it must be highlighted that it is likely that the disease prevalence in the studied population rather than the etiology of liver disease might have accounted for the reported differences.[29] In fact, the attenuation of the US beam is directly related to the liver fat content that has the same histological appearance in the majority of cases no matter what the etiology of liver disease is.

The data of an individual patient data metaanalysis have shown that CAP was unable to satisfactorily grade steatosis.[48]

Studies performed in children to evaluate the diagnostic performance of CAP are generally underpowered, including small numbers of subjects. As observed in adults, the cutoff value for the diagnosis of steatosis ranges from 225 dB/m in an unselected pediatric population to 277 dB/m in a series of severely obese children.[51,52] This difference is likely due to the disease prevalence in the studied cohorts.

CAP has been used as a tool to noninvasively assess the prevalence of NAFLD in groups at risk or in the general population. It should be highlighted that different CAP cutoffs for the detection of steatosis (S >0) were used in different studies, and this limits the robustness of the findings. Apart from the uncertainty regarding the optimal cutoff of CAP for detection of steatosis, it is likely that an overestimation or underestimation of liver steatosis prevalence might have occurred in the published studies.

CAP, alone or combined with other noninvasive indices or biomarkers, has been proposed as a tool for assessing NASH or as a noninvasive predictor of prognosis in patients with chronic liver disease. Using liver biopsy as the reference, a score (FAST score) that combined liver stiffness, CAP, and aspartate aminotransferase (AST) was derived.[53] The FAST score cutoffs were 0.35 and 0.67 for ruling out and ruling in NASH, an elevated NAFLD activity score, and significant fibrosis, respectively. The positive predictive value ranged from 33% to 81% and the negative predictive value from 73% to 100% in the external validation cohorts.

Of note, in several NAFLD/NASH cases with advanced liver disease, small amounts of fat in the liver have been observed, and the term *burnt-out NASH* has been proposed.[54] A "protective" effect for the development of a first hepatic decompensation has been reported for CAP value ≥220 dB/m.[55-57]

It must be highlighted that, before using CAP as tool to noninvasively monitor changes of liver fat content over time, it is important to set what is a meaningful change (i.e., the one that is not the result of a mere chance). In this regard, studies that have assessed the interobserver concordance in the CAP measurements have shown that the mean difference in CAP values between two observers is up to 20 dB/m; therefore, in the follow-up of patients, this difference should be taken into account.[58]

An upgraded CAP algorithm named SmartExam is able to acquire much more data with respect to the previous algorithm and may lead to an improvement in accuracy. This new method uses US signals acquired continuously during the A-mode phase of the examination with the FibroScan device.[59] The major improvements of this new CAP method are the higher number of individual US attenuation measurements (20 times more data) in a larger volume of liver tissue and an automatically adapted measurement depth. The final CAP result is expressed as the mean with the standard deviation.

Attenuation Imaging (Canon Medical Systems, Japan)

Two-dimensional attenuation imaging (ATI) is the technique implemented in the Aplio i-series US systems. The degree of the attenuation of the US beam is color-coded and obtained in a large ROI in real time. Vessels or strong artifacts are automatically filtered out by the software and appear as colorless areas in the color map. The radiofrequency data are used; thus the influence of the gain and US beam profiles does not affect the calculation of the AC, which is given in decibels per centimeter per megahertz. In the ATI display mode, the B-mode image is shown on the left side and the corresponding ATI color-coded image is shown on the right side. A single measurement box is placed inside the ROI, guided by the B-mode image (Fig. 11.6). A dark orange area, which may be present in the proximal part of the ROI, or dark blue areas posterior to blood vessels or in the distal part of the ROI must not be included in the measurement box as these are artifacts due to reverberation or high noise with weak echo signal by less penetration (Fig. 11.7). As of early 2022, it is suggested that the final AC value is the median of five consecutive measurements. The reliability of the measurement is displayed on the monitor with a linear regression coefficient of determination, or R^2 value: an AC value of best quality is the one with an $R^2 \geq 0.90$ as recommended by the manufacturer. The font color of the ATI measurement and R^2 displayed on the monitor varies with the quality of the measurement. The white font represents high-quality measurement ($R^2 \geq 0.90$), the yellow font represents moderate-quality ($0.70 < R^2 < 0.90$) and red font represents low-quality ($R^2 < 0.70$) (Fig. 11.8).

The intraobserver and interobserver reproducibility of measurements ranges from good to excellent.[7] The cutoffs reported in the literature are 0.59–0.69 dB/cm/MHz for the detection of liver steatosis (S ≥ 1) (eight studies), 0.70–0.72 dB/cm/MHz for significant steatosis (S ≥ 2) (eight studies), and 0.73–0.86 dB/cm/MHz for severe steatosis (S = 3) (three studies).[60-67] The AUROCs were 0.84–0.93 for steatosis grade S ≥ 1; 0.86–0.93 for steatosis grade S ≥ 2, and 0.79–0.93 for steatosis grade S = 3. Literature reports that fibrosis or necroinflammatory activity is not associated with the AC.[62,63] A study reported that ATI was more accurate than the CAP for grading liver steatosis, and this improvement was statistically significant for S >1.[60]

ATI comes with two settings: ATI-Gen, which is tuned on a US frequency of 4.0 MHz and ATI-Pen which works at 3.0 MHz.[61] A study performed in a small series of subjects reported that the cutoffs for detecting steatosis (S >0) are different between the two because of the frequency dependence on the AC. In particular, the cutoff was 0.62 dB/cm/MHz with ATI-Gen and 0.69 dB/cm/MHz with ATI-Pen.

Attenuation Measurement (Fujifilm, previously Hitachi Ltd, Japan)

Attenuation measurement (iATT) estimates the AC using a dual frequency method (i.e., it calculates the amplitude difference of backscattered US signals in two frequencies and determines the slope). The dual frequency method eliminates the effects of structures along the propagation path such as microvasculature or brightness variation.

iATT quantifies steatosis in a fixed area that is not user-adjustable, and a color map is not provided; thus, there is the risk of including reverberation artifacts in subjects with large skin-to-liver capsule distance. The results are given in decibels per centimeter per megahertz together with liver

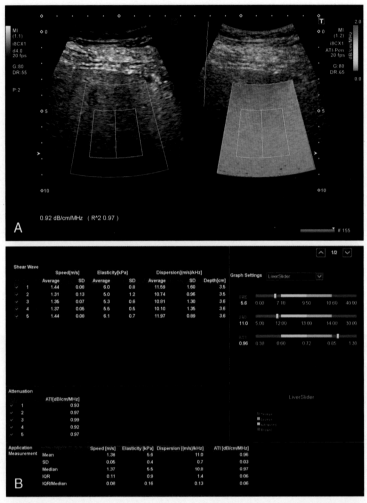

Fig. 11.6 (A) Liver fat estimate with attenuation imaging *(ATI)* in a 46-year-old female with elevated liver function tests. The system provides a quality measure for fat quantification, which is a linear regression coefficient of determination (bottom left R^2); it should be 0.90 or above for a good quality measurement. In this case the liver fat estimate with ATI gives an attenuation coefficient of 0.92 dB/cm/MHz that indicates severe steatosis. (B) Report of a multiparametric assessment of the liver in a patient with severe steatosis without liver fibrosis. The different colors of the bars in the graph are based on cutoff values suggested by the manufacturer. The dispersion value is within the normal range, and this may indicate that inflammation is absent. However, further studies are needed before using the dispersion value in the clinical practice.

stiffness measurement (Fig. 11.9). Therefore the protocol for liver stiffness measurement must be followed.[30] One study reported cutoff values of 0.62 dB/cm/MHz (72% sensitivity, 82% specificity), 0.67 dB/cm/MHz (87% sensitivity, 72% specificity), and 0.73 dB/cm/MHz (82% sensitivity, 89% specificity) for S $\geq$1, S $\geq$2, and S = 3, respectively.[68]

The interobserver agreement in fat quantification estimate seems high; however, thresholds are not well defined yet, and the use of vendor-specific thresholds is recommended.

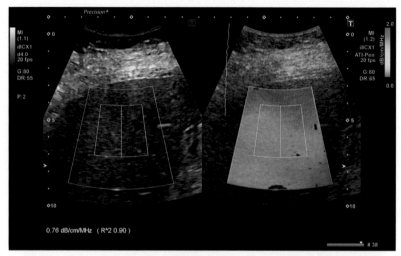

Fig. 11.7 Example of incorrect acquisition. In this case, the software gives an R^2 value of 0.90, indicating a measurement is of good quality. However, the reverberation artifact has been included in the measurement box; therefore, there is an overestimation of liver fat content. Note also a blue area in the distal part of the region of interest, which is likely due to high noise with weak echo signal. Blue areas can also be observed posterior to blood vessel. They should not be included in the measurement box.

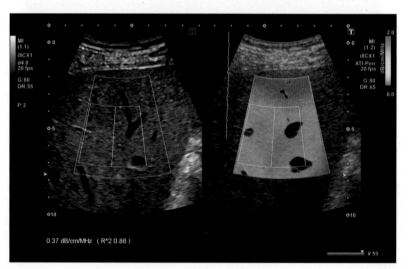

Fig. 11.8 Attenuation imaging (ATI) incorrect measurement. The R^2 value is below 0.90, indicating a suboptimal quality of the acquisition (the font color in *yellow* is a visual warning). A patchy blue area, likely due to high noise, has been included in the measurement box.

Ultrasound-Guided Attenuation Parameter (GE Healthcare, USA)

To compensate for the characteristics of transmitting and receiving beamforming of the US system, the AC value is calculated according to a reference phantom method integrated into the US system, with known attenuation and BSCs[30] (Fig. 11.10).

The result is given in decibels per centimeter per megahertz. As observed with the other algorithms based on the AC, there is a high agreement between measurements. In the two published

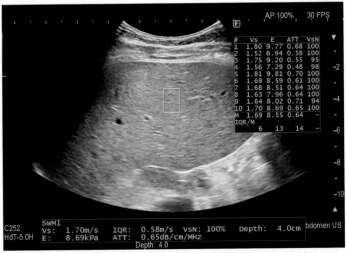

Fig. 11.9 Estimation of liver fat content with the attenuation measurement *(iATT)* (Fujifilm previously Hitachi, Japan). The attenuation coefficient is computed in a fixed area along the same axis of liver stiffness measurement. As per point shear wave elastography acquisition protocol, 10 measurements are performed, and the median value is used. The system automatically gives the interquartile range/median *(IQR/M)* for both liver stiffness and iATT.

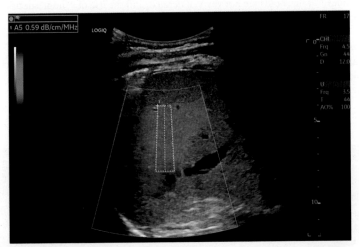

Fig. 11.10 Implementation of attenuation coefficient estimation on the GE system. The *yellow measurement box* is the area of measurement. Vessels and other artifacts are not included in the measurement. The attenuation coefficient is 0.59 dB/cm/MHz corresponding to S0.

studies the thresholds were 0.53–0.60 dB/cm/MHz for S ≥1, 0.60–0.70 dB/cm/MHz for S ≥2, and 0.65–0.70 dB/cm/MHz for S = 3.[69,70] A GE white paper, based on a Japanese cohort of 1010 patients with mixed etiologies of liver disease and using MRI-PDFF as the reference standard, reported thresholds of 0.65 dB/cm/MHz for S ≥1, 0.71 dB/cm/MHz for S ≥2, and 0.77 dB/cm/MHz for S = 3.[71]

In a study, US-guided attenuation parameter performed significantly better than CAP for identifying S ≥2 and S = 3 steatosis.[69] In another study, the AC values were not affected by liver stiffness.[72]

Attenuation (Hologic, USA)

The attenuation algorithm (Att PLUS) implemented on Hologic SuperSonic MACH systems is a method that uses the ultrafast technology that theoretically allows dynamic transmit and receive focusing with a minimal diffraction effect (Fig. 11.11). The AC is estimated in an ROI at a fixed depth, and the result is displayed in decibels per centimeter per megahertz. A training dataset with known attenuation is implemented in this proprietary algorithm. Att PLUS is obtained together with the sound speed estimate, and this may help in identifying wrong acquisitions when there is a discrepancy between the two parameters. As of early 2022, no published studies are available. Thresholds are not yet defined, and the use of vendor-specific thresholds is recommended.

Tissue Attenuation Imaging (Samsung Medison, Korea)

Tissue attenuation imaging (TAI) quantifies attenuation based on changes in the center frequency (Fig. 11.12). As of early 2022, there are no published studies aimed at assessing the performance of the technique. Therefore, cutoffs for detecting and grading liver steatosis are not yet defined, and the use of vendor-specific thresholds is recommended.

Ultrasound-Derived Fat Fraction (Siemens Healthineers, Germany)

The ultrasound-derived fat fraction (UDFF) combines attenuation and BSC, and the value is given as a percentage of liver steatosis (Fig. 11.13). Reference phantom data are integrated into the US system and a fixed-acquisition ROI is used.

A study reported a high correlation of UDFF with MRI-PDFF without any influence by the body mass index.[73] Thresholds are not yet well defined, and the use of vendor-specific thresholds is recommended. The values are provided as percentage fat correlated to MRI-PDFF.

Attenuation (Philips Medical Systems, The Netherlands)

Philips Ultrasound has just released an attenuation algorithm that provides liver fat estimates in decibels per centimeter per megahertz (Fig. 11.14). As of early 2022, thresholds are not well defined yet, and the use of vendor-specific thresholds is recommended.

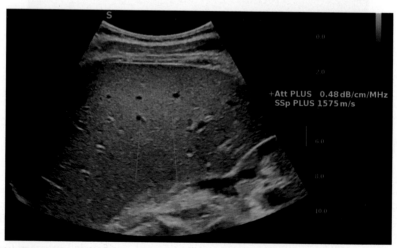

Fig. 11.11 The Hologic (previous SuperSonic Imagine) system calculated the attenuation coefficient *(Att PLUS)* within the yellow measurement box. The system can also calculate the speed of sound *(SSp PLUS)* at the same time. The attenuation coefficient is 0.48 dB/cm/MHz corresponding to S0.

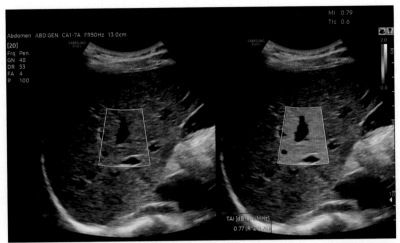

Fig. 11.12 Estimation of the attenuation coefficient using the Samsung system. In this case the attenuation coefficient *(TAI)* is 0.77 dB/cm/MHz suggesting S2. The R^2 value is 0.76 suggesting good quality. The R^2 value is a quality assessment and when the numbers are red suggests a poor quality.

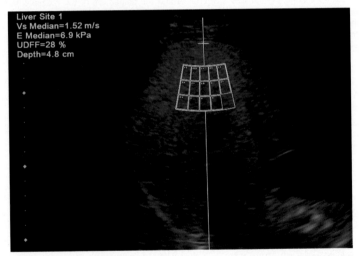

Fig. 11.13 The Siemens system calculates both the attenuation coefficient and the backscatter coefficient and combines them into one measurement. The reported value is on percent fat content correlated to magnetic resonance imaging–derived proton density fat fraction. The system can also take 15 point shear wave elastography measurements at the same time. The perpendicular line above the measurement box is used to standardize the depth of measurement. The line should be placed at the liver capsule. The fat content of the liver is 28% representing S2.

Backscatter Coefficient

Backscatter coefficient (BSC) is a measure of the fraction of US energy returned to the transducer from tissue.[74] It is calculated from a custom-derived software, and the computation is obtained offline by using an open-source software tool. An external reference phantom that has acoustic properties similar to average human liver tissue is used to reduce sources of variability due to system setting or operators. Consecutive frames are recorded from the same region of the liver.

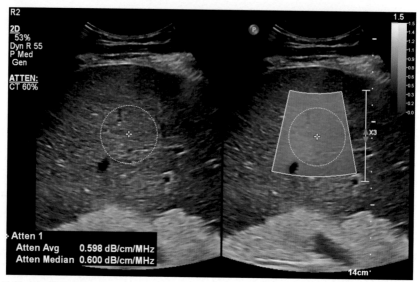

Fig. 11.14   The Philips algorithm calculated the attenuation coefficient in the area of the *dotted white circle*. The system allows for adjusting the size of the circle and the placement of the measurement box at any depth. Reverberation artifact will appear as orange color in the near field of the larger box (not present in this case) and should be avoided. A large measurement circle is recommended for the measurement (default) and should be placed in an area with minimal artifacts. The system does not include vessels and other artifacts in the measurement. The attenuation coefficient is 0.60 dB/cm/MHz corresponding to S0.

Thereafter, without changing any scanner settings, consecutive frames are recorded in the external phantom.

As of early 2022, the software is not commercially available, and all the published studies were performed using the Acuson S3000 US system (Siemens Healthineers, Germany) with a direct US research interface option (Fig. 11.15).[75-80]

The reproducibility of measurements is high and independent from the operator or the settings of the US system.

The accuracy of BSC in diagnosing and quantifying hepatic steatosis was evaluated in a series of 204 individuals, with and without NAFLD, using MRI-PDFF as the reference standard.[79] The AUROC, sensitivity, specificity, and accuracy for the diagnosis of steatosis were above 0.90 in the training group, with an optimal cutoff value of 0.0038 1/cm-steradian. The sensitivity and specificity in the validation group were 87% and 91%, respectively.

Speed of Sound

An increase of fat in the liver causes a decrease in the speed of the sound. Different methods to measure the speed of sound in the liver are being developed.[81-84] Among them, speed of sound estimation using the assessment of the spatial coherence function of the backscattered echoes, which result from a US beam focusing in the medium, has been tested in a proof-of-concept study.[81] The quantification of the speed of sound was obtained by an offline analysis of raw data using an in-house software. The method was tested using the Aixplorer US system (Hologic, formerly SuperSonic Imagine) in a pilot study: speed of sound estimation was highly reproducible, and cutoffs ≤1.537 mm/μs and ≤1.511 mm/μs were identified for the detection of any steatosis grade (S1–S3) and significant steatosis (S2–S3), respectively[83] (Fig. 11.16).

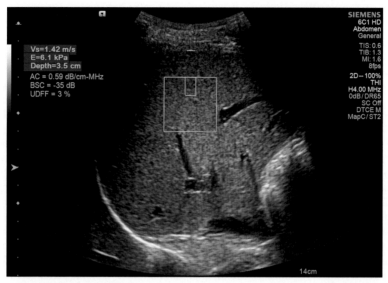

Fig. 11.15 Presently the only FDA-approved system using backscatter coefficient *(BSC)* is the Siemens system. The backscatter measurement is included in the ultrasound-derived fat fractuib *(UDFF)* measurement (combination of backscatter and attenuation). This is an example of the backscatter measurement (not available on released systems). The BSC is -35dB, and the attenuation coefficient is 0.59 dB/cm/MHz. The two coefficients are combined, and the value is reported as a percentage fat based on correlation to magnetic resonance imaging–derived proton density fat fraction. In this case it is 3% corresponding to S0.

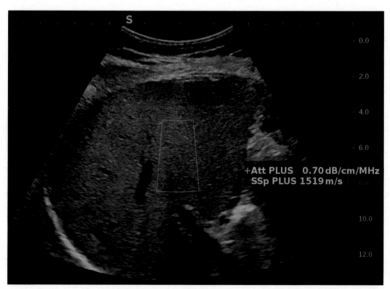

Fig. 11.16 Presently, the only system that estimates the speed of sound calculation is the Hologic (previous SuperSonic Imagine). The system calculates both the attenuation coefficient (*Att PLUS*) as well as the speed of sound *(SSp PLUS)*. In this case the SSp PLUS is 1519 m/s.

Does Steatosis Affect Liver Stiffness Values?

There are conflicting results in the literature. A multicenter study performed in patients with NAFLD using liver biopsy as the reference standard reported that the presence of severe steatosis, as assessed with CAP, overestimated liver fibrosis assessed by VCTE.[49] The risk of overestimation was low for CAP values lower than 300 dB/m. Based on these findings, the authors proposed an algorithm to identify the risk of false positive results in F2–F4 fibrosis and F3–F4 fibrosis and recommended using another noninvasive test or liver biopsy in these cases.[49] A major weakness of this study is that all measurements were performed with the M probe; therefore it is unclear whether the inclusion of the subcutaneous fat in some cases may have led per se to the overestimation of liver stiffness.[85]

The influence of steatosis on liver stiffness assessment was not confirmed in another study.[44] Likewise, the data from an individual patient data metaanalysis showed that the negative predictive value for ruling out significant fibrosis improved just slightly when the CAP values were taken into account; however, the CAP dependency was not significant.[86]

A single center study that included 1306 chronic hepatitis B patients with histology results and that used a two-dimensional shear wave elastography technique for the stiffness assessment, found that the performance of the technique was not affected by different grades of liver steatosis at the stage of liver cirrhosis. For the detection of significant fibrosis (F ≥2), the performance was significantly higher in cases of no steatosis or mild steatosis.[87] Higher liver stiffness values were found in patients with no/mild fibrosis (F0–F1) who had moderate or severe steatosis.

Of note, conflicting results are also reported with magnetic resonance elastography.[88-91] Therefore a definitive answer to this question is not available yet. Steatosis causes increased attenuation of the acoustic push-pulse generating shear waves of lower amplitude, resulting in decreased signal-to-noise that may account for the variability seen.

KEY POINTS

1. The biopsy specimen is obtained from a very small part of liver, and fatty infiltration could be heterogenous. Moreover, a substantial intraobserver and interobserver variability between readings has been reported.
2. Considering the obesity epidemic, biopsy is not a practical approach for screening in patients with MAFLD who may have simple steatosis in the majority of cases.
3. Liver steatosis is a dynamic process that may change in short periods of time (weeks), requiring a noninvasive technique that can be repeated at multiple times to accurately assess progression or regression of disease.
4. Conventional B-mode US gives an estimate of the degree of fatty infiltration in the liver but has low sensitivity for the detection of mild steatosis.
5. CAP is able to quantify liver steatosis: however, there is a large overlap of CAP values between consecutive grades of liver steatosis, thus limiting its use in follow-up studies evaluating changes over time.[7,30,92] Moreover, the cutoffs are not clearly defined.
6. MRI-PDFF is an accurate biomarker for the estimate of liver fat content and can be used as a noninvasive reference standard for evaluating the performance of the new liver fat quantification techniques, whereas CAP must not be used because it has a suboptimal performance in quantifying liver fat content.[7,30]
7. The AC estimates available on US systems seem to have good accuracy in quantifying hepatic steatosis. Until there is standardization of the procedures and better interpretation for the results, the vendor's recommendations must be used to acquire the measurements, assess their quality, and interpret the values.[7,30]

References

1. Obesity and overweight. Available at: https://www.who.int/news-room/fact-sheets/detail/obesity-and-overweight.
2. Asrani SK, Devarbhavi H, Eaton J, Kamath PS. Burden of liver diseases in the world. *J Hepatol.* 2019;70:151-171.
3. Younossi ZM. Non-alcoholic fatty liver disease - a global public health perspective. *J Hepatol.* 2019;70:531-544.
4. Harrison SA, Gawrieh S, Roberts K, et al. Prospective evaluation of the prevalence of non-alcoholic fatty liver disease and steatohepatitis in a large middle-aged US cohort. *J Hepatol.* 2021;75(2):284-291.
5. Chalasani N, Younossi Z, Lavine JE, et al. The diagnosis and management of nonalcoholic fatty liver disease: practice guidance from the American Association for the Study of Liver Diseases. *Hepatology.* 2018;67:328-357.
6. Younossi ZM, Koenig AB, Abdelatif D, Fazel Y, Henry L, Wymer M. Global epidemiology of nonalcoholic fatty liver disease - meta-analytic assessment of prevalence, incidence, and outcomes. *Hepatology.* 2016;64:73-84.
7. Ferraioli G, Berzigotti A, Barr RG, et al. Quantification of liver fat content with ultrasound: a WFUMB position paper. *Ultrasound Med Biol.* 2021;47(10):2803-2820.
8. Loomba R, Sanyal AJ. The global NAFLD epidemic. *Nat Rev Gastroenterol Hepatol.* 2013;10:686-690.
9. Arulanandan A, Ang B, Bettencourt R, et al. Association between quantity of liver fat and cardiovascular risk in patients with nonalcoholic fatty liver disease independent of nonalcoholic steatohepatitis. *Clin Gastroenterol Hepatol.* 2015;13:1513-1520.
10. Ajmera V, Park CC, Caussy C, et al. Magnetic resonance imaging proton density fat fraction associates with progression of fibrosis in patients with nonalcoholic fatty liver disease. *Gastroenterology.* 2018;155:307-310.
11. Simon TG, Roelstraete B, Khalili H, Hagström H, Ludvigsson JF. Mortality in biopsy-confirmed non-alcoholic fatty liver disease: results from a nationwide cohort. *Gut.* 2021;70:1375-1382.
12. McPherson S, Hardy T, Henderson E, Burt AD, Day CP, Anstee QM. Evidence of NAFLD progression from steatosis to fibrosing-steatohepatitis using paired biopsies: implications for prognosis and clinical management. *J Hepatol.* 2015;62:1148-1155.
13. Pais R, Charlotte F, Fedchuk L, et al. A systematic review of follow-up biopsies reveals disease progression in patients with non-alcoholic fatty liver. *J Hepatol.* 2013;59:550-556.
14. Adams LA, Ratziu V. Non-alcoholic fatty liver - perhaps not so benign. *J Hepatol.* 2015;62:1002-1004.
15. Simon TG, Roelstraete B, Hartjes K, et al. Non-alcoholic fatty liver disease in children and young adults is associated with increased long-term mortality. *J Hepatol.* 2021;75(5):1034-1041.
16. Eslam M, Sanyal AJ, George J. Toward more accurate nomenclature for fatty liver diseases. *Gastroenterology.* 2019;157:590-593.
17. Kleiner DE, Brunt EM, Van Natta M, et al. Design and validation of a histological scoring system for nonalcoholic fatty liver disease. *Hepatology.* 2005;41:1313-1321.
18. Seeff LB, Everson GT, Morgan TR, et al. Complication rate of percutaneous liver biopsies among persons with advanced chronic liver disease in the HALT-C trial. *Clin Gastroenterol Hepatol.* 2010;8:877-883.
19. Stotland BR, Lichtenstein GR. Liver biopsy complications and routine ultrasound. *Am J Gastroenterol.* 1996;91:1295-1296.
20. Ratziu V, Charlotte F, Heurtier A, et al. Sampling variability of liver biopsy in nonalcoholic fatty liver disease. *Gastroenterology.* 2005;128:1898-1906.
21. Vuppalanchi R, Unalp A, Van Natta ML, et al. Effects of liver biopsy sample length and number of readings on sampling variability in nonalcoholic fatty liver disease. *Clin Gastroenterol Hepatol.* 2009;7:481-486.
22. Middleton MS, Heba ER, Hooker CA, et al. Agreement between magnetic resonance imaging proton density fat fraction measurements and pathologist-assigned steatosis grades of liver biopsies from adults with nonalcoholic steatohepatitis. *Gastroenterology.* 2017;153:753-761.
23. Permutt Z, Le TA, Peterson MR, et al. Correlation between liver histology and novel magnetic resonance imaging in adult patients with nonalcoholic fatty liver disease—MRI accurately quantifies hepatic steatosis in NAFLD. *Aliment Pharmacol Ther.* 2012;36:22-29.
24. Reeder SB, Hu HH, Sirlin CB. Proton density fat-fraction: a standardized MR-based biomarker of tissue fat concentration. *J Magn Reson Imaging.* 2012;36:1011-1014.
25. Negrete LM, Middleton MS, Clark L, et al. Inter-examination precision of magnitude-based MRI for estimation of segmental hepatic proton density fat fraction in obese subjects. *J Magn Reson Imaging.* 2014;39:1265-1271.

26. Kang GH, Cruite I, Shiehmorteza M, et al. Reproducibility of MRI determined proton density fat fraction across two different MR scanner platforms. *J Magn Reson Imaging.* 2011;34:928-934.

27. Caussy C, Reeder SB, Sirlin CB, et al. Noninvasive, quantitative assessment of liver fat by MRI-PDFF as an endpoint in NASH trials. *Hepatology.* 2018;68:763-772.

28. Noureddin M, Lam J, Peterson MR, et al. Utility of magnetic resonance imaging versus histology for quantifying changes in liver fat in nonalcoholic fatty liver disease trials. *Hepatology.* 2013;58:1930-1940.

29. Ferraioli G. CAP for the detection of hepatic steatosis in clinical practice. *Lancet Gastroenterol Hepatol.* 2021;6:151-152.

30. Ferraioli G, Kumar V, Ozturk A, Nam K, de Korte C, Barr RG. Ultrasound attenuation for liver fat quantification: an AIUM-RSNA QIBA pulse echo quantitative ultrasound (PEQUS) initiative. *Radiology.* 2022;302(3):495-506.

31. Ferraioli G, Soares Monteiro LB. Ultrasound-based techniques for the diagnosis of liver steatosis. *World J Gastroenterol.* 2019;25:6053-6062.

32. Barr RG. Ultrasound of diffuse liver disease including elastography. *Radiol Clin North Am.* 2019;57:549-562.

33. Macaluso FS, Maida M, Cammà C, et al. Body mass index and liver stiffness affect accuracy of ultrasonography in detecting steatosis in patients with chronic hepatitis C virus genotype 1 infection. *Clin Gastroenterol Hepatol.* 2014;12:878-884.

34. Lee SS, Park SH, Kim HJ, et al. Non-invasive assessment of hepatic steatosis: prospective comparison of the accuracy of imaging examinations. *J Hepatol.* 2010;52:579-585.

35. Bril F, Ortiz-Lopez C, Lomonaco R, et al. Clinical value of liver ultrasound for the diagnosis of nonalcoholic fatty liver disease in overweight and obese patients. *Liver Int.* 2015;35:2139-2146.

36. Hernaez R, Lazo M, Bonekamp S, et al. Diagnostic accuracy and reliability of ultrasonography for the detection of fatty liver: a meta-analysis. *Hepatology.* 2011;54:1082-1090.

37. European Association for the Study of the Liver (EASL); European Association for the Study of Diabetes (EASD); European Association for the Study of Obesity (EASO). EASL-EASD-EASO Clinical Practice Guidelines for the management of non-alcoholic fatty liver disease. *J Hepatol.* 2016;64:1388-1402.

38. Hamaguchi M, Kojima T, Itoh Y, et al. The severity of ultrasonographic findings in nonalcoholic fatty liver disease reflects the metabolic syndrome and visceral fat accumulation. *Am J Gastroenterol.* 2007;102:2708-2715.

39. Ballestri S, Lonardo A, Romagnoli D, et al. Ultrasonographic fatty liver indicator, a novel score which rules out NASH and is correlated with metabolic parameters in NAFLD. *Liver Int.* 2012;32:1242-1252.

40. Webb M, Yeshua H, Zelber-Sagi S, et al. Diagnostic value of a computerized hepatorenal index for sonographic quantification of liver steatosis. *AJR Am J Roentgenol.* 2009;192:909-914.

41. Nam K, Rosado-Mendez IM, Wirtzfeld LA, et al. Comparison of ultrasound attenuation and backscatter estimates in layered tissue-mimicking phantoms among three clinical scanners. *Ultrason Imaging.* 2012;34:209-221.

42. Barr RG, Cestone A, De Silvestri A. A pre-release algorithm with a confidence map for estimating the attenuation coefficient for liver fat quantification. *J Ultrasound Med.* 2021. doi:10.1002/jum.15870.

43. de Lédinghen V, Vergniol J, Capdepont M, et al. Controlled attenuation parameter (CAP) for the diagnosis of steatosis: a prospective study of 5323 examinations. *J Hepatol.* 2014;60:1026-1031.

44. Eddowes PJ, Sasso M, Allison M, et al. Accuracy of FibroScan controlled attenuation parameter and liver stiffness measurement in assessing steatosis and fibrosis in patients with nonalcoholic fatty liver disease. *Gastroenterology.* 2019;156:1717-1730.

45. Vuppalanchi R, Siddiqui MS, Van Natta ML, et al. Performance characteristics of vibration-controlled transient elastography for evaluation of nonalcoholic fatty liver disease. *Hepatology.* 2018;67:134-144.

46. Ferraioli G, Tinelli C, Lissandrin R, et al. Interobserver reproducibility of the controlled attenuation parameter (CAP) for quantifying liver steatosis. *Hepatol Int.* 2014;8:576-581.

47. Wong VW, Petta S, Hiriart JB, et al. Validity criteria for the diagnosis of fatty liver by M probe-based controlled attenuation parameter. *J Hepatol.* 2017;67:577-584.

48. Petroff D, Blank V, Newsome PN, et al. Assessment of hepatic steatosis by controlled attenuation parameter using the M and XL probes: an individual patient data meta-analysis. *Lancet Gastroenterol Hepatol.* 2021;6:185-198.

49. Petta S, Wong VW, Cammà C, et al. Improved noninvasive prediction of liver fibrosis by liver stiffness measurement in patients with nonalcoholic fatty liver disease accounting for controlled attenuation parameter values. *Hepatology.* 2017;65:1145-1155.

50. Ferraioli G, Tinelli C, Lissandrin R, et al. Controlled attenuation parameter for evaluating liver steatosis in chronic viral hepatitis. *World J Gastroenterol.* 2014;20:6626-6631.
51. Desai NK, Harney S, Raza R, et al. Comparison of controlled attenuation parameter and liver biopsy to assess hepatic steatosis in pediatric patients. *J Pediatr.* 2016;173:160-164.
52. Runge JH, van Giessen J, Draijer LG, et al. Accuracy of controlled attenuation parameter compared with ultrasound for detecting hepatic steatosis in children with severe obesity. *Eur Radiol.* 2021;31:1588-1596.
53. Newsome PN, Sasso M, Deeks JJ, et al. FibroScan-AST (FAST) score for the non-invasive identification of patients with non-alcoholic steatohepatitis with significant activity and fibrosis: a prospective derivation and global validation study. *Lancet Gastroenterol Hepatol.* 2020;5:362-373.
54. van der Poorten D, Samer CF, Ramezani-Moghadam M, et al. Hepatic fat loss in advanced nonalcoholic steatohepatitis: are alterations in serum adiponectin the cause? *Hepatology.* 2013;57:2180-2188.
55. Mendoza Y, Cocciolillo S, Murgia G, et al. Noninvasive markers of portal hypertension detect decompensation in overweight or obese patients with compensated advanced chronic liver disease. *Clin Gastroenterol Hepatol.* 2020;18:3017-3025.
56. Scheiner B, Steininger L, Semmler G, et al. Controlled attenuation parameter does not predict hepatic decompensation in patients with advanced chronic liver disease. *Liver Int.* 2019;39:127-135.
57. Liu K, Wong VW, Lau K, et al. Prognostic value of controlled attenuation parameter by transient elastography. *Am J Gastroenterol.* 2017;112:1812-1823.
58. Ferraioli G. The clinical value of the controlled attenuation parameter in the follow-up of HIV-infected patients. *HIV Med.* 2017;18:444.
59. Audière S, Labourdette A, Miette V, et al. Improved ultrasound attenuation measurement method for the non-invasive evaluation of hepatic steatosis using FibroScan. *Ultrasound Med Biol.* 2021;47(11):3181-3195.
60. Ferraioli G, Maiocchi L, Raciti MV, et al. Detection of liver steatosis with a novel ultrasound-based technique: a pilot study using MRI-derived proton density fat fraction as the gold standard. *Clin Transl Gastroenterol.* 2019;10:e00081.
61. Ferraioli G, Maiocchi L, Savietto G, et al. Performance of the attenuation imaging technology in the detection of liver steatosis. *J Ultrasound Med.* 2021;40:1325-1332.
62. Bae JS, Lee DH, Lee JY, et al. Assessment of hepatic steatosis by using attenuation imaging: a quantitative, easy-to-perform ultrasound technique. *Eur Radiol.* 2019;29:6499-6507.
63. Dioguardi Burgio M, Ronot M, Reizine E, et al. Quantification of hepatic steatosis with ultrasound: promising role of attenuation imaging coefficient in a biopsy-proven cohort. *Eur Radiol.* 2020;30:2293-2301.
64. Lee DH, Cho EJ, Bae JS, et al. Accuracy of two-dimensional shear wave elastography and attenuation imaging for evaluation of patients with nonalcoholic steatohepatitis. *Clin Gastroenterol Hepatol.* 2021;19:797-805.
65. Sugimoto K, Moriyasu F, Oshiro H, et al. The role of multiparametric US of the liver for the evaluation of nonalcoholic steatohepatitis. *Radiology.* 2020;296:532-540.
66. Tada T, Iijima H, Kobayashi N, et al. Usefulness of attenuation imaging with an ultrasound scanner for the evaluation of hepatic steatosis. *Ultrasound Med Biol.* 2019;45:2679-2687.
67. Jeon SK, Lee JM, Joo I, et al. Prospective evaluation of hepatic steatosis using ultrasound attenuation imaging in patients with chronic liver disease with magnetic resonance imaging proton density fat fraction as the reference standard. *Ultrasound Med Biol.* 2019;45:1407-1416.
68. Tamaki N, Koizumi Y, Hirooka M, et al. Novel quantitative assessment system of liver steatosis using a newly developed attenuation measurement method. *Hepatol Res.* 2018;48:821-828.
69. Fujiwara Y, Kuroda H, Abe T, et al. The B-mode image-guided ultrasound attenuation parameter accurately detects hepatic steatosis in chronic liver disease. *Ultrasound Med Biol.* 2018;44:2223-2232.
70. Tada T, Kumada T, Toyoda H, et al. Utility of attenuation coefficient measurement using an ultrasound-guided attenuation parameter for evaluation of hepatic steatosis: comparison with MRI-determined proton density fat fraction. *AJR Am J Roentgenol.* 2019;212:332-341.
71. GE White Paper. Ultrasound-Guided Attenuation Parameter. Available at: https://www.gehealthcare.com.au/-/jssmedia/47190c9b8b2748c2886e072f8cc397e0.pdf?la=en-au.
72. Tada T, Kumada T, Toyoda H, et al. Liver stiffness does not affect ultrasound-guided attenuation coefficient measurement in the evaluation of hepatic steatosis. *Hepatol Res.* 2020;50:190-198.
73. Labyed Y, Milkowski A. Novel method for ultrasound-derived fat fraction using an integrated phantom. *J Ultrasound Med.* 2020;39:2427-2438.

74. Coila A, Oelze ML. Effects of acoustic nonlinearity on pulse-echo attenuation coefficient estimation from tissue-mimicking phantoms. *J Acoust Soc Am.* 2020;148:805.
75. Han A, Andre MP, Deiranieh L, et al. Repeatability and reproducibility of the ultrasonic attenuation coefficient and backscatter coefficient measured in the right lobe of the liver in adults with known or suspected nonalcoholic fatty liver disease. *J Ultrasound Med.* 2018;37:1913-1927.
76. Han A, Byra M, Heba E, et al. Noninvasive diagnosis of nonalcoholic fatty liver disease and quantification of liver fat with radiofrequency ultrasound data using one-dimensional convolutional neural networks. *Radiology.* 2020;295:342-350.
77. Han A, Labyed Y, Sy EZ, et al. Inter-sonographer reproducibility of quantitative ultrasound outcomes and shear wave speed measured in the right lobe of the liver in adults with known or suspected non-alcoholic fatty liver disease. *Eur Radiol.* 2018;28:4992-5000.
78. Han A, Zhang YN, Boehringer AS, et al. Assessment of hepatic steatosis in nonalcoholic fatty liver disease by using quantitative US. *Radiology.* 2020;295:106-113.
79. Lin SC, Heba E, Wolfson T, et al. Noninvasive diagnosis of nonalcoholic fatty liver disease and quanti-fication of liver fat using a new quantitative ultrasound technique. *Clin Gastroenterol Hepatol.* 2015;13: 1337-1345.
80. Paige JS, Bernstein GS, Heba E, et al. A pilot comparative study of quantitative ultrasound, conventional ultrasound, and MRI for predicting histology-determined steatosis grade in adult nonalcoholic fatty liver disease. *AJR Am J Roentgenol.* 2017;208:W168-W177.
81. Imbault M, Faccinetto A, Osmanski BF, et al. Robust sound speed estimation for ultrasound-based hepatic steatosis assessment. *Phys Med Biol.* 2017;62:3582-3598.
82. Jaeger M, Held G, Peeters S, Preisser S, Grunig M, Frenz M. Computed ultrasound tomography in echo mode for imaging speed of sound using pulse-echo sonography: proof of principle. *Ultrasound Med Biol.* 2015;41:235-250.
83. Stahli P, Kuriakose M, Frenz M, Jaeger M. Improved forward model for quantitative pulse-echo speed-of-sound imaging. *Ultrasonics.* 2020;108:106168.
84. Dioguardi Burgio M, Imbault M, Ronot M, et al. Ultrasonic adaptive sound speed estimation for the diagnosis and quantification of hepatic steatosis: a pilot study. *Ultraschall Med.* 2019;40:722-733.
85. Eddowes P, Sasso M, Fournier C, Vuppalanchi R, Newsome P. Steatosis and liver stiffness measurements using transient elastography. *Hepatology.* 2016;64:700.
86. Karlas T, Petroff D, Sasso M, et al. Impact of controlled attenuation parameter on detecting fibrosis using liver stiffness measurement. *Aliment Pharmacol Ther.* 2018;47:989-1000.
87. Huang Z, Zhou J, Lu X, et al. How does liver steatosis affect diagnostic performance of 2D-SWE.SSI: assessment from aspects of steatosis degree and pathological types. *Eur Radiol.* 2021;31:3207-3215.
88. Joshi M, Dillman JR, Singh K, et al. Quantitative MRI of fatty liver disease in a large pediatric cohort: correlation between liver fat fraction, stiffness, volume, and patient-specific factors. *Abdom Radiol (NY).* 2018;43:1168-1179.
89. Leitao HS, Doblas S, Garteiser P, et al. Hepatic fibrosis, inflammation, and steatosis: influence on the MR viscoelastic and diffusion parameters in patients with chronic liver disease. *Radiology.* 2017;283:98-107.
90. Loomba R, Wolfson T, Ang B, et al. Magnetic resonance elastography predicts advanced fibrosis in patients with nonalcoholic fatty liver disease: a prospective study. *Hepatology.* 2014;60:1920-1928.
91. Chen J, Talwalkar JA, Yin M, et al. Early detection of nonalcoholic steatohepatitis in patients with non-alcoholic fatty liver disease by using MR elastography. *Radiology.* 2011;259:749-756.
92. Ferraioli G, Wong VW, Castera L, et al. Liver ultrasound elastography: an update to the World Federa-tion for Ultrasound in Medicine and Biology Guidelines and Recommendations. *Ultrasound Med Biol.* 2018;44:2419-2440.

CHAPTER 12

Shear Wave Dispersion

Katsutoshi Sugimoto ■ Giovanna Ferraioli ■
Richard G. Barr

Introduction

Acoustic radiation force impulse (ARFI) is a continually developing technology that provides biomechanical information concerning tissue elasticity (stiffness) by emitting a push pulse, which generates laterally propagating shear waves (SWs).[1-3] In addition to elasticity, viscosity provides biomechanical information concerning the pathologic state of tissue, which is a different property than elasticity alone.[4-6] However, most ultrasound (US) elastographic models use a linear elastic model to describe tissue mechanical properties, and only tissue elasticity is quantified. Dispersion is related to the frequency dependence of the shear wave speed (SWS) and is affected by the attenuation of SWs because of the viscous component of the tissue.[7] If a tissue is dispersive, the SWS and the attenuation of SWs will increase with frequency.[7] Analysis of the dispersion properties of SWs can therefore serve as an indirect method for measuring viscosity. As of early 2022, dispersion imaging, a new imaging technology, has been developed by a few US vendors including Shear Wave Dispersion Imaging (SWD; Canon Medical Systems, Japan), Viscosity PLUS (Vi PLUS; Hologic, U.S.A.) and Elastance (Columbus, Ohio, U.S.A.).[8,9] In this chapter, the feasibility of liver viscosity evaluation is reviewed based on the findings of both animal studies and clinical evaluation in humans.

Physics

A homogeneous biological tissue can be modeled using viscoelastic models such as the Voigt and Maxwell models,[10] which consist of a spring and a damper, and the Zener model,[11] which consists of two springs and a damper. Using the Voigt model as an example to illustrate the frequency dependence of SWS, the SWS c_s at SW frequency ω calculated by the Voigt model is as shown below[12,13]:

$$c_s(\omega) = \sqrt{\frac{2\left(\mu^2 + \omega^2 \cdot \eta^2\right)}{\rho\left(\mu + \sqrt{\mu^2 + \omega^2 \cdot \eta^2}\right)}},\qquad (1)$$

where ρ, μ, and η are the density, shear elasticity, and shear viscosity of the medium, respectively.

When zero is substituted for shear viscosity η in equation (1), that is, a perfectly elastic tissue is assumed and viscosity is ignored, SWS c_s can be transformed to a simple relationship with shear elasticity:

$$c_s(\omega) = \sqrt{\frac{\mu}{\rho}}.\qquad (2)$$

On the other hand, as shown in equation (1), SWS depends on the frequency of the SWs in a viscoelastic tissue and therefore exhibits frequency dispersion.[13,14] The gradient of SWS, that is,

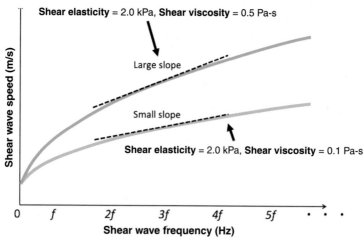

Fig. 12.1 In perfectly elastic tissue, shear wave speed is constant regardless of shear wave frequency. However, in viscoelastic tissue such as that found in the human body, shear wave speed does vary depending on shear wave frequency. The graph shows the relationship between shear wave speed and shear wave frequency in viscoelastic tissue. The charts are written based on the Voight model. If shear elasticity is fixed at 2.0 kPa and shear viscosity varies from 0.1–0.5 Pa-s, the slope becomes larger according to the shear viscosity level. The slopes are not the viscosity coefficient itself but correlate with the viscosity coefficient. (f), Frequency.

the slope of the graph of SWS versus frequency, varies according to the shear viscosity value. Therefore the shear viscosity value can be estimated from the slope over the SW frequency bandwidth (Fig. 12.1). It should be noted that the slope does not measure viscosity directly, but this method provides the quantification of a parameter that is directly related to viscosity without the need to use a rheological model. It must be highlighted that the shear wave dispersion slope (SWDS) value is based on the frequency range; hence different ranges give different values.

For a uniform and device-independent set of measurements, it is necessary to address differences and sources of disagreement, including the different shear wave frequencies used to measure the SWD along with other experimental factors.[15]

Review of Systems with Dispersion Imaging

CANON MEDICAL SYSTEMS

How the Shear Wave Dispersion Map Is Obtained

A SWD map can be created using an imaging technique that has been incorporated into commercially available US systems (Aplio i-series). This technique can be used to estimate the dispersion slope of SWS versus frequency to evaluate changes in tissue viscosity.

SWD processing involves four steps (Fig. 12.2). In the first step the displacements induced by the SWs are obtained using a technique based on color-Doppler US scanning. Second, the displacement at each location is transformed from the time domain to the frequency domain by a Fourier transform to estimate the phase changes in the SWs at several frequencies. Third, SWS is calculated using the phase-difference method. SWS at each frequency c_s (ω) is as shown below:

$$c_s(\omega) = \omega\sqrt{\frac{\Delta L}{\Delta\phi(\omega)}} \qquad (3)$$

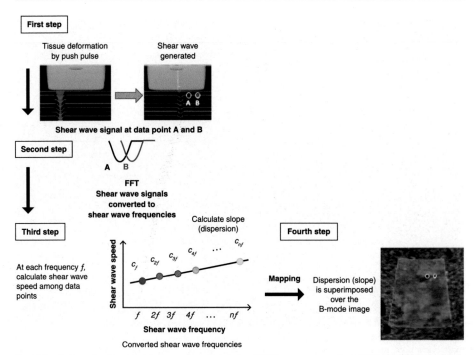

Fig. 12.2 Schematic diagram of shear wave dispersion (SWD) map processing. SWD processing involves four steps. First, the displacement induced by the shear waves is obtained using a technique based on color-Doppler scanning. Second, the displacement at each location is converted from the time domain to the frequency domain by fast Fourier transform *(FFT)* to estimate the phase changes of the shear waves at several frequencies *(f)*. Third, shear wave speed (SWS) is calculated using the phase-difference method. Fourth, the gradient of SWS is calculated based on the distribution of SWS versus frequency. The gradient value is then superimposed on the measurement locations to create a dispersion map.

where $\Delta\phi(\omega)$ is the phase change over the distance traveled *(ΔL)* between two measurement locations in the direction of SW propagation. Fourth, the gradient of SWS is calculated based on the distribution of SWS versus frequency. The calculated gradient values are then superimposed on the measurement locations to create a dispersion map.

Shear Wave Dispersion Imaging

The details of the actual acquisition using the Aplio i-series are as follows. SWD can be activated automatically in shear wave elastography (SWE) mode. The dispersion map shows the dispersion slope, which is a parameter directly related to viscosity. The calculated dispersion slope value ([m/s]/kHz) and its standard deviation are displayed. In SWE quad view mode, SWS or stiffness (speed map, elasticity map), SW arrival time contours (propagation map), gray scale, and dispersion slope (dispersion map) can be displayed simultaneously (Fig. 12.3).

Examination Technique

Due to the absence of guidelines in the literature for ensuring proper SWD measurements as of early 2022, the recommended two-dimensional SWE (2D-SWE) protocol[16] should be employed because proper SWS measurement is required for dispersion slope measurement. The protocol for obtaining dispersion measurements based on SWS measurements is described below and it is the same for a proper SWS measurement (see Chapter 4).

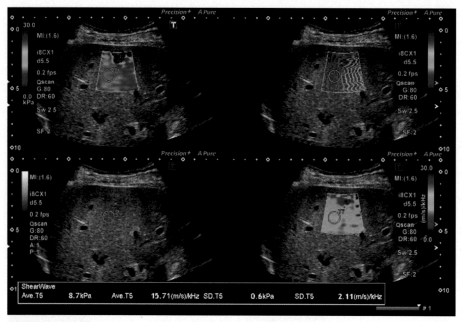

Fig. 12.3 Quad view for shear wave elastography/shear wave dispersion quantification. *Upper left:* elasticity map; *upper right:* propagation map; *lower left:* gray scale; *lower right:* dispersion map.

The patient is placed in the supine or slight left lateral decubitus position. The right arm is raised above the head to expand the intercostal acoustic window. The transducer is placed in an intercostal location. The B-mode image is optimized for the best acoustic window. The measurement is made while the patient is holding their breath for a few seconds. The patient should avoid deep inspiration/expiration or the Valsalva maneuver, which can affect stiffness measurements.[17] A region of interest (ROI) is placed 1.0–1.5 cm below the Glisson capsule to avoid reverberation artifacts and increased subcapsular stiffness. Within the ROI (usually an ROI of 3 × 3 cm), a single circular measurement box (usually with a diameter of 1.0 cm) is placed manually, avoiding areas of color drop-out, color hot spots, and blood vessels within the reference propagation map. Currently, no specific recommendations regarding the size of the measurement box have been given, but a relatively small measurement box (1.0 cm in diameter) is used to avoid the above-mentioned artifacts. Further research is required to determine optimal size and position of the measurement box for optimal accuracy.

Although five 2D-SWE measurements are recommended,[16] no reports have presented guidance on the optimal number of measurements for dispersion measurements. Thus for the time being, the recommendation of 10 or 5 SWD measurements should be followed. Furthermore, there are no quality criteria for dispersion slope measurements, and the interquartile range/median (IQR/M) value for stiffness measurements is used. The IQR/M being ≤30% in kilopascals or ≤15% in meters per second suggests that a dataset may be acceptable.[15] Based on the guideline and previous studies,[18] a value ≤30% in meters per second per kilohertz may also be suitable for dispersion measurement.

HOLOGIC

The software, Vi PLUS displays information about the viscosity calculated from the SWDS, assuming the liver is a viscoelastic Voigt model in terms of viscoelastic properties, where μ is the elastic modulus and η is the viscosity coefficient. The extent of change in SWS between frequencies is qualitatively represented in an easy-to-interpret color-coded image and quantitatively expressed in Pascal-second (Pa-s) over a range of values (Fig. 12.4). In the system configuration the user can select to display SWDS in meters per second per kilohertz or viscosity in Pa-s. With respect to SWDS, viscosity has a narrower range of values.

Since Vi PLUS is combined with the SWE mode (Fig. 12.5), acquisitions are made simultaneously with the SWE measurements using the same protocol (see Chapter 4).

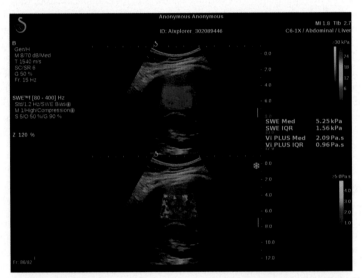

Fig. 12.4 Image from a healthy patient using the Hologic system. The liver stiffness is presented in the upper image with a liver stiffness value *(SWE Med)* of 5.25 kPa. The dispersion image converted to viscosity is presented in the lower image; here with a viscosity *(Vi PLUS Med)* of 2.09 Pa-s.

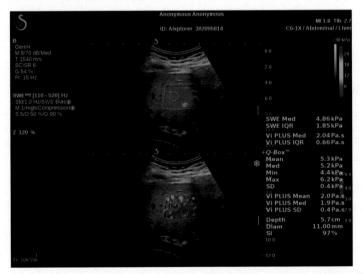

Fig. 12.5 Image from the Hologic system. The upper image displays the elasticity map with a stiffness value *(Mean)* of 5.3 kPa, and the lower image is the viscosity measurement *(Vi PLUS Mean)* of 2.04 Pa-s.

ELASTANCE

A relatively new approach analyzes the limiting case of shear waves established as a reverberant field (Fig. 12.6). In this framework it is assumed that a distribution of shear waves exists, oriented across all directions in 3D and continuous in time. The simultaneous multifrequency application of reverberant shear wave fields can be accomplished by applying an array of external sources that can be excited by multiple frequencies within a bandwidth, for example 50, 100, 150, ..., 500 Hz, all contributing to the shear wave field produced in the liver or other target organ. This enables the analysis of the dispersion of SWS as it increases with frequency, indicating the viscoelastic and lossy nature of the tissue under study (Fig. 12.7). Furthermore, dispersion images can be created and displayed alongside the SWS images (Fig. 12.8).

In preliminary studies on breast and liver tissues using the multifrequency reverberant shear wave technique, which employs frequencies up to 700 Hz in breast tissue, robust reverberant patterns of SWs across the entire liver and kidney in obese patients were obtained. Dispersion images are shown to have contrast between tissue types and with quantitative values that align with previous studies. No published data on the intra- or interobserver reproducibility is published nor on formal clinical studies.

Reproducibility Studies

CANON MEDICAL SYSTEMS

A study investigated the intraobserver repeatability of SWDS for evaluation of nonalcoholic fatty liver disease (NAFLD) and assessed interobserver repeatability in asymptomatic volunteers.[19] The intraclass correlation coefficient (ICC) was 0.95 for interobserver repeatability and 0.80 for intraobserver repeatability.

Another study also investigated the intraobserver and interobserver reliability of multiparametric US such as SWS, SWDS, attenuation coefficient (AC), normalized local variance, and echo intensity ratio of liver to kidney for evaluation of normal and steatotic livers using magnetic resonance imaging-proton density fat fraction as the reference standard.[20] Although ICCs for intraobserver repeatability and interobserver reproducibility in measuring multiple US parameters in both normal and fatty livers were above 0.75, 95% confidence interval for measuring SWD in all livers ranged from 0.38 to 0.90. Therefore it seems that SWDS has a relatively poor intra- and interobserver repeatability compared with other parameters.

HOLOGIC

In a study performed long before the commercial release of the application, the average estimated intraoperator variability for viscosity of the liver was 10.6%. Interoperator correlation was weak (ICC: 0.45). There was no statistically significant difference in liver viscosity measurements in different intercostal spaces.[21]

Association between Dispersion Measurement and Liver Inflammation

A study of 25 male Sprague Dawley rats investigated SWS and SWDS measurements in rat livers with various degrees of necroinflammation and fibrosis.[8] SWDS was significantly higher in the necroinflammation model rats (median: 6.11 (m/s)/kHz, IQR: 5.16–7.43) than in the

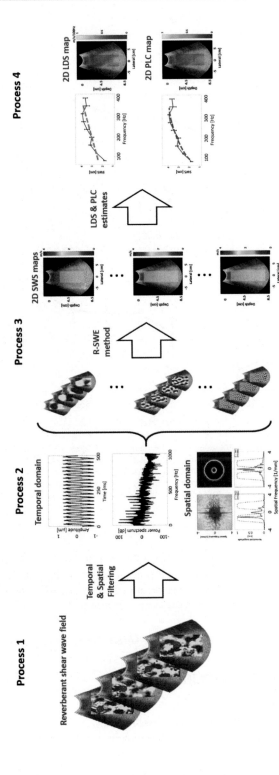

Fig. 12.6 Illustration of the reverberant technique. Process 1 is obtaining images from the reverberant field obtained at multiple frequencies. Process 2 evaluates the results in both a temporal domain and a spatial domain. Process 3 converts the results to images of the shear wave speed (SWS) maps at the various frequencies used in the reverberant field. Process 4 plots the SWS obtained at the various frequencies and generates dispersion maps. 2D, Two-dimensional; LDS, linear dispersion slope; PLC, power law coefficient; R-SWE, reverberant shear wave elastography.

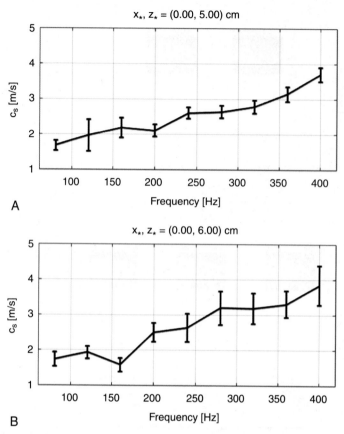

Fig. 12.7 The reverberant process allows the analysis of the dispersion of shear wave speed (SWS) as it changes with frequency, indicating the viscoelastic and lossy nature of the tissue under study. SWS versus frequency plots for the Computerized Imaging Reference Systems, Inc. (CIRS) breast phantom (A) and viscoelastic phantoms (B). C_s, Shear wave speed; (Copied with permission from Ormachea J, Parker KJ, Barr RG. An initial study of complete 2D shear wave dispersion images using a reverberant shear wave field. *Phys Med Biol.* 2019 Jul 16;64(14):145009.)

fibrosis model rats (G4) (median: 4.90 (m/s)/kHz, IQR: 4.39–4.97) ($P < 0.05$). In the multivariable analysis conducted using histologic features as independent variables, SWS was significantly related to fibrosis stage ($P < 0.05$) and SWDS was significantly related to necrosis grade ($P < 0.05$). The possible influence of other factors such as steatosis was not evaluated.

Clinical Significance of Dispersion Quantification in the Liver

COMMERCIALLY AVAILABLE APPLICATIONS

Canon Medical Systems

A study investigated the usefulness of the SWDS for assessing allograft damage (hepatic parenchymal damage) after liver transplantation.[22] The results showed that the median liver stiffness

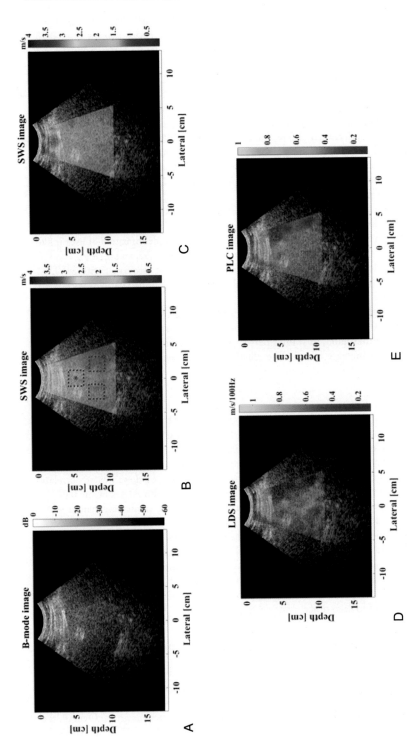

Fig. 12.8 The dispersion images can be created and displayed alongside the shear wave speed (*SWS*) images. (A) B-mode images in an obese subject. (B) and (C) SWS images superimposed on their corresponding B-mode image, obtained with the reverberant shear wave elastography approach at two different vibration frequencies, 80 Hz and 200 Hz, respectively. (D) and (E) Linear dispersion slope (*LDS*) and power law coefficient (*PLC*) images using an 80–320 Hz frequency range. The *dashed-line squares* in (B) illustrate the selected regions of interest (ROIs) (only shown in one image for reference purposes) to calculate mean and standard deviation values. The asterisk(*) illustrates the center point of one ROI that was used to plot dispersion curves in (A) obtained at different frequencies. (Copied with permission from Ormachea J, Parker KJ, Barr RG. An initial study of complete 2D shear wave dispersion images using a reverberant shear wave field. *Phys Med Biol.* 2019 Jul 16;64(14):145009.)

(8.2 kPa vs. 6.3 kPa; $P < 0.01$) and SWDS (14.4 [m/s]/kHz vs. 10.4 [m/s]/kHz; $P < 0.01$) were higher in participants with allograft damage than in those without damage. Meanwhile, SWDS showed a diagnostic performance significantly higher than liver stiffness (area under the curve [AUC]: 0.86 vs. 0.75, respectively; $P < 0.01$).

Another study investigated the diagnostic performance of SWDS in assessing inflammation for the noninvasive diagnosis of nonalcoholic steatohepatitis (NASH) in Japanese patients suspected of having NAFLD.[18] It reported that, in biopsy-proven NAFLD, SWDS enabled the identification of liver inflammation with an AUC of 0.95 for lobular inflammation grade $\geq$A1 (mild), 0.81 for $\geq$A2 (moderate), and 0.85 for $\geq$A3 (marked). SWDS (odds ratio = 1.06) and AC (odds ratio = 1.50) were significantly associated with lobular inflammation grade. They were also associated with steatosis grade (odds ratio = 1.04 for SWDS and 3.51 for AC). For the diagnosis of NASH, the AUC of SWDS was suboptimal (0.76). Combining SWDS, AC, and SWS improved performance (AUC: 0.81).

A study in Korean patients suspected of having NAFLD investigated the diagnostic performance of SWDS in assessing inflammation and in the noninvasive diagnosis of NASH.[23] The results showed that, in biopsy-proven NAFLD, SWDS enabled the identification of liver inflammation with AUCs of 0.89 for lobular inflammation $\geq$A1, 0.85 for $\geq$A2, and 0.78 for $\geq$A3. On multivariate analysis, lobular inflammation grade was the only factor associated with SWDS. A risk score to predict NASH, obtained combining AC and SWDS, identified patients with NASH with an AUC of 0.93.

It must be highlighted that a study reported a high correlation with fibrosis of SWDS ($r = 0.85$, $P < 0.0001$),[24] which was in agreement with studies performed using different methods.[9,21] On the other hand, in studies performed with magnetic resonance elastography, there was a consistent increase in both the elasticity and viscosity values with the stage of liver fibrosis.[25]

Hologic

A clinical study performed long before the commercial release of the application for the evaluation of SWDS and viscosity estimated the SWD applying the shear wave spectroscopy technique and the 2D-SWE technique implemented on the Aixplorer system.[21] It reported that the performance of both viscosity and SWDS in estimating necroinflammation was not clinically adequate, particularly for SWDS for which the highest AUC was 0.64. Moreover, there was no correlation between steatosis and viscosity or the slope of the dispersion curve with AUCs below 0.65. Viscosity was able to stage fibrosis, with AUCs lower but not statistically significant than 2D-SWE or vibration controlled transient elastography (VCTE).

A study of 215 patients with NAFLD assessed the relationships between the Vi PLUS values and the following parameters: body mass index (BMI), abdominal circumference, aspartate aminotransferase, alanine aminotransferase, liver stiffness by VCTE, and liver stiffness by 2D-SWE.[9] In multivariate regression analysis, BMI ($P < 0.0001$) and liver stiffness ($P < 0.0001$) were independently associated with Vi PLUS values. This study further confirms that viscosity and liver stiffness are related to each other.

METHODS AT THE RESEARCH STAGE (AS OF EARLY 2022)

By using a Samsung US system, a study measured the shear wave (group and phase velocity, dispersion, and attenuation) for a complete viscoelastic characterization of the liver tissue in 20 adults (mean age: 55.1 years; mean BMI: 30.5 kg/m²).[15] Liver histology was used as the reference standard. SWDS and shear wave attenuation increased with steatosis grade. Overall, there was a better performance for SWS as a function of fibrosis scores and of SWDS and shear wave attenuation as a function of steatosis grades. In the same study, measurements were also carried out in seven different concentrations of oil-in-gelatin phantoms. Of note, there was a subtle increase in SWDS and shear wave attenuation for low concentrations of oil, whereas the changes were more evident at higher concentrations. This finding is similar to that of a previous study[26] and suggests that the measurement of these parameters could be useful for higher viscosity levels or fatty liver grades, but it could be more difficult for distinguishing early low grades.[15]

A method called shear-wave dispersion ultrasound vibrometry (SDUV) has been developed, but it is still at the research stage. Harmonic radiation force, induced by modulating the energy density of incident US, is used to generate cylindrical shear waves of various frequencies in a homogeneous medium. The SWS is measured from phase shift detected over the distance propagated. Measurements of SWS at multiple frequencies are fit with the Voigt model to solve for the complex stiffness of the medium. Therefore both elasticity and viscosity are estimated.[27] It is important to note that ARFI uses transient shear waves, whereas SDUV uses periodic shear waves, and this leads to two main differences between the two methods: SWS is estimated from the arrival time of the shear wave front in ARFI but from phase differences in SDUV, and SWS is estimated from a transient wave front in ARFI as opposed to multiple cycles of shear wave vibration in SDUV.[28] Hence, SDUV may have some advantages when tissue displacement or signal-to-noise ratio is low. However, SDUV uses high-intensity US in the push beam, and potential risks associated with this method need to be assessed.

In a small series of individuals with chronic liver disease, it was demonstrated that, after adjusting for Voigt elasticity, Voigt viscosity was not significantly associated with fibrosis stage at multivariate logistic regression analysis.[29] The follow-up data available for the two outliers with lower elasticity but high viscosity showed that one patient had acute liver disease and the other had iron overload caused by hereditary hemochromatosis.

CONCLUSIONS

Altogether, the conflicting results in the literature indicate that further studies in larger cohorts are needed to clarify the clinical value of SWD in the evaluation of diffuse liver disease.

KEY POINTS

1. SWDS is a US parameter that is only recently commercially available and that seems to provide additional information than SWE alone.
2. SWDS is the change in SWS at different ARFI frequencies.
3. For a uniform and device-independent set of measurements, it is necessary to address differences and sources of disagreement, including the different shear wave frequencies used to measure the SWDS along with other factors.[15]
4. It seems that several cofactors may affect SWDS values, and the clinical implications of these intricate interrelationships need to be better clarified in future studies.
5. As of early 2022 it is unknown how many biological cofactors may increase or decrease SWD.[15]
6. Additional studies are required to assess exactly what SWDS is measuring and how it can be used clinically.
7. Additional studies are required to determine the optimal acquisition settings and how to assess the quality of the measurement.

References

1. Palmeri ML, Wang MH, Dahl JJ, Frinkley KD, Nightingale KR. Quantifying hepatic shear modulus in vivo using acoustic radiation force. *Ultrasound Med Biol.* 2008;34:546-558.
2. Boursier J, Isselin G, Fouchard-Hubert I, et al. Acoustic radiation force impulse: a new ultrasonographic technology for the widespread noninvasive diagnosis of liver fibrosis. *Eur J Gastroenterol Hepatol.* 2010;22:1074-1084.
3. Bavu E, Gennisson JL, Couade M, et al. Noninvasive in vivo liver fibrosis evaluation using supersonic shear imaging: a clinical study on 113 hepatitis C virus patients. *Ultrasound Med Biol.* 2011;37:1361-1373.
4. Huwart L, Sempoux C, Salameh N, et al. Liver fibrosis: noninvasive assessment with MR elastography versus aspartate aminotransferase-to-platelet ratio index. *Radiology.* 2007;245:458-466.
5. Deffieux T, Montaldo G, Tanter M, Fink M. Shear wave spectroscopy for in vivo quantification of human soft tissues visco-elasticity. *IEEE Trans Med Imaging.* 2009;28:313-322.
6. Barry CT, Hah Z, Partin A, et al. Mouse liver dispersion for the diagnosis of early-stage fatty liver disease: a 70-sample study. *Ultrasound Med Biol.* 2014;40:704-713.
7. Chen S, Urban MW, Pislaru C, Kinnick R, Greenleaf JF. Liver elasticity and viscosity quantification using shearwave dispersion ultrasound vibrometry (SDUV). *Annu Int Conf IEEE Eng Med Biol Soc.* 2009;2009:2252-2255.
8. Sugimoto K, Moriyasu F, Oshiro H, et al. Viscoelasticity measurement in rat livers using shear-wave US elastography. *Ultrasound Med Biol.* 2018;44:2018-2024.
9. Popa A, Bende F, Şirli R, et al. Quantification of liver fibrosis, steatosis, and viscosity using multiparametric ultrasound in patients with non-alcoholic liver disease: a "real-life" cohort study. *Diagnostics (Basel).* 2021;11:783.
10. Catheline S, Gennisson JL, Delon G, et al. Measuring of viscoelastic properties of homogeneous soft solid using transient elastography: an inverse problem approach. *J Acoust Soc Am.* 2004;116:3734-3741.
11. Djabourov M, Leblond J, Papon P. Gelation of aqueous gelatin solutions. II. Rheology of the sol-gel transition. *J Phys France.* 1988;49:333-343.
12. Yamakoshi Y, Sato J, Sato T. Ultrasonic imaging of internal vibration of soft tissue under forced vibration. *IEEE Trans Ultrason Ferroelectr Freq Control.* 1990;37:45-53.
13. Oestreicher HL. Field and impedance of an oscillating sphere in a viscoelastic medium with an application to biophysics. *J Acoust Soc Am.* 1951;23:707-714.
14. Chen S, Fatemi M, Greenleaf JF. Quantifying elasticity and viscosity from measurement of shear wave speed dispersion. *J Acoust Soc Am.* 2004;115:2781-2785.
15. Ormachea J, Parker KJ. Comprehensive viscoelastic characterization of tissues and the inter-relationship of shear wave (group and phase) velocity, attenuation and dispersion. *Ultrasound Med Biol.* 2020;46:3448-3459.
16. Barr RG, Ferraioli G, Palmeri ML, et al. Elastography assessment of liver fibrosis: Society of Radiologists in Ultrasound consensus conference statement. *Radiology.* 2015;276:845-861.
17. Yun MH, Seo YS, Kang HS, et al. The effect of the respiratory cycle on liver stiffness values as measured by transient elastography. *J Viral Hepat.* 2011;18:631-636.
18. Sugimoto K, Moriyasu F, Oshiro H, et al. The role of multiparametric US of the liver for the evaluation of nonalcoholic steatohepatitis. *Radiology.* 2020;296:532-550.
19. Yoo J, Lee JM, Joo I, et al. Prospective validation of repeatability of shear wave dispersion imaging for evaluation of non-alcoholic fatty liver disease. *Ultrasound Med Biol.* 2019;45:2688-2696.
20. Gao J, Lee R, Trujillo M. Reliability of performing multiparametric ultrasound in adult livers. *J Ultrasound Med.* 2021;41:699-711.
21. Deffieux T, Gennisson JL, Bousquet L, et al. Investigating liver stiffness and viscosity for fibrosis, steatosis and activity staging using shear wave elastography. *J Hepatol.* 2015;62:317-324.
22. Lee DH, Lee JY, Bae JS, et al. Shear-wave dispersion slope from US shear-wave elastography: detection of allograft damage after liver transplantation. *Radiology.* 2019;293:327-333.
23. Lee DH, Cho EJ, Bae JS, et al. Accuracy of two-dimensional shear wave elastography and attenuation imaging for evaluation of patients with nonalcoholic steatohepatitis. *Clin Gastroenterol Hepatol.* 2021;19:797-805.
24. Ferraioli G, Maiocchi L, Dellafiore C, Tinelli C, Above E, Filice C. Performance and cutoffs for liver fibrosis staging of a two-dimensional shear wave elastography technique. *Eur J Gastroenterol Hepatol.* 2021;33:89-95.

25. Urban MW, Chen S, Fatemi M. A review of shearwave dispersion ultrasound vibrometry (SDUV) and its applications. *Curr Med Imaging Rev.* 2012;8:27-36.
26. Bernard S, Kazemirad S, Cloutier G. A frequency-shift method to measure shear-wave attenuation in soft tissues. *IEEE Trans Ultrason Ferroelectr Freq Control.* 2017;64:514-524.
27. Chen S, Fatemi M, Greenleaf JF. Quantifying elasticity and viscosity from measurement of shear wave speed dispersion. *J Acoust Soc Am.* 2004;115:2781-2785.
28. Chen S, Urban MW, Pislaru C, et al. Shearwave dispersion ultrasound vibrometry (SDUV) for measuring tissue elasticity and viscosity. *IEEE Trans Ultrason Ferroelectr Freq Control.* 2009;56:55-62.
29. Chen S, Sanchez W, Callstrom MR, et al. Assessment of liver viscoelasticity by using shear waves induced by ultrasound radiation force. *Radiology.* 2013;266:964-970.

CHAPTER 13

Focal Liver Lesions in the Setting of Chronic Liver Disease

Christina D. Merrill ■ Anna S. Samuel ■ Richard G. Barr ■
Stephanie R. Wilson

Introduction

Any discussion of chronic liver disease (CLD) would be remiss if a detailed description of hepatocellular carcinoma (HCC) were not included.

In 2018 primary liver cancer was projected to be the sixth most diagnosed and fourth most common cause of cancer death worldwide, with HCC making up 75%–85% of all primary liver cancers.[1] CLD or cirrhosis is recognized as the most important precursor of HCC. Although only 1%–4% of people with cirrhosis develop HCC, 80%–90% of patients with HCC have underlying CLD or cirrhosis as a well-established risk factor.[2]

Tumors in at-risk livers are predominantly HCC, but intrahepatic cholangiocarcinoma (ICC) has also been shown to have increased occurrence within the same at-risk population.[3,4] Therefore, as health care providers, we know where to look for those at risk for the development of these aggressive tumors—HCC and ICC—within the cirrhotic population.

HCC is a tumor of the liver hepatocytes. It develops by the process of hepatocarcinogenesis, which is the transformation of liver nodules from benign to malignant. Alternately, it can develop de novo or spontaneously in the liver. However, identification of spontaneous tumors is rare, and they have an unknown explanation.[5,6]

The prognosis of patients with HCC is extremely poor, with a 5-year survival rate below 20%.[7] Early detection of HCC is important as tumors detected in their early stages are more amenable to treatment, leading to increased survival rates and reduced disease-related mortality.[8]

Liver imaging and the contrast-enhanced ultrasound (CEUS) algorithm, with a focus on its role in the determination of malignancy, is an important step in lesional analysis in all livers, including those with CLD and normal livers. However, recommendations for management and treatment of lesions in at-risk livers include the important classification system of the liver imaging reporting and data system (LI-RADS).

LI-RADS published on the American College of Radiology (ACR) website[9] includes an algorithm created by a specialized team in the field of ultrasound (US) and CEUS to standardize performance, observation, and subsequent management of liver lesions. It includes US LI-RADS for detection of liver nodules and CEUS-LI-RADS for their characterization postdetection. The LI-RADS algorithm covers benign lesions, nonhepatocellular malignant tumors, and a spectrum of precursor and malignant hepatocellular tumors.

The focus of this chapter is to look at HCC and its development and the important role that US and CEUS can play as part of today's aggressive management of HCC.

Bubble Specific Imaging

Following a standard gray-scale US, a lesion is located and optimally positioned for CEUS so it remains in the imaging plane during respiration. The contrast agents utilized for CEUS are lipid-encapsulated, gas-filled microspheres. The contrast agent and saline bolus are administered via intravenous injection. These bubbles have low toxicity and are thus introducible to the vascular system and remain for the duration of the diagnostic examination. The bubbles are sparse in circulation, therefore only a small amount of contrast (0.2–2.5 mL) is required per injection.[10]

CEUS uses a contrast-specific software that has a dual display, with a low mechanical indexgray-scale image on one side and a microbubble-only image on the other. This gives superior sensitivity to microbubble signal detection. After adding a dual caliper, the lesion can be located on the gray-scale side and correlated with the precise location on the microbubble-only image (or vice versa).

Microbubbles are purely intravascular. They are approximately the same size as red blood cells and therefore can move through capillary beds, but their size does not permit them to pass through the vascular endothelium. They remain in the circulation without diffusing into the interstitium,[11] unlike the contrast agents used in computed tomography (CT) and magnetic resonance (MR), which have a well-recognized interstitial phase.

As the microbubbles are purely intravascular, the contrast display reflects the volume of microbubbles exclusively within blood vessels in the organ and/or lesions. This allows for a sensitive depiction of tumor vascularity in all phases of contrast enhancement.

THE UNIQUE CAPABILITIES OF CONTRAST-ENHANCED ULTRASOUND IMPORTANT TO LIVER IMAGING

For the diagnosis of HCC and its evolving nodules, CEUS has special imaging capabilities distinct from CT and MR that are invaluable. These include real-time scanning, high spatial resolution, narrow scan plane, and pulse-inversion imaging technique (i.e., the ability to create a microbubble-only image).

Microbubble imaging utilizes specialized techniques that alter the US pulses, including their number, phase, or amplitude. One of the earliest successful techniques is pulse-inversion imaging.

Pulse-Inversion Imaging

In pulse-inversion imaging, two pulses are sent from the US probe, the second pulse a mirror image of the first (180 degrees out of phase). For tissue that behaves in a linear manner, the sum of the pulses is 0, and imaging information from the tissue is subtracted. For echo with nonlinear components, such as oscillating microbubbles, the sum is additive. A signal is detected from the oscillating spheres and is subsequently enhanced. The linear liver echoes are subtracted, creating a microbubble-only image and an environment in which visualizing the smallest of vessels within an organ can be achieved.[10,12]

Real-Time Scanning

Acquisition of images for CEUS utilizes dynamic real-time imaging performed at frame rates of about 10 per second, providing the highest temporal resolution available today in abdominal imaging. CEUS shows enhancement regardless of the arrival time of the microbubble contrast or the dynamic changes, including how fast the contrast arrives. Alternatively, MR and CT imaging have a predetermined timing protocol and therefore have static and fixed time points. Real-time scanning on CEUS overcomes this obstacle and shows vascular characteristics within the lesion that may be missed by either CT or MR, related to their timing or speed.[13] Focal nodular hyperplasia (FNH) and hemangiomas with rapidly changing filling patterns are easily detected on CEUS. In particular, flash filling hemangiomas are of great importance when speaking about HCC as they are frequently found within cirrhotic livers.

Excellent Spatial Resolution

CEUS can observe contrast enhancement caused by the bubble oscillations as finite dots as small as 1–2 mm. This is a unique feature in comparison with all other contrast modalities. This allows CEUS to see blood flow within thin septations and small nodules, which is essential for the accurate classification of growing tumors.[14]

Narrow Scan Plane

Thin slice thickness for CEUS improves characterization of septations and nodularity and detection of their enhancement.

Contrast-Enhanced Ultrasound Arterial Phase and Portal Venous Phase

Approximately 20% of the liver's blood supply comes from the hepatic artery and 80% from the portal vein. In liver contrast imaging, this creates the opportunity to observe an arterial phase (AP) involving the hepatic artery, and a portal venous phase (PVP) created by the portal vein. It is a unique environment for the observation of liver lesions, as tumors are mostly supplied by newly evolving arteries, and liver perfusion or parenchymal enhancement, the majority of which is supplied by the portal vein.

In CEUS, AP enhancement of a mass is assessed for its intensity relative to the enhancement of the background liver parenchyma. The intensity of intravascular contrast agents is determined by two important factors: (1) the volume of contrast in the blood vessels and (2) the rate of perfusion or time of uptake of contrast within the lesion or area of interest.[15] Enhancement observations are generally classified into three groups in the AP relative to the background liver: isoenhancing, identical to; hypoenhancing, less than; and hyperenhancing, increased enhancement.

Arterial changes and documentation of the blood flow in evolving liver nodules are best recorded as cine clips and can be saved as high-quality movies in audio video interleave format. Movies are utilized to show the wash-in of the contrast agent from bubble arrival to peak enhancement. Still frames stored for future review are best acquired from the original movie clip.[16] The added benefit of a microbubble-only image and pulse-inversion imaging gives CEUS the benefit of exceptional visualization of lesion enhancement without interference from background liver echoes, which have been subtracted from the microbubble-only image.

In addition to documentation of the arterial supply of identified nodules, subsequent imaging is focused on identification of wash-out in the PVP. Wash-out refers to a decline in the enhancement of the nodule to less than the enhancement of the adjacent liver parenchyma, following the initial AP enhancement.[17] The process of wash-out is poorly understood, but it is believed that the normal venous supply of the liver is eliminated in tumor formation as a precursor and cause of wash-out.

Perfusion of the liver parenchyma and enhancement increase progressively through the AP and PVP lasting until 2 minutes. The start of the PVP is generally around the 40-second mark. In the late phase (LP) (>2 minutes) there is a steady decline in enhancement as the contrast leaves the liver parenchyma.[18] The PVP and LP are best imaged by intermittent scanning at 1-, 2-, 3-, and 4-minute intervals to avoid bubble destruction by applying a consistent US beam.

An invaluable technique for PVP and LP, imaging is referred to as a liver sweep whereby the patient maintains full suspended inspiration while the probe is swept to include large portions of the liver in sagittal and axial planes. Wash-out areas show as small or large areas of decreased enhancement within the liver. The wash-out area can be optimally positioned using the contrast software, and another injection with contrast is done "on top" of the wash-out area to observe AP enhancement specific to the wash-out zone.

Contrast-Enhanced Ultrasound Algorithm

CEUS integrates the CEUS algorithm for diagnosis of liver lesions. It was described in the early work of Wilson and Burns published in 2006 and then expanded in 2017 by Burrowes et al.[18,19] It provides a comprehensive observational guide to the diagnosis and characterization of liver lesions, using their classic enhancement patterns (Fig. 13.1).

The CEUS algorithm is important in lesion analysis in all livers including those with CLD and those with no risk factors. However, its ability to determine malignancy and direct lesion diagnosis relates directly to HCC and ICC (i.e., the focus of this chapter).

Although in reality we observe the enhancement patterns of lesions from the AP sequentially prior to the PVP, the most valuable way to interpret the liver lesions is to first determine if there is wash-out to assess for malignancy. Wash-out is the biggest and most important observation of malignancy. It can occur anytime, rapid in the AP but very often in PVP and in the LP.[18,19]

Wash-out is invaluable for differentiating nonhepatocellular and hepatocellular malignancy and is classified according to its timing of onset and intensity[19]: rapid vs. late wash-out and weak vs. marked.

Timing criteria for rapid wash-out are evaluated as a decrease in enhancement of the lesion before 1 minute, whereas in late wash-out the lesion begins to show decreased enhancement after 1 minute.

On all contrast-enhanced imaging, it is common to use the descriptive terms *AP* and *PVP* to define the time intervals following the contrast injection, with LP or delayed phase for images beyond 2 minutes. However, on CEUS, because of the dynamic real-time performance of the scan, there are multiple thresholds used in an algorithmic determination in which it is more suitable to use precise intervals in terms of seconds and minutes displayed on a clock.

Intensity description includes marked wash-out that must occur before 2 minutes following injection of the flush and appears as a black punched hole. Mild wash-out shows enhancement of the nodule less than the adjacent liver but continues to show evidence of bubbles within the nodule.[20]

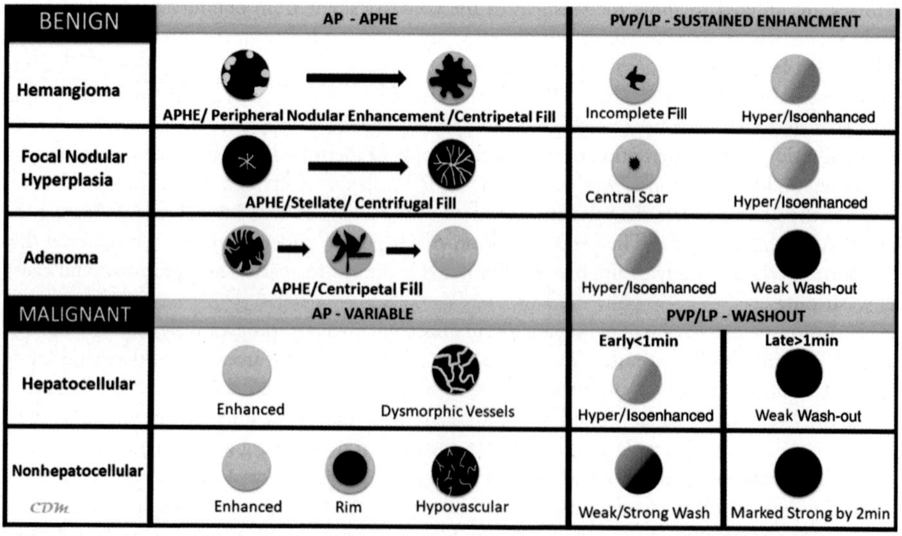

Fig. 13.1 Lesion analysis showing enhancement patterns and wash-out in the arterial and portal venous phase for common benign and malignant tumors. *AP,* Arterial phase; *APHE,* arterial phase hyperenhancement; *LP,* late phase; *PVP,* portal venous phase. (Reproduced from Wilson SR, Burns PN, Kono Y. Contrast-enhanced ultrasound of focal liver masses: a success story. *Ultrasound Med Biol* 2020;46:1059-1070.)

Late, weak wash-out after 1 minute is indicative of a hepatocellular malignancy or HCC. However, it is important to look for wash-out for up to 5 minutes, as delayed wash-out is an important feature to diagnose HCCs. Alternatively, rapid wash-out before 1 minute and/or marked wash-out are suggestive of a nonhepatocellular malignancy, including metastases, lymphoma, and cholangiocarcinoma.

Wash-out has been shown to occur in 97% of malignant lesions and 37% of benign lesions evaluated with CEUS. Of the benign lesions that showed wash-out, many can be accurately characterized in the AP.[17]

Imaging with CEUS has value in the AP in which classic patterns contribute to diagnosis. The AP shows blood from the hepatic artery lasting to approximately 40 seconds. Timing begins at the start of the saline bolus, and the AP usually starts at 10–20 seconds and lasts up to 30–45 seconds following contrast injection.[9] Its evaluation interval is from the arrival of the first bubble within the field of view until peak enhancement is achieved. The arrival of microbubbles in the AP is referred to as wash-in.

Rapidly changing dynamic patterns of AP enhancement and their observations are hugely important in diagnosis of benign lesions. Benign lesions show specific and reproducible AP enhancement patterns such as peripheral nodular enhancement. The direction of fill, such as centripetal and centrifugal filling, are also identifiable features of benign lesions. These characteristics are all easily recognized in CEUS during the AP.[18]

The CEUS algorithm defines standard enhancement patterns for hepatocellular and nonhepatocellular malignancies. These enhancement patterns can vary considerably in the AP. Hepatocellular malignancies often have arterial phase hyperenhancement (APHE), which is globular or diffuse. More importantly, late- weak wash-out that occurs later than 1 minute is suggestive of HCC. Nonhepatocellular malignancies including cholangiocarcinoma, metastasis, and lymphoma also show variable AP enhancement patterns, including rim, diffuse, and hypoenhancement. However, rim APHE and strong wash-out before 1 minute are the most characteristic features for ICC.[21]

The Importance of Liver Imaging Reporting and Data System in at-Risk Livers

The CEUS algorithm is an important step in the classification of all lesions, from malignant to benign, in all livers. However, it is deficient for classification of lesions within a chronically diseased liver, because the spectrum of observations and the breadth of possibilities are much greater. LI-RADS provides detection of lesions within US LI-RADS and categorization of lesions according to a probabilistic scale within CEUS LI-RADS. All information on US and CEUS LI-RADS can be found on the ACR website.[9]

TUMOR DETECTION HEPATOCELLULAR CARCINOMA

Gray-Scale Surveillance and Ultrasound Liver Imaging Reporting and Data System

Gray-scale US has become the cornerstone of surveillance programs for detection of tumors in patients with CLD. The recommended guidelines from American Association for the Study of Liver Disease (AASLD) suggest US every 6 months to fulfill this objective.[22]

Surveillance US should include a thorough gray-scale US evaluation assessing for nodules and morphologic features of cirrhosis. Elastography is invaluable to measure liver stiffness, especially in patients with a liver nodule and unknown liver status and in those with moderate to severe fatty liver, allowing for a predetermination of the risk for potential HCC.[23] Surveillance US requires excellent equipment and a high skill level for the performance of the scan. Familiarity with the wide range of background nodularity that can be shown in a cirrhotic liver is essential

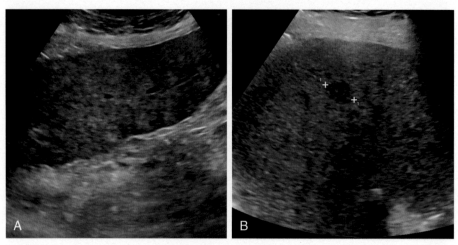

Fig. 13.2 Two different livers in two separate patients with cirrhosis. (A) Gray-scale image shows a coarse liver with a nodular contour. There is no dominant nodule. (B) Gray-scale image in a cirrhotic liver with a dominant nodule *(calipers)* superimposed on a background liver with tiny hypoechoic nodules. The dominant nodule measures 1.2 cm and therefore requires contrast-enhanced imaging for its diagnosis.

to allow for distinguishing the frequently larger and more conspicuous dominant nodules that require characterization with a contrast-enhanced imaging technique (Fig. 13.2).

US LI-RADS helps make the distinction of a nodule from surveillance, necessitating further investigation using the three following criteria:

1. US-1 negative, no nodule detected;
2. US-2 subthreshold, an indeterminate US in which an observation of a nodule less than 10 mm is detected that is not definitely benign and may warrant short-term surveillance; and
3. US-3 positive, a US study in which an observation of a nodule greater than or equal to 10 mm or a new thrombus in the vein is identified for which diagnostic contrast material–enhanced imaging or multiphase contrast imaging is recommended with either CT, MR, or US technique.[24]

TUMOR CHARACTERIZATION HEPATOCELLULAR CARCINOMA

Hepatocarcinogenesis

Prior to tumor characterization, knowledge about hepatocarcinogenesis and the associated change in vascular supply to evolving nodules is essential. Hepatocarcinogenesis is a multistep process of nodular evolution from a benign to a malignant nodule within a chronically diseased liver. HCC development is poorly understood but is believed to be caused by the inflammatory response created in CLD, inciting repeated cycles of cellular injury, death, and regeneration.[25] This creates an insult to the normal liver cell, causing cirrhosis and possible genetic change to its DNA.

During hepatocarcinogenesis, liver hepatocytes create regenerative nodules (RNs) that enlarge and develop cellular atypia as they transform from low-grade to high-grade dysplastic nodules (DNs) before becoming HCC.[26] Vascular changes accompanying hepatocarcinogenesis include the reduction of the normal paired arteries and hepatic veins, as well as neoangiogenesis, the formation of new blood vessels stimulated by an evolving tumor (Fig. 13.3).[27] Understanding the vascular alterations during hepatocarcinogenesis in evolving nodules and their gray-scale US

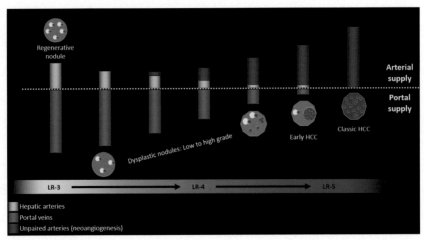

Fig. 13.3 The nodules show transformation of regenerative nodules to low-grade and then to high-grade dysplastic nodules before HCC develops through hepatocarcinogenesis. Associated vascular changes include progressive reduction in paired arteries, and venous blood supply as neoangiogenesis stimulates new arteries to supply the malignant tumor. Classic HCC has exclusively arterial blood supply. *HCC,* Hepatocellular carcinoma. (Adapted with permission from Kobayashi S, Kozaka K, Gabata T, Matsui O, Minami T. Intraarterial and intravenous contrast enhanced CT and MR imaging of multi-step hepatocarcinogenesis defining the early stage of hepatocellular carcinoma development. *Hepatoma Res* 2020;6:36.)

appearance is essential to detect and characterize the many variations in morphology and vascularity that are possible in transforming nodules.

The changing vasculature in hepatocarcinogenesis can create a wide variation of enhancement patterns. Fortunately, CEUS, with its exquisite spatial resolution and the option to have a dynamic real-time display, can play a unique and new role in imaging of liver tumors with the ability to observe the smallest of vessels and the most subtle of RN, DN, and HCC. CEUS LI-RADS addresses this inadequacy, allowing for a wide categorization of nodules and their variable enhancement pattern in the process of hepatocarcinogenesis.

TUMOR CHARACTERIZATION

Contrast-Enhanced Ultrasound Liver Imaging Reporting and Data System and Hepatocarcinogenesis

LI-RADS was created to standardize the reporting and data collection of CT, MR, and CEUS imaging for HCC. This method of categorizing liver findings for patients with risk factors for developing HCC allows the radiology community to apply consistent terminology, reduce imaging interpretation variability and errors, enhance communication with referring clinicians, and facilitate quality assurance and research.[9]

All information on US and CEUS LI-RADS can be found on the ACR website.[9] We would like to acknowledge the work of the CEUS working group, as it was integral in the development of the following information.[13,28]

Developed by a panel of CEUS experts, LI-RADS is strictly used on patients who are at risk for HCC, and it is valid for CEUS studies performed with pure blood pool agents. Risk factors can include any one or a combination of cirrhosis, hepatitis B or C, fatty liver, and alcohol-related liver disease, among others. Rigid criteria for at-risk patients are defined in published guidelines by all international liver organizations, such as the AASLD, European Association for the Study of the Liver (EASL), and Asian Pacific Association for the Study of the Liver.

CEUS LI-RADS categorizes nodules according to a probabilistic scale, ranging from LR-1 (benign nodules with no probability of malignancy) to LR-5 (100% probability for HCC).[29] LR-5 has a high specificity for HCC within this category. The high confidence level in the LR-5 category eliminates the need for more invasive procedures such as biopsy.

Although HCC can also be found within the LR-2, LR-3, and LR-4 classifications, this is less likely. Nodules undergoing hepatocarcinogenesis benefit from the CEUS LI-RADS algorithm and intermediate classifications, as they include a method for characterizing multiple enhancement patterns and the changing vasculature in evolving nodules.

The LR-M category (probably or definitely malignant, but not HCC-specific) includes malignancies of nonhepatocellular origin. This allows CEUS LI-RADS to detect all malignancies without any reduction in the specificity of the LR-5 category for HCC.

The CEUS LI-RADS algorithm (Fig. 13.4) has a place for categorization for all nodules seen in an at-risk liver, including HCC, hepatocarcinogenic nodules and benign tumors, and other malignant tumors such as ICC and metastases.

It includes a diagnostic table that addresses the characterization of nodules developing by hepatocarcinogenesis. The categories within this branch of the algorithm include CEUS LR-3 (intermediate malignancy probability), CEUS LR-4 (probably HCC), and CEUS LR-5 (definitely HCC).

LR-5: Definitely Hepatocellular Carcinoma
The main objective of CEUS LI-RADS is the highly specific LR-5 category. It has three essential criteria including:

- size of the nodule that is ≥10 mm,
- APHE (not rim or peripheral discontinuous globular), and
- late-weak wash-out present >1 minute postcontrast injection (Fig. 13.5).

The LR-5 category must meet all criteria in an at-risk liver.

Due to the high specificity of the category, biopsy confirmation of LR-5 nodules is not necessary. A confidently diagnosed HCC can be treated, be resected, or undergo transplantation without the requirement for invasive biopsy.

CEUS has a unique ability to document the diverse enhancement and wash-out characteristics of nodules undergoing hepatocarcinogenesis in real time. Refer to Fig. 13.3 for a visual representation of these features.

In coordination with CEUS LI-RADS, observers can classify intermediate nodules that are not benign but are also not confirmed HCC. CEUS LR-3 and CEUS LR-4 nodules have an increasing chance of developing into HCC and can be classified accordingly using CEUS LI-RADS. The diagnostic capabilities of CEUS allow radiologists to carefully follow nodules suspicious for HCC in at-risk patients and create opportunities for the early detection of these lesions.

LR-3: Intermediate Malignancy Probability
The benefit of CEUS LI-RADS is that it incorporates a range of possible enhancement patterns that represent the variable vascular changes in hepatocarcinogenesis. Many are found in the LR-3 category. These include:

- AP hypoenhancing/isoenhancing nodules of any size with no wash-out present (Fig. 13.6),
- AP hypoenhancing/isoenhancing nodules <20 mm with late-weak wash-out >1 minute in the PVP (Fig. 13.7), and
- nodules <10 mm with APHE and no wash-out present.

The presentation of CEUS LR-3 nodules is highly variable; most patients continue to have surveillance at specified intervals and some cases necessitate biopsy confirmation. As APHE and wash-out are signs of malignancy, depending on the nodule enhancement characteristics, management can range from surveillance at variable intervals to biopsy.

CEUS LI-RADS® v2017 ESSENTIALS
(For CEUS with Pure Blood Pool Agents)

Untreated observation visible on precontrast US and without pathologic proof in patient at high risk for HCC

- If cannot be categorized due to image degradation or omission → **CEUS LR-NC**
- If definite tumor in vein (TIV) → **CEUS LR-TIV**
- If definitely benign → **CEUS LR-1**
- If probably benign → **CEUS LR-2**
- If probably or definitely malignant but not HCC specific (i.e., if meets CEUS LR-M criteria [a]) → **CEUS LR-M**

Otherwise, use CEUS diagnostic table below

- If intermediate malignancy probability → **CEUS LR-3**
- If probably HCC → **CEUS LR-4**
- If definitely HCC → **CEUS LR-5**

CEUS Diagnostic Table

Arterial phase hyperenhancement (APHE)	No APHE		APHE (not rim [b], not peripheral discontinuous globular [c])	
Nodule size (mm)	< 20	≥ 20	< 10	≥ 10
No washout of any type	CEUS LR-3	CEUS LR-3	CEUS LR-3	CEUS LR-4
Late and mild wash-out	CEUS LR-3	CEUS LR-4	CEUS LR-4	CEUS LR-5

a. CEUS LR-M criteria – any of following:
- **rim APHE OR**
- **early (<60s) wash-out OR**
- **marked wash-out**

b. rim APHE indicates CEUS LR-M
c. peripheral discontinuous globular indicates hemangioma (CEUS LR-1)

If unsure about the presence of any major feature, characterize that feature as absent

Fig. 13.4   Contrast-enhanced ultrasound *(CEUS)* liver imaging reporting and data system *(LI-RADS)* algorithm and diagnostic table. (Reproduced from ACR.org with permission.)

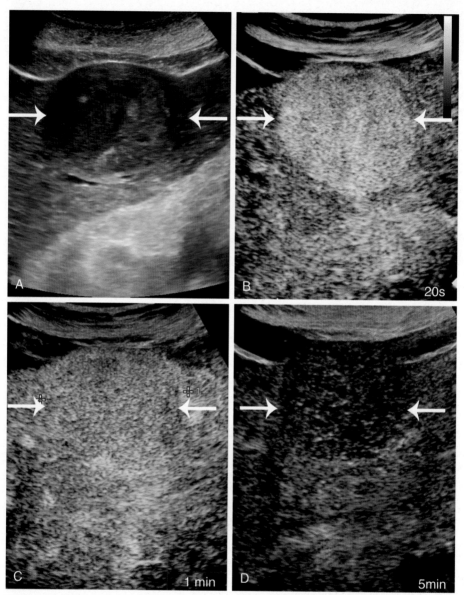

Fig. 13.5 LR-5 nodule, hepatocellular carcinoma in 68-year-old female with hepatitis C virus, autoimmune hepatitis, and alcoholic liver disease cirrhosis. (A) Gray-scale image shows a hypoechoic exophytic solid mass with a hypoechoic halo in segments 2/3 of the liver *(arrows)*. (B) In the arterial phase at 20 seconds, the mass is homogenously hyperenhancing and brighter than the adjacent liver parenchyma. (C) At 1 minute in the portal venous phase, the mass shows sustained enhancement. (D) At 5 minutes, there is evidence of microbubbles still present within the mass, but there is a definite decline in enhancement relative to the adjacent liver parenchyma. This is considered late-weak wash-out. These characteristics are typical of an LR-5 mass and allow for a confident hepatocellular carcinoma diagnosis. Treatment may be performed without biopsy.

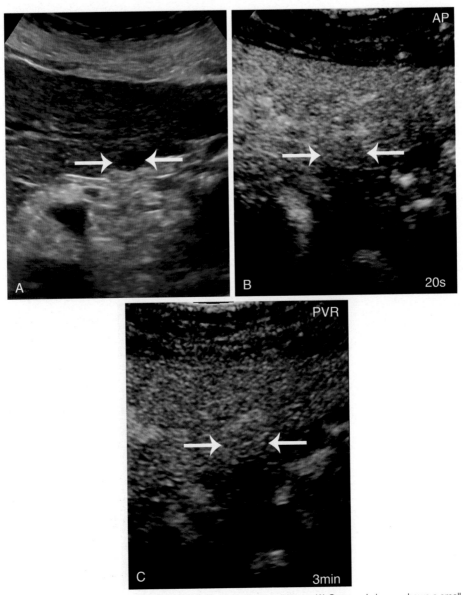

Fig. 13.6   LR-3 mass in a 59-year-old female with alcoholic liver disease. (A) Gray-scale image shows a small hypoechoic mass in segment 3 of this cirrhotic and heterogeneous liver *(arrows)*. At 20 seconds in the arterial phase (B), and 3 minutes in the portal venous phase (C), the mass is isoenhancing relative to the liver parenchyma. Isovascularity in all phases indicates an LR-3 classification and thus an intermediate probability of developing hepatocellular carcinoma from this mass. Historically, this would be called a regenerative nodule.

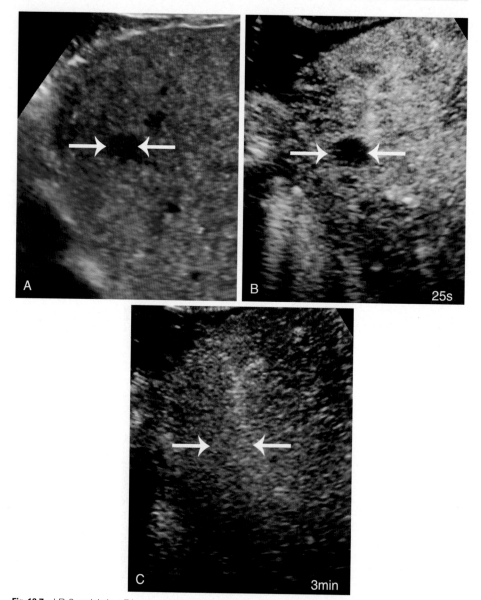

Fig. 13.7 LR-3 nodule in a 74-year-old male with nonalcoholic steatohepatitis cirrhosis. (A) Gray-scale image reveals a hypoechoic nodule in segment 2 of the liver *(arrows)*. (B) At 25 seconds in the arterial phase, the nodule is devoid of microbubbles and is hypovascular to the surrounding tissue. (C) At 3 minutes in the portal venous phase, the mass is isovascular to the liver parenchyma and does not wash. Hypovascularity followed by no wash-out indicates an LR-3 categorization. Historically, this would be called a dysplastic nodule.

LR 4: Highly Suspicious for Hepatocellular Carcinoma

Nodules on the pathway to becoming HCC are more concerning and have increased cellular atypia with neoangiogenesis. The CEUS LI-RADS algorithm describes their enhancement patterns as:

■ AP hypoenhancing/isoenhancing nodules ≥20 mm with late-weak wash-out >1 minute (Fig. 13.8),

■ nodules ≥10 mm with APHE (not rim or peripheral discontinuous globular) and no wash-out (Fig. 13.9), and

■ nodules <10 mm with APHE (not rim or peripheral discontinuous globular) and late-weak wash-out >1 minute.

As these nodules cannot be confirmed as HCC on CEUS LI-RADS alone, biopsy can be requested based on the degree of suspicion, especially APHE alone or wash-out alone.

There are also key CEUS LI-RADS categories that do not appear on the diagnostic table but are still equally important. These include LR-M, LR-TIV, LR-1, LR-2, and LR-NC.

LR-M: Probably or Definitely Malignant, Not Specific for Hepatocellular Carcinoma

LR-M nodules are malignancies of nonhepatocellular origin and can include some poorly differentiated HCC that do not follow the criteria for LR-5 classification. ICC (Fig. 13.10) and metastases (Fig. 13.11) typically make up the majority of the LR-M category, but LR-M can also include HCC if the tumors have any of the characteristics mentioned in the next list (Fig. 13.12). Nodules are classified as LR-M if they have one or any combination of the following:

■ rapid wash-out <1 minute postcontrast injection,

■ marked wash-out <2 minutes, creating a "punched out" appearance, and

■ AP rim enhancement and wash-out of any degree.

LR-M does not need to meet all criteria, as any one of these features categorizes a nodule as LR-M. Due to the variety of nodules within the LR-M category, these nodules often require biopsy confirmation for resolution of pathology.

LR-TIV: Tumor-in-Vein

Soft tissue masses identified within the vein lumen are highly suspicious for LR-TIV, or tumor-in-vein (TIV). CEUS is utilized to distinguish these tumor masses from bland thrombi. When avascularity is observed in all CEUS enhancement phases, the mass is classified as a bland thrombus. Alternatively, diagnostic features of TIV include APHE and wash-out. Although the majority of LR-TIV are HCC, TIVs can also be associated with LR-3, LR-4, and nonhepatocellular malignancies. LR-TIV classifications usually require multidisciplinary discussion and can require further imaging or biopsies. CEUS is also utilized to classify lesions that are definitely or probably benign.

LR-1: Definitely Benign

On the other end of the probabilistic scale, CEUS can use key enhancement and wash-out characteristics to identify nodules that are definitely benign and have 0% probability of becoming HCC. These nodules are classified under the LR-1 category. The AP enhancement pattern is the primary diagnostic feature used to classify LR-1 lesions (see Fig. 13.1). Examples of lesions include hemangiomas, FNH (Fig. 13.13), adenomas, focal fat deposition and sparing, and simple cysts.

LR-2: Probably Benign

LR-2 lesions were historically referred to as RN. Nodules assigned to the LR-2 category are identified by the following criteria:

■ distinct solid nodule <10 mm that isoenhances in all phases,

■ nondistinct solid nodule of any size (not hepatic fat deposition/sparing),

■ LR-3 nodules that have remained the same observational size for ≥2 years (interval size stability), and

■ LR-3 nodules with decreased interval observational size (interval size reduction).

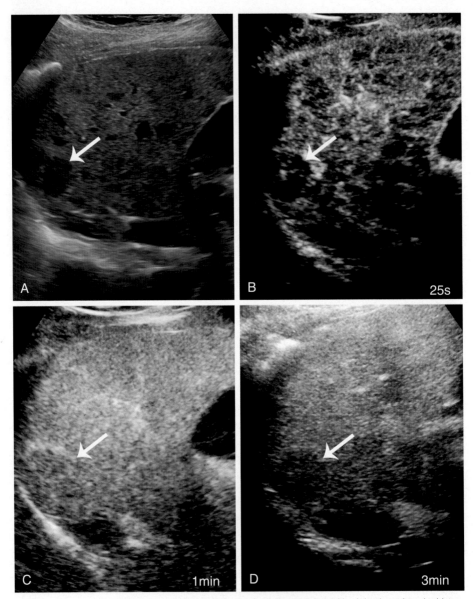

Fig. 13.8   LR-4 nodule in an 81-year-old female with nonalcoholic steatohepatitis cirrhosis and a prior history of hepatocellular carcinoma (HCC) and lung cancer. (A) Gray-scale imaging reveals a hypoechoic nodule in segment 7 of the liver in a posterior and subcapsular location *(arrows)*. (B) At 25 seconds, contrast-enhanced ultrasound shows arterial phase hypovascularity. (C) At 1 minute in the portal venous phase, the nodule is isovascular to the adjacent liver parenchyma. (D) At 3 minutes, wash-out is observed. This nodule is classified as LR-4 and is therefore likely HCC. Pathology confirms that this mass is a moderately differentiated HCC.

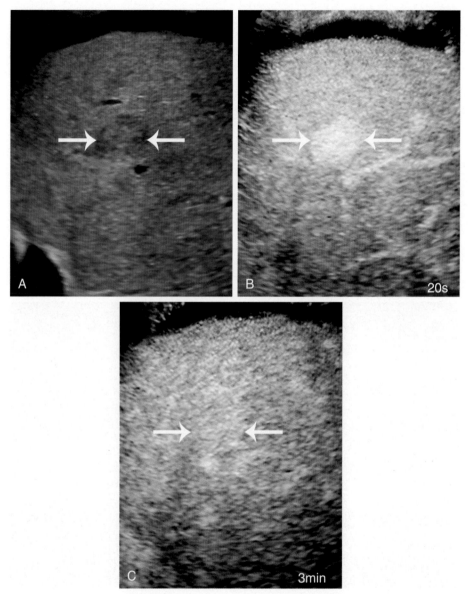

Fig. 13.9 LR-4 mass in a 64-year-old male with alcoholic liver disease cirrhosis and portal hypertension. (A) Gray-scale imaging reveals a hypoechoic lesion in segment 8 of the liver *(arrows)*. (B) At 20 seconds in the arterial phase, the lesion uniformly hyperenhances and is brighter than the surrounding liver parenchyma. (C) At 3 minutes in the portal venous phase, the lesion shows sustained enhancement with no evidence of wash-out. These characteristics indicate an LR-4 classification.

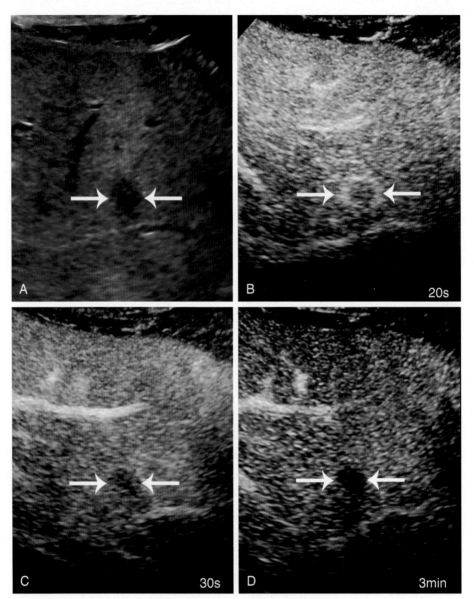

Fig. 13.10   Intraphepatic cholangiocarcinoma (ICC) in a 71-year-old male with nonalcoholic steatohepatitis. (A) Gray-scale image shows a well-defined hypoechoic mass in segments 2/3 of the liver *(arrows)*. (B) At 20 seconds, there is arterial phase hyperenhancement with a bright rim pattern. (C) Before 30 seconds, the mass exhibits rapid wash-out, manifesting as disappearance of the rim. (D) The mass shows marked wash-out at 3 minutes. Rapid wash-out and rim enhancement pattern are both indicative of an LR-M classification suspicious for nonhepatocellular malignancy. This is a pathologically proven ICC.

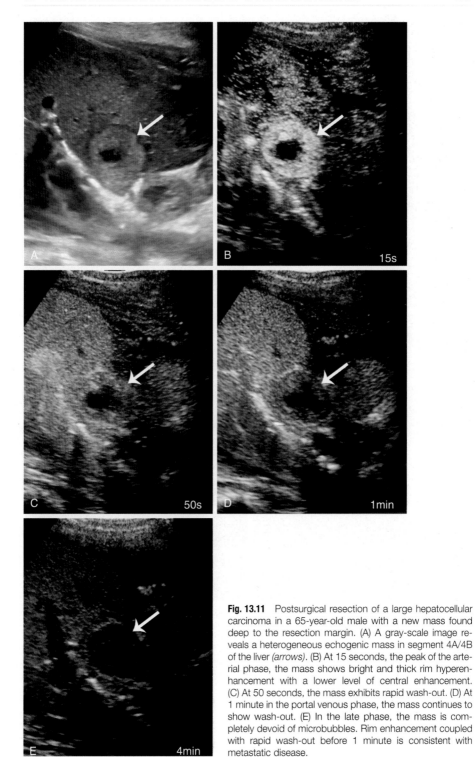

Fig. 13.11 Postsurgical resection of a large hepatocellular carcinoma in a 65-year-old male with a new mass found deep to the resection margin. (A) A gray-scale image reveals a heterogeneous echogenic mass in segment 4A/4B of the liver *(arrows)*. (B) At 15 seconds, the peak of the arterial phase, the mass shows bright and thick rim hyperenhancement with a lower level of central enhancement. (C) At 50 seconds, the mass exhibits rapid wash-out. (D) At 1 minute in the portal venous phase, the mass continues to show wash-out. (E) In the late phase, the mass is completely devoid of microbubbles. Rim enhancement coupled with rapid wash-out before 1 minute is consistent with metastatic disease.

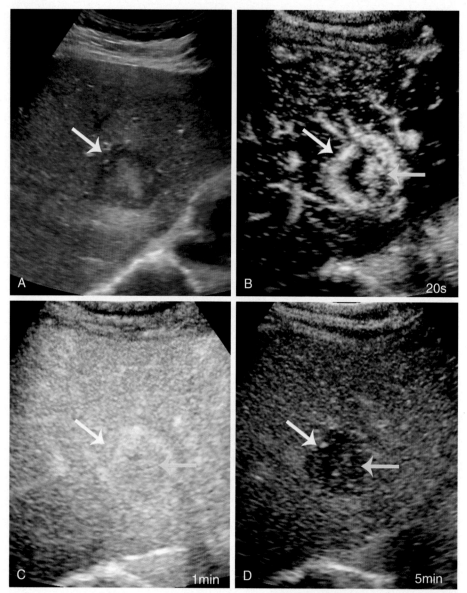

Fig. 13.12   A 78-year-old male with hepatitis B virus and a noncirrhotic liver. (A) Gray-scale imaging reveals a focal mass in segments 8/4A of the liver *(white arrow)*. (B) At 20 seconds, the mass shows arterial phase hyperenhancement (APHE) of the rim with a central enhancing nodule *(yellow arrow)*; a nodule-in-nodule appearance. (C) At 1 minute in the portal venous phase, there is uniform hyperenhancement of the entire mass. (D) There is unequivocal late-weak wash-out at 5 minutes. APHE of the rim indicates an LR-M classification. Thus this nodule is a proven hepatocellular carcinoma within the LR-M category.

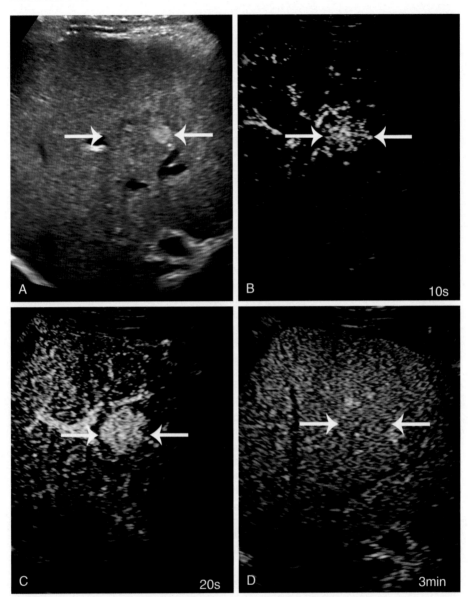

Fig. 13.13   Focal nodular hyperplasia (FNH), LR-1, in a 36-year-old female with hepatitis B virus and a fatty, noncirrhotic liver. (A) Gray-scale image reveals a mass in segment 8 of the liver that is partially echogenic and partially hypoechoic *(arrows)*. (B) At 10 seconds in the arterial phase, bubble tracking techniques show enhancement of the mass with a centrifugal filling pattern and stellate vessels. (C) By 20 seconds, the mass shows homogenous arterial phase hyperenhancement. (D) There is sustained enhancement of the mass at 5 minutes in the portal venous phase. The absence of wash-out combined with a centrifugal enhancement pattern confirms a benign FNH diagnosis.

LR-NC: Not Categorizable

An essential step in the CEUS LI-RADS evaluation is to assess the quality of the CEUS examination. Equipment failure or flawed technique may render a CEUS examination inconclusive. As sufficient diagnostic observations are not collected, a typical LI-RADS category cannot be assigned. These cases are thus classified as LR-NC, or not categorizable. In such cases, physicians can turn to other imaging modalities like CT or MR to achieve a resolution of pathology.

Ancillary Features

Although ancillary features are common components of CT and MR LI-RADS score, there are very few features that allow adjustment of categories on CEUS. They include (1) growth, definite size increase, and stability and reduction; (2) nodule-in-nodule; and (3) mosaic architecture. The only exception to the system is that features of malignancy cannot be used to upgrade LR-4 nodules to LR-5 nodules; this is to maintain the high specificity of the LR-5 category.

Integration to Liver Imaging

Worldwide, national liver organizations such as AASLD and EASL make recommendations for imaging of livers at risk for HCC. Currently, MR is the cornerstone imaging recommendation in North America, with triphasic CT scan as a valuable alternative.

With its high sensitivity and specificity and unique features, CEUS should play a greater role in focal liver lesion assessment. The temporal and spatial resolution and capabilities of CEUS are unmatched by other imaging modalities. The CEUS algorithm in combination with CEUS LI-RADS has shown such high specificity for the LR-5 category and HCC that it eliminates the need for pathologic confirmation or invasive procedures such as biopsy.[29,30]

When used in conjunction with MR, CEUS and its unique capabilities is a tremendous integrated modality. CEUS in conjunction with CT and MR is an excellent problem solver, especially in the case of indeterminate MR. Indeterminate results on MR are common. CEUS can provide alternate information about blood flow that aids in tumor diagnosis, including resolution of arterial shunts, benign lesions, and HCC in which CEUS has been shown to have high specificity and sensitivity.[31]

CEUS, as part of a surveillance program that includes MR, can be especially useful in the detection of ICC. More specifically, the two modalities show discordance in the PVP. MR shows sustained enhancement of ICC and CEUS due to the intravascular contrast agent and wash-out of the lesion. This distinction is attributed to the difference in contrast agents. Although MR contrast agents have an interstitial phase, CEUS agents are intravascular and show true wash-out. Discordance between modalities can be utilized to provide a convincing diagnosis of ICC. Not only can CEUS function as an incredibly useful independent imaging modality, it is also especially powerful when used in conjunction with MR.[32]

Elastography of Liver Masses

Shear wave elastography is widely used today in the measurement of liver stiffness and is valuable in assessing the risk level in patients when evaluating liver masses. As per the current Society of Radiologists in Ultrasound guidelines,[23] a normal liver would be indicated by a speed of <1.3 m/s, and a stiff liver >2.1 m/s indicates cirrhosis. A stiff liver indicated by elastography would increase the likelihood that an observed nodule in an at-risk liver would be malignant.

Although there was some initial interest in the elastography of liver masses, it is not widely used today. The premise of elastography in liver masses was that malignant lesions would appear stiff, and benign lesions such as hemangiomas would be softer. However, we know that in CLD, the liver stiffness changes, and as it does, so does the stiffness of the liver lesion.

Stiffness values have shown a statistically significant difference between benign (1.73 [SD, 0.8] m/s) and malignant (2.57 [SD, 1.01] m/s) ($P \geq 0.001$). However, they suggest only fair accuracy due to the wide range of values obtained.[33] For example, a benign lesion such as a hemangioma is soft, but a sclerosed hemangioma can show marked increased stiffness.

With the addition of two-dimensional shear wave elastography, visualization of stiffness in lesions is apparent (Fig. 13.14). Elastography of liver masses still remains interesting, but is not a guide in management of patients. The CEUS and CEUS LI-RADS algorithms are proven and reliable diagnostic tools that can arrive at a confirmed diagnosis.

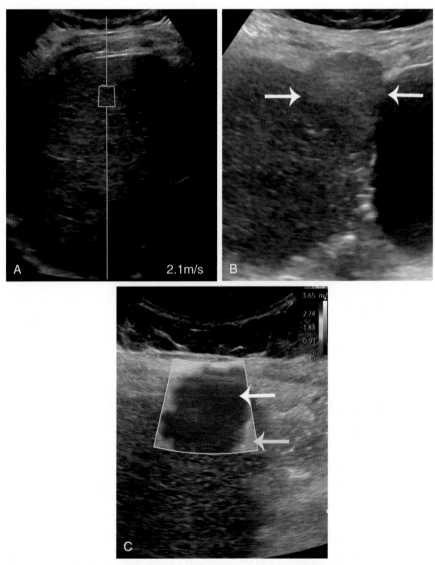

Fig. 13.14 Shear wave elastography of a hepatocellular carcinoma in a cirrhotic liver. (A) A gray-scale image using point shear wave elastography with a value of 2.1 m/s, indicating a cirrhotic liver. (B) *White arrows* pointing to a slightly exophytic isoechoic nodule. (C) Two-dimensional shear wave elastography of the mass with a small stiffness indicator in the top right. The red denotes increased stiffness in the mass *(white arrow)*. Liver tissue *(yellow arrow)* with a lighter color indicates that the liver is less stiff than the focal mass. This is a confirmed malignant lesion (hepatocellular carcinoma).

Conclusions

CLD predisposes patients to develop HCC. CEUS plays an important role in the detection and characterization of liver masses in at-risk livers. US LI-RADS leads to early detection of liver masses. CEUS LI- RADS is an important tool as an integrated modality with CT and MR and leads to reduced disease-related mortality and improved patient outcomes. With increasing expertise and use, CEUS in conjunction with CEUS LI-RADS is becoming an ever-increasing independent modality that is competitive with CT and MR.

KEY POINTS

1. Dynamic real-time scanning with CEUS allows for increased capacity for visualization of blood flow changes associated with hepatocarcinogenesis.
2. Purely intravascular microbubble contrast agents accurately show wash-out with malignancy, whereas CT/MR contrast agents have a recognized interstitial phase, which may show sustained or increasing pseudoenhancement instead.
3. Software for CEUS imaging creates a unique microbubble-only image, which is sensitive to subtle vascular changes that occur as tumors evolve.
4. The CEUS algorithm is an important tool in classifying all liver lesions from benign to malignant.
5. CEUS LI-RADS is specific for the characterization of masses in at-risk livers.
6. CEUS LI-RADS LR-5 category has high specificity for HCC, removing the necessity for biopsy before treatment.
7. CEUS resolves indeterminate MR, which shows APHE only in patients with arterial shunts.
8. CEUS is important as a multimodality imaging tool and is quickly becoming a competitive independent modality.

References

1. Bray F, Ferlay J, Soerjomataram I, Siegel RL, Torre LA, Jemal A. Global cancer statistics 2018: GLOBOCAN estimates of incidence and mortality worldwide for 36 cancers in 185 countries. *CA Cancer J Clin.* 2018;68:394-424.
2. Mittal S, El-Serag HB. Epidemiology of hepatocellular carcinoma: consider the population. *J Clin Gastroenterol.* 2013;47(suppl 0):S2-S6.
3. Welzel TM, Graubard BI, El-Serag HB, et al. Risk factors for intrahepatic and extrahepatic cholangiocarcinoma in the United States: a population-based case-control study. *Gastroenterol Hepatol.* 2007;5:1221-1228.
4. Khan SA, Tavolari S, Brandi G. Cholangiocarcinoma: epidemiology and risk factors. *Liver Int.* 2019;39(suppl 1):19-31.
5. Park YN, Kim MJ. Hepatocarcinogenesis: imaging-pathologic correlation. *Abdominal Imaging.* 2011;36:232-243.
6. Choi JY, Lee JM, Sirlin CB. CT and MR imaging diagnosis and staging of hepatocellular carcinoma. Part II. Extracellular agents, hepatobiliary agents, and ancillary imaging features. *Radiology.* 2014;273:30-50.
7. Allemani C, Weir HK, Carreira H, et al. Global surveillance of cancer survival 1995–2009: analysis of individual data for 25 676 887 patients from 279 population-based registries in 67 countries (CONCORD-2). *Lancet.* 2015;385:977-1010.
8. Kim DH, Choi J. Current status of image-based surveillance in hepatocellular carcinoma. *Ultrasonography.* 2021;40:45-56.
9. American College of Radiology. *CEUS LI-RADS v2017 CORE* [Internet]. Reston, VA: American College of Radiology; 2017. Available at: https://www.acr.org/-/media/ACR/Files/RADS/LI-RADS/CEUS-LIRADS-2017-Core.pdf?la=e.
10. Burns PN, Wilson SR. Microbubble contrast for radiological imaging: 1. Principles. *Ultrasound Q.* 2006;22:5-13.

11. Yang HK, Burns PN, Jang HJ, et al. Contrast-enhanced ultrasound approach to the diagnosis of focal liver lesions: the importance of washout. *Ultrasonography.* 2019;38:289-301.
12. Burns PN, Wilson SR, Simpson DH. Pulse inversion imaging of liver blood flow: improved method for characterizing focal masses with microbubble contrast. *Invest Radiol.* 2000;35(1):58-71.
13. Wilson SR, Lyshchik A, Piscaglia F, et al. CEUS LI-RADS: algorithm, implementation, and key differences from CT/MRI. *Abdom Radiol.* 2018;43:127-142.
14. Nguyen S, Merrill C, Burrowes D, Medellin A, Wilson SR. Hepatocellular carcinoma (HCC) in evolution. *Radiographics.* 2022 (in press).
15. Wilson SR, Burns PN, Kono Y. Contrast-enhanced ultrasound of focal liver masses: a success story. *Ultrasound Med Biol.* 2020;46:1059-1070.
16. Burns PN, Wilson SR. Focal liver masses: enhancement patterns on contrast-enhanced images—concordance of US scans with CT scans and MR images. *Radiology.* 2007;242:162-174.
17. Bhayana D, Kim TK, Jang HJ, Burns PN, Wilson SR. Hypervascular liver masses on contrast-enhanced ultrasound: the importance of washout. *Am J Roentgenol.* 2010;194:977-983.
18. Burrowes DP, Medellin A, Harris AC, Milot L, Wilson SR. Contrast-enhanced US approach to the diagnosis of focal liver masses. *Radiographics.* 2017;37:1388-1400.
19. Wilson SR, Burns PN. An algorithm for the diagnosis of focal liver masses using microbubble contrast-enhanced pulse-inversion sonography. *Am J Roentgenol.* 2006;186:1401-1412.
20. Lyshchik A, Kono Y, Dietrich CF, et al. Contrast-enhanced ultrasound of the liver: technical and lexicon recommendations from the ACR CEUS LI-RADS working group. *Abdom Radiol.* 2018;43:861-879.
21. Leoni S, Piscaglia F, Granito A, et al. Characterization of primary and recurrent nodules in liver cirrhosis using contrast-enhanced ultrasound: which vascular criteria should be adopted? *Ultraschall Med.* 2013;34:280-287.
22. Heimbach JK, Kulik LM, Finn RS, et al. AASLD guidelines for the treatment of hepatocellular carcinoma. *Hepatology.* 2018;67:358-380.
23. Barr RG, Wilson SR, Rubens D, Garcia-Tsao G, Ferraioli G. Update to the Society of Radiologists in ultrasound liver elastography consensus statement. *Radiology.* 2020;296:263-274.
24. American College of Radiology. *US LI-RADS v2017 CORE* [Internet]. Reston, VA: American College of Radiology; 2017. https://www.acr.org/Clinical-Resources/Reporting-and-Data-Systems/LI-RADS/Ultrasound-LI-RADS-v2017.
25. Brody RI, Theise ND. An inflammatory proposal for hepatocarcinogenesis. *Hepatology.* 2012;56:382-384.
26. International Working Party. Terminology of nodular hepatocellular lesions. *Hepatology.* 1995;22:983-993.
27. Matsui O, Gabata T, Kobayashi S, et al. Imaging of multistep human hepatocarcinogenesis. *Hepatol Res.* 2007;37(suppl 2):S200-S205.
28. Vezeridis AM, Kono Y. Contrast-enhanced ultrasound liver reporting and data system for hepatocellular carcinoma diagnosis. *Hepatoma Res.* 2020;6:53.
29. Makoyeva A, Kim TK, Jang HJ, Medellin A, Wilson SR. Use of CEUS LI-RADS for the accurate diagnosis of nodules in patients at risk for hepatocellular carcinoma: a validation study. *Radiol Imaging Cancer.* 2020;2:e190014.
30. Terzi E, Iavarone M, Pompili M, et al. Contrast ultrasound LI-RADS LR-5 identifies hepatocellular carcinoma in cirrhosis in a multicenter restropective [sic] study of 1,006 nodules. *J Hepatol.* 2018;68:485-492.
31. Hu J, Bhayana D, Burak KW, Wilson SR. Resolution of indeterminate MRI with CEUS in patients at high risk for hepatocellular carcinoma. *Abdom Radiol.* 2020;45:123-133.
32. Wilson SR, Caine B, Saransh G, Burrowes D. Portal venous phase discordance between CEUS and MRI: a valuable predictor of intrahepatic cholangiocarcinoma. (submitted for publication).
33. Yu H, Wilson SR. Differentiation of benign from malignant liver masses with acoustic radiation force impulse technique. *Ultrasound Q.* 2011;27:217-223.

CHAPTER 14

Conclusions (Multiparametric Ultrasound for the Work-Up of Chronic Liver Disease)

Giovanna Ferraioli ■ Richard G. Barr

Overview

Chronic liver disease (CLD) is a significant cause of morbidity and mortality worldwide, and in Chapter 1 the extent of the problem is fully discussed. There are now effective treatments for liver disease caused by hepatitis B or hepatitis C virus, and these causes are expected to continue to decrease in incidence over time. Nonalcoholic fatty liver disease (NAFLD) is a worldwide problem, and the incidence is expected to increase worldwide. The only treatment at this time is lifestyle intervention.

B-mode ultrasound (US) plays a major role in the diagnostic imaging armamentarium for CLD. Because it is widely available, repeatable, relatively inexpensive, cost effective, and poses no exposure to ionizing radiation, US is usually the first imaging modality in the evaluation of liver disease. In patients with advanced CLD, a surveillance program for hepatocellular carcinoma (HCC) with B-mode US performed every 6 months, with or without alpha-fetoprotein, is recommended by guidelines issued by several scientific societies.[1-3]

However, even combined with Doppler, B-mode US is not able to adequately characterize focal liver lesions (FLLs). Contrast-enhanced US (CEUS) provides information on tissue perfusion and allows excellent differential diagnosis of FLLs based on arterial phase enhancement patterns and assessment of the timing and intensity of wash-out. It has an accuracy similar to computed tomography and magnetic resonance imaging, which are the established imaging methods for an accurate diagnosis of FLLs. CEUS liver imaging reporting and data system (LI-RADS) provides a detailed methodology for the characterization of FLLs in patients with CLD.

Doppler US coupled with B-mode US may help in the diagnosis of portal hypertension (PH). Doppler parameters, especially of the portal vein, correlate with PH and were largely used in the past; however, they represent additional findings and should be integrated with other data rather than used independently for PH diagnosis. The presence of typical signs might allow the diagnosis, but the absence of these signs cannot exclude it. Newer methods of quantifying PH are being evaluated but remain at the research phase as of early 2022.

Over the past several years, other US-based techniques have been introduced, leading to the possibility of a US-based multiparametric approach for the evaluation of diffuse liver disease.

With the availability of shear wave elastography (SWE) techniques, the number of liver biopsies performed for staging liver fibrosis in several clinical scenarios has drastically decreased. It must be considered that SWE techniques were validated using liver histology as the reference standard. However, elastography measures the stiffness, not fibrosis, and therefore it is inappropriate to report and interpret the values using a histological classification. Moreover, stiffness is a quantitative estimate, whereas the histological scoring systems for liver fibrosis staging are based on categorical scales. Therefore, even in "ideal" conditions, an overlap between consecutive stages of liver fibrosis is inevitable when using liver stiffness (LS) as a surrogate marker of liver fibrosis. It is recommended that LS values be interpreted as the probability of compensated advanced chronic liver disease (cACLD), which is what is most clinically relevant.

Before performing liver elastography, the patient should be evaluated clinically. As highlighted by guidelines/consensus on liver SWE, the interpretation of LS measurement (LSM) depends on the specific clinical scenario, the prevalence of disease in the population under investigation, the current patient's comorbidities, and the cause of the liver disease.

For all US SWE techniques, adherence to a strict protocol when assessing LS is required for obtaining the most reliable measurement. Factors that affect the reproducibility of the measurement are similar across the different techniques and are related to the operator's experience and to factors dependent on the subject being examined.

To-date, most studies have been performed in patients with viral hepatitis or NAFLD. However, evidence is growing about the use of SWE techniques in other causes of liver disease, mainly alcohol-related, cholestatic, and autoimmune liver disease.

For patients with virus-related chronic hepatitis or with NAFLD, guidelines have suggested to interpret LSMs by vibration controlled transient elastography (VCTE) and acoustic radiation force impulse (ARFI)–based techniques by using the "rule of 5" and "rule of 4," respectively.[4,5]

In monitoring fibrosis over time, it should be kept in mind that there is a rapid decline of LS in patients with chronic hepatitis C who have been successfully treated with direct-acting antiviral (DAA) agents. This is mainly because of its positive effect on reducing liver inflammation. Therefore the use of LS cutoff values obtained in untreated patients can underestimate liver fibrosis in patients who have achieved sustained virologic response with DAA agents. In this setting, the Society of Radiologists in Ultrasound consensus has proposed to use the delta change of LSM over time instead of the absolute value as the best method to assess progression or regression of CLD and to consider as baseline stiffness value the one obtained at the end of the treatment in patients with hepatitis C virus.[5] Obtaining an LSM before DAA agent treatment is helpful. If the patients have cACLD before treatment, they are still at elevated risk, although to a lesser extent, for the complications including HCC, PH, and varices and thus require continued monitoring for complications.

Elastography has been used for evaluating the longitudinal changes in LSMs in patients with chronic hepatitis undergoing antiviral treatment, and a significant decline of LS in the long-term follow-up has been reported. However, without histological confirmation with paired liver biopsies, whether the decrease in LSMs is associated with regression of liver fibrosis, improvement in necroinflammation, or both is unclear.

Elastography has been proposed as a tool to predict the risk of death or complications in patients with CLD. In patients with cACLD, the risk of liver decompensation increases with increasing LSM. LSM by VCTE combined with platelets count is a validated noninvasive method for varices screening with very good results in terms of invasive procedures being spared (see Chapter 8). ARFI-based techniques also show promising results in this setting (see Chapter 8).

In patients with chronic viral hepatitis, the risk of developing liver-related events cannot be completely eliminated, even in those who achieve complete virological response; this risk is mainly related to the degree of liver fibrosis before starting the treatment. Some models that include LSM have been developed to predict the risk of HCC in patients with chronic hepatitis B treated with antivirals (see Chapter 7).

Screening for liver fibrosis in the general population is not recommended by guidelines; however, because of the high prevalence of CLD and the development of cirrhosis and HCC as major causes of death worldwide, such possibility in subjects at risk is gaining interest.

The diagnosis and quantification of hepatic fat can predict future development of diabetes and other cardiovascular events. Moreover, it has been shown that significant steatosis is associated with fibrosis progression in patients with NAFLD; therefore the quantitative assessment of the fat in the liver is of great interest. B-mode US gives a subjective estimate of fatty infiltration and has low sensitivity for mild steatosis. There is also a substantial intra- and interobserver variability. Moreover, the presence of an underlying CLD may reduce the accuracy of US in the diagnosis of hepatic steatosis. To improve the quantification of liver fat with B-mode US, some indices and scoring systems, including the hepatorenal index, have been proposed. However, they are impacted by the operator's experience and lack validation in large cohorts.

As of early 2022, quantitative US parameters for liver fat estimate are attenuation coefficient (AC), backscatter coefficient, and speed of sound. Most of the commercially available algorithms are those that estimate the AC. Controlled attenuation parameter (CAP), which was the first commercially available, needs a dedicated device that does not allow a morphological evaluation of the liver. It is obtained together with LSM and has become a point-of-care technique that is easy to use in the hepatologist's office. A large overlap of CAP values between consecutive grades of liver steatosis has been reported, thus limiting its use in follow-up studies that evaluate changes over time. Moreover, the cutoffs are not clearly defined. The AC algorithms available on US systems seem to have good accuracy in quantifying hepatic steatosis. The major advantage on using them is that the fat quantification is obtained together with B-mode evaluation and other US parameters. These algorithms have only recently been introduced, and their use needs to be standardized.

Ultrasound Multiparametric Approach

There are now several US parameters that can be obtained for evaluation of CLD in a fast, relatively inexpensive, widely available, reproducible manner using a nonradiation technique. These include evaluation with conventional B-mode US, LS evaluation with SWE, fat quantification using quantitative US, dispersion imaging, Doppler US, and CEUS for the characterization of FLLs.

As of early 2022, not all the new techniques are implemented in all US systems, but it is expected that they will be in the near future, at least on high-end systems. Fortunately, attenuation imaging does not require expensive hardware or software and should be available on mid-range and low-range US systems soon. The ability to quantify liver fat is needed worldwide to identify patients with NAFLD in screening programs who are at risk for nonalcoholic steatohepatitis (NASH) so these patients can be triaged for appropriate treatment and follow-up. Liver elastography either by the VCTE or ARFI-based techniques continues to improve, and there is a trend for better standardization between vendors as well as improved quality of measurements. Both VCTE and ARFI-based techniques have matured, and appropriate guidelines for how to acquire LSMs as well as interpret the results are available. The confounding factors and artifacts are well defined as presented in Chapters 4 and 6.

SWE provides biomechanical information regarding tissue elasticity. However, all tissues are viscoelastic. Dispersion is related to the frequency dependence of the shear wave speed (SWS) and is affected by the attenuation of shear waves because of the viscous component of the tissue. If a tissue is dispersive, the SWS and the attenuation of the shear waves will increase with frequency. Analysis of the dispersion properties of the shear waves can therefore serve as an indirect method for measuring viscosity. Shear wave dispersion is a US parameter that is only recently commercially available and that seems to provide more information than SWE alone. Dispersion imaging is still a relatively new technique, and more studies are needed to understand the extent of the additional information that can be obtained for evaluating CLD. Early research from a small number of centers suggests it may be helpful in assessing liver inflammation. Nevertheless, other factors that may influence the dispersion slope results are not yet well understood. This technique, which evaluates the change of SWS at different frequencies, should provide information related to the viscosity of tissue. However, it is not known what the best range of frequencies is to obtain information on CLD. The dispersion parameter is usually acquired at the same time as the LS value. Another interesting feature of the use of dispersion is that a reference frequency may be selected that can be used to better standardize the various systems acquiring LS.

Ideally, multiparametric ultrasound (MP-US) will help identify patients at risk of CLD at an earlier stage of disease, prompting earlier treatment intervention so they do not progress to cACLD. With low cost, rapid fat quantitation screening for fatty liver disease can detect patients at risk, and intervention can be started at an early stage to decrease the progression to NASH and its consequences. Whether the use of LSMs and dispersion will allow assessing the probability of NASH and monitoring the patient's progression or regression of disease, as well as monitoring treatment, still remains to be defined by futures studies. If a patient has progressed to cACLD, US screening for development of the complications (HCC, PH, varices) is advised. If a focal lesion is identified, it can be characterized with CEUS using the CEUS LI-RADS scoring system. Early detection of HCC is necessary to impact the survival of the patient. CEUS can be used to guide treatment interventions as well as follow-up treatment for HCC.

Future Advancements

LIVER STIFFNESS MEASUREMENTS

One problem with MP-US is evaluation of patients with high body mass index (BMI). The accuracy of LSM decreases in these patients because of the attenuation of the ARFI pulse and poorer B-mode image to track the shear waves. One method of improving evaluation of patients with a high BMI is to use a US system equipped with a lower frequency transducer that allows for stronger ARFI pulses at depth at the expense of B-mode image resolution. This has been adopted by one vendor, and the transducer is also able to evaluate the liver deeper in B-mode and color-Doppler US but with some decrease in resolution. The transducer also allows for CEUS image improvement at depth in the liver. There is some interest in having the power limit for ARFI increased so that more energy deposition will create larger shear waves, especially at a depth where there is presently a problem.

Another method in the research phase is using external vibration sources to generate shear waves similar to that in magnetic resonance elastography. This can be done having a "shaker" incorporated in the scanning table or using speakers (sound waves) incorporated into the scanning table or placed on the patient.[7,8] A US algorithm can then be applied to determine the LS. The system can only generate one frequency at a time but is able to have adequate shear waves present throughout the liver. Artifacts are not well defined at this stage of development. This could allow for better LS at depth and may not be influenced by the frequency bandwidth associated with the ARFI techniques.

A technique called *time-harmonic ultrasound elastography (THE)* that is based on US and continuous vibrations produced by a loudspeaker integrated in the patient bed has been developed.[7] THE employs continuous harmonic shear vibrations at several frequencies from 30 to 60 Hz in a single examination and determines the elasticity and the viscosity of the liver from the dispersion of the SWS within the applied frequency range. The mechanical excitation is able to reach a deeper part of the liver, allowing assessment of stiffness in morbidly obese individuals.[9] THE is not commercially available yet, and the published studies so far have been performed by a single center.

Elastance is a method that uses multiple acoustic speakers that are either placed on the scanning table beneath the patient or other acoustic speakers that can be placed appropriately on the patient near the area to be assessed. The technology allows for multiple frequencies from 50 to 2000 Hz to be utilized at the same time, creating a reverberant field (a complex pattern of waves).[8]

The US transducer can be used to acquire the information from all the applied frequencies and generate a dispersion curve over the frequencies that were applied. At each frequency, a LS value can be obtained. The acquisition of the data can be performed in less than 1 minute. Preliminary work on patients with a high BMI confirmed that the reverberant field is present throughout the liver, allowing for measurements at various depths, and is not limited by patient body habitus. The artifacts using this system are still not well understood.

MEASURING OF PORTAL PRESSURE

Presently the most accurate method of measuring the portal pressure is the hepatic venous pressure gradient, which is an invasive and expensive technique that has some risks and is not widely available. A noninvasive test that allows for quantifying PH and is able to monitor changes with treatment would be extremely helpful in the assessment and treatment of PH. Spleen stiffness studies suggest it may be a biomarker of portal pressures. This is more developed for VCTE than ARFI techniques, and more research is needed as of early 2022.

The use of subharmonic CEUS is at a very early research stage as of early 2022, and its accuracy is not known. In this technique, US contrast bubbles are injected into the vascular system, and subharmonic imaging is used to assess the response of the bubbles. The response of the bubbles can be then correlated with pressure.[6]

Another possible method to compute the volume flow is in very early development by the Quantitative Imaging Biomarker Alliance (QIBA) Volume Blood Flow Biomarker Committee. This technique combines standard Doppler measurements and gray-scale decorrelation. Using steered Doppler to determine the in-plane velocities, out-of-plane velocities from the temporal A-line decorrelation can be estimated. The result is a three-dimensional vector flow field computed over the imaging plane without using the vessel orientation. The volume flow is computed by integrating the out-of-plane flow over the vessel cross-section.[10]

ASSESSMENT OF INFLAMMATION

The use of dispersion imaging, which assesses how the LS changes when the ARFI frequency is changed, theoretically can provide information on the tissue viscosity as discussed previously. Inflammation should change the tissue viscosity, and therefore dispersion imaging may provide some information on inflammation. However, it seems that several cofactors may affect the shear wave dispersion values, and the clinical implications of these intricate interrelationships need to be better clarified in future studies. The use of present ARFI modalities only allows for a small range of ARFI frequencies. It is not known which frequency ranges would provide the most information on CLD. The research systems using external vibratory methods may be able to allow for a much greater range of frequencies and could provide more information than the present approved systems.[7,8]

Conclusions

The US techniques presently available for clinical use when taken together (i.e., a multiparametric approach) allow for assessment of CLD from any cause. MP-US is a nonradiation technique, relatively inexpensive, that is widely available but does require adequate training to obtain accurate results. New improvements to existing technology and new techniques in the research phase as of early 2022 should only improve the ability to assess CLD with MP-US, providing a complete assessment of the patient's condition in a rapid and noninvasive manner[11] that can be used to follow patients over time. The assessment of LS, dispersion, and biomarkers of portal pressure for the near future will require a high-end system for accurate measurements. However, the techniques to quantify liver fat content will likely be implemented on low-end systems, allowing for screening for NAFLD and, if these techniques prove to be accurate and reproducible, for triaging patients at risk for NASH for further evaluation.

References

1. Heimbach JK, Kulik LM, Finn RS, et al. AASLD guidelines for the treatment of hepatocellular carcinoma. *Hepatology.* 2018;67:358–380.
2. European Association for the Study of the Liver. EASL clinical practice guidelines: management of hepatocellular carcinoma. *J Hepatol.* 2018;69:182–236.
3. Omata M, Cheng AL, Kokudo N, et al. Asia-Pacific clinical practice guidelines on the management of hepatocellular carcinoma: a 2017 update. *Hepatol Int.* 2017;11:317-370.
4. Ferraioli G, Wong VW, Castera L, et al. Liver ultrasound elastography: an update to the World Federation for Ultrasound in Medicine and Biology Guidelines and Recommendations. *Ultrasound Med Biol.* 2018;44:2419-2440.
5. Barr RG, Wilson SR, Rubens D, Garcia-Tsao G, Ferraioli G. Update to the Society of Radiologists in ultrasound liver elastography consensus statement. *Radiology.* 2020;296:263-274.
6. Machado P, Gupta I, Gummadi S, et al. Hepatic vein contrast-enhanced ultrasound subharmonic imaging signal as a screening test for portal hypertension. *Dig Dis Sci.* 2021;66:4354-4360.
7. Tzschätzsch H, Ipek-Ugay S, Guo J, et al. In vivo time-harmonic multifrequency elastography of the human liver. *Phys Med Biol.* 2014;59:1641-1654.
8. Ormachea J, Parker KJ, Barr RG. An initial study of complete 2D shear wave dispersion images using a reverberant shear wave field. *Phys Med Biol.* 2019;64:145009.
9. Hudert CA, Tzschätzsch H, Guo J, et al. US time-harmonic elastography: detection of liver fibrosis in adolescents with extreme obesity with nonalcoholic fatty liver disease. *Radiology.* 2018;288:99-106.
10. Rubin JM, Tuthill TA, Fowlkes JB. Volume flow measurement using Doppler and grey-scale decorrelation. *Ultrasound Med Biol.* 2001;27:101-109.
11. Aitharaju V, De Silvestri A, Barr RG. Assessment of chronic liver disease by multiparametric ultrasound: results from a private practice outpatient facility. *Abdom Radiol (NY).* 2021;46:5152-5161.